Critical Care SBA Questions

A Companion for Intensive Care Exams

By Dr Catherine Anderson MBChb FRCA FFICM
Consultant in Anaesthesia and Intensive Care
Rotherham District General Hospital, Rotherham, UK

Edited by
Dr Ajay Raithatha MBChB MRCP FRCA FFICM EDIC
Consultant in Anaesthesia and Intensive Care Medicine
Sheffield Teaching Hospitals NHS Foundation Trust, Sheffield, UK

Dr Steven Lobaz MBBS BMedSci FRCA FFICM PGCertMedEd
Consultant Anaesthetics and Intensive Care Medicine
Barnsley Hospital NHS Foundation Trust, Barnsley, UK

Dr Alastair Glossop BMedSci BMBS MRCP FRCA DICM FFICM RCPathME
Consultant in Anaesthesia and Critical Care
Sheffield Teaching Hospitals NHS Foundation Trust, Sheffield, UK

tfm Publishing Limited, Castle Hill Barns, Harley, Shrewsbury, SY5 6LX, UK
Tel: +44 (0)1952 510061; Fax: +44 (0)1952 510192
E-mail: info@tfmpublishing.com; Web site: www.tfmpublishing.com

Editing, design & typesetting: Nikki Bramhill BSc (Hons), Dip Law
Cover photos © iStock.com: lungs, credit: magicmine; heart, credit: yodiyim; brain, credit: imaginima; kidneys, credit: ttsz; digestive system, credit: libre de droit

First edition:	© 2026
Paperback	ISBN: 978-1-913755-57-7
E-book editions:	© 2026
ePub	ISBN: 978-1-913755-58-4
Web pdf	ISBN: 978-1-913755-60-7

The entire contents of *Critical Care SBA Questions — A Companion for Intensive Care Exams* is copyright tfm Publishing Ltd. Apart from any fair dealing for the purposes of research or private study, or criticism or review, as permitted under the Copyright, Designs and Patents Act 1988, this publication may not be reproduced, stored in a retrieval system or transmitted in any form or by any means, electronic, digital, mechanical, photocopying, recording or otherwise, without the prior written permission of the publisher.

Neither the authors nor the publisher can accept responsibility for any injury or damage to persons or property occasioned through the implementation of any ideas or use of any product described herein. Neither can they accept any responsibility for errors, omissions or misrepresentations, howsoever caused.

Whilst every care is taken by the authors and the publisher to ensure that all information and data in this book are as accurate as possible at the time of going to press, it is recommended that readers seek independent verification of advice on drug or other product usage, surgical techniques and clinical processes prior to their use.

The authors and publisher gratefully acknowledge the permission granted to reproduce the copyright material where applicable in this book. Every effort has been made to trace copyright holders and to obtain their permission for the use of copyright material. The publisher apologises for any errors or omissions and would be grateful if notified of any corrections that should be incorporated in future reprints or editions of this book.

Printed by Gutenberg Press Ltd., Gudja Road, Tarxien, GXQ 2902, Malta
Tel: +356 2398 2201; Fax: +356 2398 2290
E-mail: info@gutenberg.com.mt; Web site: www.gutenberg.com.mt

Contents

	Page
Preface	iv
Acknowledgements	v
Introduction	vi
Dedication	vii
Abbreviations	viii
Normal adult ranges for blood tests	xxi
Paper 1: Questions	1
Paper 1: Answers	29
Paper 2: Questions	87
Paper 2: Answers	115
Paper 3: Questions	181
Paper 3: Answers	207
Paper 4: Questions	269
Paper 4: Answers	301
Paper 5: Questions	369
Paper 5: Answers	401
Index	481

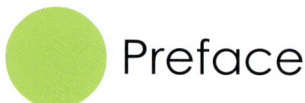
Preface

Intensive care is a specialty that has a wide scope of topics to cover in examination. When I was undertaking my Faculty of Intensive Care Medicine (FFICM) exams, I found that writing questions was a very useful way of deepening my understanding of the subject matter. I have continued to write questions as a form of continuing professional development and now have created this question book that covers the majority of the curriculum encountered in intensive care exams. My hope is that this book will be useful as both a source of information for revision as well as practising exam technique.

Catherine Anderson MBChb FRCA FFICM
Consultant in Anaesthesia and Intensive Care
Rotherham District General Hospital, Rotherham, UK

Acknowledgements

We would like to thank Nikki Bramhill at tfm publishing for her help and support during the whole process.

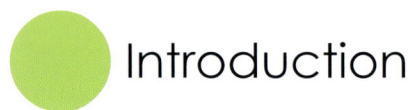

Introduction

This book comprises 5 exams each consisting of 20 long single best answers and 30 short single best answer questions. The long questions test clinical knowledge and application, whereas the short questions cover more fact-based topics such as scoring systems. At the end of each exam there are the answers to each question, along with a full explanation to help with revision of the topics.

The format of the questions is designed as practice for those undertaking the FFICM written exam, but the questions aim to cover the entirety of the intensive care curriculum, providing a good resource for anyone undertaking intensive care exams around the world.

Dr Catherine Anderson MBChb FRCA FFICM
Consultant in Anaesthesia and Intensive Care
Rotherham District General Hospital, Rotherham, UK

Dr Ajay Raithatha MBChB MRCP FRCA FFICM EDIC
Consultant in Anaesthesia and Intensive Care Medicine
Sheffield Teaching Hospitals NHS Foundation Trust, Sheffield, UK

Dr Steven Lobaz MBBS BMedSci FRCA FFICM PGCertMedEd
Consultant Anaesthetics and Intensive Care Medicine
Barnsley Hospital NHS Foundation Trust, Barnsley, UK

Dr Alastair Glossop BMedSci BMBS MRCP FRCA DICM FFICM RCPathME
Consultant in Anaesthesia and Critical Care
Sheffield Teaching Hospitals NHS Foundation Trust, Sheffield, UK

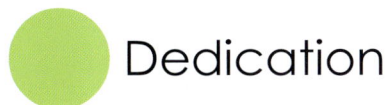
Dedication

This book is dedicated to my daughters Isobel and Charlotte and my husband Tom. You kept me going through my revision for the FFICM exam which is where the inspiration for writing this book came from. Isobel and Charlotte, you continue to amaze me every day and I am very proud of the kind young ladies you are.

Dr Catherine Anderson MBChb FRCA FFICM

Abbreviations

AAA	Abdominal aortic aneurysm
AAV	ANCA-associated vasculitis
ABG	Arterial blood gas
ACCP	Advanced critical care practitioner
ACEi	Angiotensin-converting enzyme inhibitor
ACh	Acetylcholine
AChE	Acetylcholinesterase
ACLF	Acute-on-chronic liver failure
ACR	Albumin-creatinine ratio
ACS	Abdominal compartment syndrome
ACV	Above cuff vocalisation
AED	Automated external defibrillator
AF	Atrial fibrillation
AFE	Amniotic fluid embolism
AFLP	Acute fatty liver of pregnancy
AGP	Aerosol-generating procedure
AIDP	Acute inflammatory demyelinating polyneuropathy
AIDS	Acquired immunodeficiency syndrome
AIN	Acute interstitial nephritis
AKD	Acute kidney disease
AKI	Acute kidney injury
AKIN	Acute Kidney Injury Network
ALD	Alcoholic liver disease
ALF	Acute liver failure
ALI	Acute lung injury
ALL	Acute lymphoblastic leukaemia
ALP	Alkaline phosphatase
ALS	Advanced Life Support
ALT	Alanine transaminase

Abbreviations

AMAN	Acute motor axonal neuropathy
AMSAN	Acute motor and sensory axonal neuropathy
ANA	Antinuclear antibody
ANCA	Antineutrophilic cytoplasmic antibody
AoA	Association of Anaesthetists
AoMRC	Academy of Medical Royal Colleges
AP	Action potential
APACHE	Acute Physiology and Chronic Health Evaluation
APH	Antepartum haemorrhage
APP	Abdominal perfusion pressure
APRV	Airway pressure release ventilation
APS	Antiphospholipid syndrome
APTT	Activated partial thromboplastin time
ARA	Angiotensin receptor antagonist
ARB	Angiotensin receptor blocker
ARDS	Acute respiratory distress syndrome
ART	Anti-retroviral therapy
ARVC	Arrhythmogenic right ventricle cardiomyopathy
ASD	Atrial septal defect
ASPEN	American Society for Parenteral and Enteral Nutrition
ASRA	American Society of Regional Anesthesia and Pain
AST	Aspartate aminotransferase
ASTCT	American Society for Transplantation and Cellular Therapy
AT	Anaerobic threshold
ATN	Acute tubular necrosis
AUROC	Area under the receiver operating characteristic curve
AV	Aortic valve
AVP-D	Arginine vasopressin deficiency
AVP-R	Arginine vasopressin resistance
AVR	Aortic valve replacement
BAL	Bronchoalveolar lavage
BCG	Bacillus Calmette-Guérin
BD	Twice a day
BE	Base excess
BIS	Bispectral Index
BISAP	Bedside Index of Severity in Acute Pancreatitis
BMI	Body Mass Index
BNF	British National Formulary
BNO	Bowels not open
BNP	Brain natriuretic peptide
BP	Blood pressure

BPF	Bronchopleural fistula
BSDT	Brainstem death testing
BTF	Brain Trauma Foundation
BTS	British Thoracic Society
BUN	Blood urea nitrogen
Ca^{2+}	Calcium
CAM-ICU	Confusion Assessment Method for the Intensive Care Unit
cAMP	Cyclic adenosine monophosphate
CAP	Community-acquired pneumonia
CARS	Compensatory anti-inflammatory response
CAR-T	Chimeric antigen receptor T
CBRN	Chemical, biological, radioactive or nuclear
CCB	Calcium channel blocker
CDI	*Clostridioides difficile* infection
CFT	Clot formation time
CHB	Complete heart block
CHCC	Chapel Hill Consensus Conference
CI	Cardiac index
CI-AKI	Contrast-induced acute kidney injury
CIDP	Chronic inflammatory demyelinating polyneuropathy
CIED	Intracardiac implantable electronic device
CIM	Critical illness myopathy
CINM	Critical illness polyneuromyopathy
CIP	Critical illness polyneuropathy
CIS	Clinically isolated syndrome
CJD	Creutzfeldt-Jakob disease
CK	Creatine kinase
CKD	Chronic kidney disease
Cl^-	Chloride
CLD	Chronic liver disease
CMAP	Compound motor action potential
CMV	*Cytomegalovirus*
CNS	Central nervous system
CO	Carbon monoxide; cardiac output
CO_2	Carbon dioxide
CO_{2e}	Carbon dioxide equivalent
COHb	Carboxyhaemoglobin
COPD	Chronic obstructive pulmonary disease
COX	Cyclooxygenase
CPAP	Continuous positive airway pressure
CPET	Cardiopulmonary exercise testing

Abbreviations

CpK	Creatine phosphokinase
CPM	Central pontine myelinolysis
CPP	Cerebral perfusion pressure
CPR	Cardiopulmonary resuscitation
Cr	Creatinine
CRP	C-reactive protein
CRRT	Continuous renal replacement therapy
CRS	Cytokine release syndrome
CRT	Capillary refill time
CSF	Cerebrospinal fluid
CT	Computed tomography; clotting time
CTPA	Computed tomography pulmonary angiogram
CVC	Central venous catheter
CVS	Cardiovascular
CVVH	Continuous veno-venous haemofiltration
CVVHD	Continuous veno-venous haemodialysis
CVVHDF	Continuous veno-venous haemodiafiltration
CXR	Chest X-ray
DAI	Diffuse axonal injury
DAPT	Dual antiplatelet therapy
DAS	Difficult Airway Society
DBD	Donation after brainstem death
DBP	Diastolic blood pressure
DCCV	Direct current cardioversion
DCD	Donation after circulatory death
DCI	Delayed cerebral ischaemia
DCM	Dilated cardiomyopathy
DI	Diabetes insipidus
DIC	Disseminated intravascular coagulopathy
DKA	Diabetic ketoacidosis
DM	Diabetes mellitus
DOAC	Direct oral anticoagulant
DOLS	Deprivation of Liberty Safeguards
DPG	Diphosphoglycerate
DRESS	Drug reaction with eosinophilia and systemic symptoms
DVT	Deep vein thrombosis
EBV	Epstein-Barr virus
ECG	Electrocardiogram
ECHO	Echocardiogram
ECMO	Extracorporeal membrane oxygenation

ED	Emergency department
EEG	Electroencephalography
EF	Ejection fraction
eGFR	Estimated glomerular filtration rate
EGPA	Eosinophilic granulomatosis with polyangiitis
EN	Enteral nutrition
EPALS	European Paediatric Advanced Life Support
ERCP	Endoscopic retrograde cholangiopancreatography
ESBL	Extended-spectrum beta-lactamase
ESICM	European Society of Intensive Care Medicine
ESP	Erector spinae plane
ESPEN	European Society for Clinical Nutrition and Metabolism
ESR	Erythrocyte sedimentation rate
ESRA	European Society of Regional Anaesthesia
ETT	Endotracheal tube
EUS	Endoscopic ultrasound
EVAR	Endovascular aneurysm repair
EVD	External ventricular drain
FAHR	Febrile, allergic and hypotensive reaction
FEES	Fibreoptic endoscopic evaluation of swallow
FENa$^+$	Fractional excretion of sodium
FES	Fat embolus syndrome
FFP	Fresh frozen plasma
FICM	Faculty of Intensive Care Medicine
FiO$_2$	Fraction of inspired oxygen
FONA	Front-of-neck access
FSGS	Focal segmental glomerulosclerosis
FTc	Corrected flow time
FVC	Forced vital capacity
G6PD	Glucose-6-phosphate deficiency
GA	General anaesthesia
GABA	Gamma-aminobutyric acid
GBS	Guillain-Barré syndrome
GCS	Glasgow Coma Scale
GCSF	Granulocyte colony-stimulating factor
GDH	Glutamate dehydrogenase
GI	Gastrointestinal
GMC	General Medical Council
GORD	Gastro-oesophageal reflux disease

Abbreviations

GP	General practitioner
GPIIb/IIIa	Glycoprotein IIb/IIIa
GPICS	Guidelines for the Provision of Intensive Care Services
GRACE	Global Registry of Acute Coronary Events
GTN	Glyceryl trinitrate
GVHD	Graft vs. host disease
H^+	Hydrogen
HAGMA	High anion gap metabolic acidosis
Hb	Haemoglobin
HbAS	Sickle cell trait
HBOT	Hyperbaric oxygen therapy
HbS	Sickle cell haemoglobin
HbSS	Sickle cell anaemia
HCO_3^-	Bicarbonate
HD	Haemodialysis
HE	Hepatic encephalopathy
HF	Heart failure
HFNO	High-flow nasal oxygen
HFOV	High-frequency oscillation ventilation
HFpEF	Heart failure with preserved ejection fraction
HFrEF	Heart failure with reduced ejection fraction
HHS	Hyperosmolar hyperglycaemic state
HHV	Human herpes virus
HIET	Hyperinsulinaemic euglycaemic therapy
HIT	Heparin-induced thrombocytopaenia
HIV	Human immunodeficiency virus
HLH	Haemophagocytic lymphohistiocytosis
HOCM	Hypertrophic obstructive cardiomyopathy
HR	Heart rate
HRS	Hepatorenal syndrome
HRS-AKI	Hepatorenal syndrome — acute kidney injury
HRS-NAKI	Hepatorenal syndrome — no acute kidney injury
HSV	Herpes simplex virus
HTN	Hypertension
HUS	Haemolytic uraemic syndrome
IABP	Intra-aortic balloon pump
IAH	Intra-abdominal hypertension
IAP	Intra-abdominal pressure
IBW	Ideal body weight
IC	Invasive candidiasis

ICD	Implantable cardioverter defibrillator
ICH	Intracranial haemorrhage
ICNARC	Intensive Care National Audit & Research Centre
ICP	Intracranial pressure
ICS	Intra-abdominal compartment syndrome; Intensive Care Society
ICU	Intensive care unit
ICU-AW	Intensive care unit-acquired weakness
I:E	Inspiratory to expiratory ratio
IE	Infective endocarditis
Ig	Immunoglobulin
IHD	Intermittent haemodialysis
IJV	Internal jugular vein
IM	Intramuscular
INSTI	Integrase strand transfer inhibitor
IO	Intraosseous
IP	Inspiratory pressure
ISHEN	International Society for Hepatic Encephalopathy and Nitrogen Metabolism
ISTH	International Society on Thrombosis and Haemostasis
ITP	Immune thrombocytopaenia
IV	Intravenous
IVIg	Intravenous immunoglobulin
JVP	Jugular venous pressure
K^+	Potassium
KCC	King's College Criteria
KDIGO	Kidney Disease: Improving Global Outcomes
KUB	Kidneys, ureters and bladder
LA	Local anaesthetic
LACS	Lacunar syndrome
LDH	Lactate dehydrogenase
LFT	Liver function test
LiDCO	Lithium dilution cardiac output
LMA	Laryngeal mask airway
LMWH	Low-molecular-weight heparin
LOS	Length of stay
LP	Lumbar puncture
LPR	Lactate pyruvate ratio
LPS	Lipopolysaccharide
LRINEC	Laboratory risk indicator for necrotizing fasciitis
LV	Left ventricular/left ventricle
LVAD	Left ventricular assist device
MA	Maximum amplitude

Abbreviations

MAHA	Microangiopathic haemolytic anaemia
MALA	Metformin-associated lactic acidosis
MALDI-TOF	Matrix-assisted laser desorption/ionisation time-of-flight
MAOI	Monoamine oxidase inhibitor
MAP	Mean arterial pressure
MCA	Middle cerebral artery
MCD	Minimal change disease
MCF	Maximum clot firmness
MCV	Mean corpuscular volume
MD	Myotonic dystrophy
MDMA	3,4-methylenedioxymethamphetamine
MDT	Multi-disciplinary team
MELD	Model for End-Stage Liver Disease
MEN	Multiple endocrine neoplasia
Mg^{2+}	Magnesium
MG	Myasthenia gravis
MH	Malignant hyperpyrexia
MI	Myocardial infarction
MILA	Metformin-induced lactic acidosis
MND	Motor neurone disease
MOH	Major obstetric haemorrhage
mPAP	Mean pulmonary artery pressure
MR	Mitral regurgitation
MRI	Magnetic resonance imaging
MRSA	Methicillin-resistant *Staphylococcus aureus*
MS	Multiple sclerosis
MSSA	Methicillin-sensitive *Staphylococcus aureus*
MUAC	Middle upper arm circumference
MUAP	Motor unit action potential
MULA	Metformin-unrelated lactic acidosis
MUST	Malnutrition Universal Screening Tool
MV	Minute ventilation
Na^+	Sodium
NAC	N-acetylcysteine
NADPH	Nicotinamide adenine dinucleotide phosphate
NAGMA	Normal anion gap metabolic acidosis
$NaHCO_3$	Sodium bicarbonate
NAI	Non-accidental injury
NAP4	National Audit Project 4
NF	Necrotising fasciitis
NG	Nasogastric

NHL	Non-Hodgkin lymphoma
NICE	National Institute for Health and Care Excellence
NIHSS	National Institutes of Health Stroke Scale
NIRS	Near-infrared spectroscopy
NIV	Non-invasive ventilation
NJ	Nasojejunal
NMBD	Neuromuscular blocking drug
NMJ	Neuromuscular junction
NMS	Neuroleptic malignant syndrome
NNRTI	Non-nucleoside reverse transcriptase inhibitor
NO	Nitric oxide
NOAC	Non-vitamin K antagonist oral anticoagulant
NOMI	Non-occlusive myocardial infarction
NPV	Negative predictive value
NRB	Non-rebreathe (oxygen mask)
NRS	Nutritional Risk Screening
NRTI	Nucleoside reverse transcriptase inhibitor
NSAID	Non-steroidal anti-inflammatory drug
NSE	Neuron-specific enolase
NSTEMI	Non-ST-elevation myocardial infarction
NT-proBNP	N-terminal portion of brain natriuretic peptide
NUTRIC	Nutrition Risk in the Critically ill
OD	Once a day
O/E	On examination
OMI	Occlusive myocardial infarction
OOHCA	Out-of-hospital cardiac arrest
OR	Odds ratio
ORIF	Open reduction and internal fixation
OWV	One-way inline valve
PAC	Pulmonary artery catheter
$PaCO_2$	Partial pressure of carbon dioxide
PACS	Partial anterior circulation syndrome
PAH	Pulmonary arterial hypertension
PaO_2	Partial pressure of oxygen
PAWP	Pulmonary artery wedge pressure
PCA	Patient-controlled analgesia
PCC	Prothrombin complex concentrate
PCI	Percutaneous coronary intervention
PCR	Protein:creatinine ratio; polymerase chain reaction
PCT	Procalcitonin
PCV	Pressure-controlled ventilation

Abbreviations

PD	Peritoneal dialysis
PDP	Penicillin-binding protein
PE	Pulmonary embolus
PEA	Pulseless electrical activity
PEARL	Pupils equal and reactive to light
PEEP	Positive end-expiratory pressure
PEF	Peak expiratory flow
PERC	Pulmonary Embolism Rule-out Criteria
PESI	Pulmonary Embolism Severity Index
PFC	Pancreatic fluid collection
PFO	Patent foramen ovale
PH	Pulmonary hypertension
PICC	Peripherally inserted central catheter
PiCCO	Pulse index continuous cardiac output
PIP	Peak inspiratory pressure
PJP	*Pneumocystis jirovecii* pneumonia (sometimes referred to as PCP)
Plt	Platelets
PMH	Past medical history
PMN	Polymorphonuclear leukocyte, also known as a neutrophil
PN	Parenteral nutrition
PO_4^{3-}	Phosphate
POC	Point of care
POCS	Posterior circulation stroke syndrome
POCUS	Point of care ultrasonography
PPE	Personal protective equipment
PPH	Postpartum haemorrhage
PPI	Proton pump inhibitor
PPlat	Plateau pressure
PPV	Positive predictive value
PR	Per rectum
PRBC	Packed red blood cell
PRIS	Propofol-related infusion syndrome
PRVC	Pressure-regulated volume control
PS	Pressure support
PT	Prothrombin time
PTH	Parathyroid hormone
PTU	Propylthiouracil
PV	Peak velocity
PVL	Panton-Valentine leukocidin
QDS	Four times a day
qSOFA	Quick Sepsis-related Organ Failure Assessment

RASS	Richmond Agitation-Sedation Scale
RBBB	Right bundle branch block
RCOA	Royal College of Anaesthetists
RCT	Randomised controlled trial
REBOA	Resuscitative endovascular balloon occlusion of the aorta
REE	Resting energy expenditure
RER	Respiratory exchange ratio
RIFLE	Risk, Injury, Failure, Loss of kidney function, and End-stage kidney disease
RIS	Radiologically isolated lesion
RLL	Right lower lobe
ROSC	Return of spontaneous circulation
ROTEM	Rotational thromboelastometry
RQ	Respiratory quotient
RR	Respiratory rate
RRMS	Relapsing remitting multiple sclerosis
RRT	Renal replacement therapy
RSBI	Rapid Shallow Breathing Index
RSI	Rapid sequence induction
RTA	Renal tubular acidosis
RTC	Road traffic collision
RV	Right ventricular/right ventricle
RWMA	Regional wall motion abnormality
SAAG	Serum ascites albumin gradient
SAH	Subarachnoid haemorrhage
SAPS	Simplified Acute Physiology Score
SBP	Systolic blood pressure; spontaneous bacterial peritonitis
SBT	Spontaneous breathing trial
SC	Subcutaneous
SCI	Spinal cord injury
SCUF	Slow continuous ultrafiltration
SD	Stroke distance
SDD	Selective digestive decontamination
SE	Status epilepticus
SecBP	Secondary bacterial peritonitis
SGLT	Sodium-glucose linked transporter
SHOT	Serious Hazards of Transfusion
SI	Serious incident
SIADH	Syndrome of inappropriate anti-diuretic hormone
SIC	Sepsis-induced coagulopathy
SID	Strong ion difference
SIGN	Scottish Intercollegiate Guidelines Network

Abbreviations

SIMV	Synchronised intermittent mandatory ventilation
SIRS	Systemic inflammatory response syndrome
SjO$_2$	Jugular bulb venous oxygen saturation
SJS	Stevens-Johnson syndrome
SLE	Systemic lupus erythematosus
SNAP	Sensory nerve action potential
SNRI	Serotonin-norepinephrine reuptake inhibitor
SOB	Shortness of breath
SOD	Selective oropharyngeal decontamination
SOFA	Sequential Organ Failure Assessment
SR	Sinus rhythm
SSRI	Selective serotonin reuptake inhibitor
SSSS	Staphylococcal scalded skin syndrome
STEC	Shiga toxin-producing *Escherichia coli*
STEMI	ST-elevation myocardial infarction
SUPC	Sudden unexpected postnatal collapse
SV	Stroke volume
SVC	Superior vena cava
SVR	Systemic vascular resistance
SVRI	Systemic Vascular Resistance Index
SVT	Supraventricular tachycardia
SVV	Stroke volume variation
TACO	Transfusion-associated circulatory overload
TACS	Total anterior circulatory stroke
TA-GvHD	Transfusion-associated graft-versus-host disease
TB	Tuberculosis
TBI	Traumatic brain injury
TBSA	Total body surface area
TCA	Tricyclic antidepressant
TdP	Torsade de pointes
TDS	Three times a day
TEG	Thromboelastography
TEN	Toxic epidermal necrolysis
TINU	Tubulointerstitial nephritis and uveitis
TIPS	Transjugular intrahepatic portosystemic shunt
TIVA	Total intravenous anaesthesia
TLS	Tumour lysis syndrome
TMA	Thrombotic microangiopathy
TNF-α	Tumour necrosis factor alpha
TOF	Train of four
TPE	Therapeutic plasma exchange

TPN	Total parenteral nutrition
TSH	Thyroid-stimulating hormone
TSS	Toxic shock syndrome
TTE	Transthoracic echocardiography
TTI	Transfusion-transmitted infection
TTM	Targeted temperature management
TTP	Thrombotic thrombocytopenic purpura
TRALI	Transfusion-related acute lung injury
TV	Tidal volume
TXA	Tranexamic acid
U&E	Urea and electrolyte
UKELD	United Kingdom Model for End-Stage Liver Disease
UKKA	UK Kidney Association
UO	Urine output
USS	Ultrasound scan
VAP	Ventilator-associated pneumonia
VATS	Video-assisted thoracoscopic surgery
VC	Vital capacity
VCV	Volume-controlled ventilation
VF	Ventricular fibrillation
VITT	Vaccine-induced thrombocytopaenia and thrombosis
VO_2	Oxygen consumption
VSD	Ventricular septal defect
Vt	Tidal volume
VT	Ventricular tachycardia
VTE	Venous thromboembolism
vWF	von Willebrand factor
WBC	White blood cell
WCC	White cell count
WE	Wernicke's encephalopathy
WFNS	World Federation of Neurological Societies
WIT	Warm ischaemic time
WOLST	Withdrawal of life-sustaining treatment
WPW	Wolff-Parkinson-White (syndrome)
WSACS	World Society of Abdominal Compartment Syndrome
XO	Xanthine oxidase
VZV	Varicella zoster virus

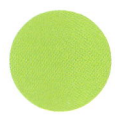

Normal adult ranges for blood tests

Table 1. Normal adult ranges for common blood tests (note: reference ranges can vary dependent on the lab).

Hb	M = 132–169g/L	Na^+	133–146mmol/L	pH	7.35–7.45
	F = 119–149g/L	K^+	3.5–5.3mmol/L	pO_2	12.0–15.0kPa
WCC	4.0–11.0 x 10^9/L	Urea	2.5–7.8mmol/L	pCO_2	4.5–6.1kPa
Platelets	150–450 x 10^9/L	Creatinine	M = 53–97µmol/L	BE	−2.0– +2.0mmol/L
Neutrophils	1.7–6.6 x 10^9/L		F = 44–71µmol/L	HCO_3^-	22–26mmol/L
Eosinophils	0.05–0.45 x 10^9/L	Serum protein	57–76g/L	Lactate	0.6–2.5mmol/L
PT	12.4–17.3 seconds	Albumin	35–50g/L	Cl^-	95–108mmol/L
APTT	28.0–42.0 seconds	Bilirubin	<21µmol/L	Glucose	7.0–11.1mmol/L
Fibrinogen	1.90–4.10g/L	ALT	10–49 IU/L	Ketones	<0.6mmol/L
INR	1.0	ALP	30–130 IU/L	AdjCa	2.2–2.6mmol/L
CRP	<5mg/L	AST	0–40 U/L	PO_4^{3-}	0.80–1.50mmol/L
PCT	<0.05ng/mL	Amylase	30–118 IU/L	Mg^{2+}	0.7–1.0mmol/L
LDH	120–246 IU/L	D-dimer	<0.5µg/L		
		Osmolality — serum	275–295mOsmol/kg		

Table 2. Normal range for other lab samples.

Urine testing

Na⁺ urine/day	40–220mmol/24h
Na⁺ spot urine	>20mmol/L
Fractional excretion Na⁺ (FENa)	<1%
Osmolality (urine)	50–1200mOsmol/kg

Normal pleural fluid

Appearance	Clear
pH	7.6–7.64
Glucose	Similar to plasma
LDH	<50% plasma level
Protein	1–2g/dL
WBC	<1000/mm^3

Lights Criteria

Pleural fluid is an exudate if one or more of the following criteria are met
- Pleural fluid protein divided by serum protein is >0.5
- Pleural fluid LDH divided by serum LDH is >0.6
- Pleural fluid LDH >2/3 the upper limit of lab normal value for serum LDH

1 SBA Paper 1: Questions

Question 1

A 44-year-old man presents with confusion and agitation. He was noted to be asleep in the morning by his wife and still in the same position when she came home later that day. He had been seen by his GP the week before because of suicidal ideation and had been taken off his olanzapine. On arrival to the emergency department (ED) observations are as follows:

A: Maintaining own airway.
B: Sats of 98% on an FiO_2 of 0.5.
C: BP 90/50mmHg, heart rate (HR) 145/min, electrocardiogram (ECG) — sinus rhythm.
D: Glasgow Coma Scale (GCS) 9 (E-2, V-3, M-4).
E: Temperature 35.5°C, no rashes.

Blood test results are shown in Table 1.1.

Table 1.1. Blood test results.

Haemoglobin (Hb)	130g/L	Na^+	131mmol/L
White cell count (WCC)	26.7 x 10^9/L	K^+	5.7mmol/L
Platelets	30 x 10^9/L	Urea	8.8mmol/L
International Normalised Ratio (INR)	7.9	Creatinine	391μmol/L
		Lactate	6.8mmol/L
Activated partial thromboplastin time (APTT)	51.8 seconds	Alanine aminotransferase (ALT)	16,813 IU/L
Fibrinogen	1g/L	Alkaline phosphatase (ALP)	228 IU/L
Glucose	0.9mmol/L	Bilirubin	95μmol/L
Paracetamol (acetaminophen)	79mg/L	Albumin	35g/L

What is the next treatment priority?

a   Referral to the local liver transplant centre.
b   250ml 10% glucose.
c   Loading dose of N-acetylcysteine (NAC).
d   Fluid resuscitation.
e   Intubation and ventilation.

● Question 2

A 55-year-old, 66kg woman presents with a vesicular rash and worsening shortness of breath. She has been looking after her grandson who has chicken pox and says she cannot recall ever having had the infection herself as a child.

She is admitted to the intensive care unit (ICU) for continuous positive airway pressure (CPAP) ventilation, but after 24 hours deteriorated requiring intubation. For the next 4 days she is stable with an FiO_2 of 0.5 before a further deterioration. She has a computed tomography (CT) scan of her chest which shows ground-glass changes in both lung bases and bilateral effusions. Her partial pressure of oxygen (PaO_2) to FiO_2 ratio (P:F ratio) is 12kPa (PaO_2 of 9.6kPa on an FiO_2 of 0.8). She is currently on pressure-controlled ventilation (PCV) with an inspiratory pressure (IP) of 30cmH_2O and a positive end-expiratory pressure (PEEP) of 12cmH_2O, achieving tidal volumes (Vt) of 400ml. Her peak inspiratory pressure (PIP) is 32cmH_2O and ventilatory rate is 20 breaths/minute. Her blood gas shows a partial pressure of carbon dioxide ($PaCO_2$) of 6.8kPa. A bedside echocardiogram (ECHO) shows a hyperdynamic well-filled heart, and 6 to 8 B-lines per pleural space. She is currently sedated on propofol 3mg/kg/hr and alfentanil 0.2µg/kg/min.

Which of the following has the best evidence for use in this patient's condition?

a   Extracorporeal membrane oxygenation (ECMO).
b   Switch to airway pressure release ventilation (APRV).
c   Prone positioning.
d   Fluid restriction and diuresis.
e   Paralysis with infusion of neuromuscular blockade.

Question 3

You are called to review a new 41-year-old patient who has been transferred to the ICU from the percutaneous coronary intervention (PCI) lab. She has a 1-month history of worsening shortness of breath and ankle swelling and presented to a local district general hospital (DGH) with an acute deterioration in her symptoms. She is normally fit and well, a non-smoker, and a non-drinker. She had a pulseless electrical activity (PEA) cardiac arrest in the DGH and after a short period of cardiopulmonary resuscitation (CPR) had return of spontaneous circulation (ROSC). A CT pulmonary angiogram (CTPA) demonstrated no pulmonary embolus (PE), so she was transferred to the PCI centre. PCI showed no disease in the coronary vessels. Her observations are as follows:

A: Endotracheal tube (ETT) *in situ*.
B: Respiratory rate (RR) 20 breaths/minute (ventilated), FiO$_2$ of 0.6 with O$_2$ saturations of 98%, volume control ventilation (VCV) Vt 400ml, PEEP of 10cmH$_2$O and P:F 14kPa.
C: BP 95/60mmHg, HR 148/min, sinus rhythm, cool peripherally, dusky fingers, noradrenaline 0.55µg/kg/min, bedside ECHO shows a severely impaired, non-dilated left ventricle (LV) and a moderately impaired right ventricle (RV).
D: Sedated on propofol and alfentanil.
E: Temperature 36.2°C, no rashes.

What is the next best treatment for this patient?

a   Milrinone infusion.
b   Milrinone bolus followed by infusion.
c   Dobutamine infusion.
d   Vasopressin infusion.
e   Adrenaline infusion.

Question 4

A 33-year-old women presents to hospital with abdominal pain, high fevers, tachycardia and hypotension. Intra-abdominal sepsis is suspected and she is started on antibiotics (cefuroxime, metronidazole and a single dose of gentamicin). She undergoes a CT abdomen with contrast. The initial blood test results are shown in Table 1.2.

Table 1.2. Blood test results.

WCC	20 x 10⁹/L	Creatinine	350µmol/L
Neutrophils	18 x 10⁹/L	Urea	12mmol/L
CRP	350mg/L		

She is given 3L of crystalloid in the ED but remains hypotensive, so she is admitted to the ICU for vasopressor support. A diagnosis of an appendix abscess is made and she has this laparoscopically removed. Given the evidence of acute kidney injury (AKI) the following tests are performed (Table 1.3).

Table 1.3. Investigations.

Urinalysis	Epithelial cell casts, protein 1+
Renal ultrasound (USS)	Normal with no hydronephrosis
Urinary sodium (Na⁺)	45mmol/L
Fractional excretion Na⁺ (FENa⁺)	2.2%
Urinary osmolality	400mOsmol/kg

Two days later her creatinine is 300µmol/L and her urine output is 30–40ml/hr (as it has been throughout her admission).

What is the most likely diagnosis?

a   Contrast-induced nephropathy.
b   Acute tubular necrosis (ATN).
c   Pre-renal AKI secondary to sepsis.
d   Acute interstitial nephritis (AIN).
e   Obstructive post-renal AKI.

Question 5

You are asked to review a 35-year-old woman who is 35 weeks pregnant (G3P1). She has previously lost a pregnancy at 22 weeks due to pre-eclampsia. On this occasion she has presented to the ED with epigastric pain and feeling generally unwell, complaining of dark urine and orange-looking eyes.

On examination:

A: Maintaining own airway.
B: O_2 saturation 99% in room air, RR 25/min.
C: BP 130/80mmHg, HR 110/min, capillary refill time (CRT) 3 seconds.
D: Alert and orientated.
E: Gravid abdomen mildly tender in the epigastrium, USS of her abdomen shows a few gallstones with a normal sized gallbladder. Nil else.

Blood test results of note are shown in Table 1.4.

Table 1.4. Blood test results.

Hb	120g/L	Creatinine	160µmol/L
WCC	22 x 10⁹/L	Urea	7.4mmol/L
Platelets	130 x 10⁹/L	ALT	350 IU/L
PT	16.5 seconds	Aspartate aminotransferase (AST)	400 U/L
APTT	30 seconds	Bilirubin	55µmol/L
Fibrinogen	1.8g/L	ALP	300 IU/L

What is the most likely diagnosis?

a   Cholecystitis.
b   HELLP syndrome.
c   Intrahepatic cholestasis of pregnancy.
d   Acute fatty liver of pregnancy.
e   Severe pre-eclampsia.

Question 6

A 65-year-old man has been on the ICU for 35 days. He was originally admitted for *Legionella* pneumonia. He spent 10 days paralysed and receiving intermittent prone ventilation. On day 20 he had a size 8 percutaneous tracheostomy without a subglottic suction port inserted. Since then, his sedation and ventilation pressures have been weaned (with a gradual reduction in pressure support [PS] approach). He is currently on PS 10cmH$_2$O over a PEEP of 5cmH$_2$O. He is achieving a Vt of around 450ml. He has had sprint weaning attempts over the last few days, but tires within a few minutes and desaturates. He has had a fibreoptic endoscopic evaluation of swallow (FEES) and has a normal upper airway with no oedema, an intact swallow, with a moderate oral secretion load. His mood is low, and his family feel that if he could talk to them, this may help improve matters.

Which of the following is the best option for enabling vocalisation in this case?

a   Not suitable for any form of vocalisation currently.
b   Periods of cuff down with external CPAP.
c   In-line speaking valve (Passy-Muir).
d   Above cuff vocalisation.
e   Change to a fenestrated tracheostomy tube.

Question 7

You attend the ED as part of the trauma team. You have been pre-alerted to a 'code red' trauma arriving via helicopter. The patient has been involved in a road traffic collision (RTC) where he was an unrestrained driver of a car which crashed into a tree at around 50mph. He was ejected through the front window of the car. There was a paramedic on scene within a few minutes who found the patient in respiratory arrest and commenced hand ventilation. On arrival of the Helimed team, the patient was immediately intubated. The crew noted at this time that he had a short period of asystole during intubation that did not require CPR or adrenaline. He had reduced air entry on the left side of his chest, so had a finger thoracostomy at scene resulting in an improvement in oxygen saturations.

SBA Paper 1: Questions

On arrival to the ED, the primary survey is as follows:

A: Intubated (no evidence of catastrophic bleeding).
B: RR 18/min, O_2 sats 99% on an FiO_2 of 0.5 synchronised intermittent mandatory ventilation (SIMV) mode: all mandatory breaths. Finger thoracostomy to the left side of the chest, with a small amount of bleeding, but equal air entry bilaterally. Extensive bruising over the left side of his chest.
C: BP 85/40mmHg, HR 60/min, warm peripherally, CRT 3–4 seconds.
D: Pupils equal and reactive, sedated. Bruising over the right side of his head.
E: Temperature 35.0°C, obviously deformed swollen right thigh.

What is the most likely predominant cause of his haemodynamic state?

a   Hypovolaemic shock.
b   Neurogenic shock.
c   Haemorrhagic shock.
d   Spinal shock.
e   Cardiogenic shock.

● Question 8

You are reviewing a patient on the ICU as part of the daily reviews. He is a 35-year-old man who has been in the ICU for 37 days with acute necrotising pancreatitis, believed to be secondary to alcohol. He was intubated on day 7 due to agitation and worsening oxygenation with intolerance of CPAP. He had a tracheostomy inserted on day 25 and is now on a slow tracheostomy and sedation wean. During his daily review, the nurses mention that they have had to increase his clonidine infusion overnight due to worsening agitation. His bloods show a small rise in inflammatory markers but he remains apyrexial and he is not currently on any antibiotics. His nasogastric (NG) aspirate volumes are increasing, having previously been absorbing NG feed well. The rest of his bloods are unremarkable, he has stable oxygen requirements and continues to wean ventilatory pressures well.

A CT scan of his abdomen is performed and shows a large-volume walled-off pancreatic pseudocyst involving the head, neck and body of the pancreas with no evidence of necrosis.

What is the best management of this complication?

a Broad-spectrum antibiotics.
b Insertion of a nasojejunal (NJ) tube for post-pyloric feeding.
c Endoscopic transmural drainage.
d Percutaneous radiologically-guided drain.
e Surgical necrosectomy and drainage.

● Question 9

You are asked to urgently review a patient in the ICU. She is a 55-year-old woman admitted 2 days prior with hyponatraemic seizures secondary to alcohol excess. Her past medical history includes chronic liver disease (CLD) secondary to alcohol (previously variceal banding), diabetes mellitus (DM) and ischaemic heart disease. You have been asked to review her as she has started vomiting large quantities of blood. She remains alert, complaining of some chest discomfort. You are in a hospital with a 8am to 6pm 'Bleed consultant' service and it is currently 7.30am.

On examination:

A: Maintaining own airway.
B: RR 24/min, O_2 sats 95% in room air.
C: BP 80/40mmHg, HR 130/min, ECG — sinus rhythm with lateral ST-segment depression.
D: Alert and orientated.
E: Epigastric tenderness. Multiple vomit bowels full of fresh blood and clots at the bedspace.

You initiate the major transfusion protocol and start to give her blood products. What else should form part of your immediate management?

a Endoscopy and banding of varices.
b Terlipressin 2mg immediately and every 4 hours.
c Octreotide bolus followed by infusion.
d Intubation to facilitate insertion of a Sengstaken-Blakemore tube.
e Arrange transfer of the patient to a hospital with a 24-hour bleed service.

Question 10

You receive a phone call from the oncology ward regarding a deteriorating patient. A 24-year-old man with relapsed B-cell acute lymphoblastic leukaemia (ALL) has received chimeric antigen receptor T (CAR T) cell therapy the day before and has now developed high fevers unresponsive to ward-based management, hypotension refractory to fluid therapy and a reduced urine output.

On examination the patient looks unwell with the following observations:

A: Maintaining own airway.
B: RR 28/min, O_2 sats 98% on an FiO_2 of 0.6 (new oxygen requirement), CXR — patchy bibasal changes.
C: BP 75/40mmHg, HR 130/min, cool fingers, CRT 3–4 seconds, urine output 20ml/hr.
D: Confused, moving all four limbs.
E: Abdomen soft and non-tender, calves equal and non-tender.

Blood test results of note are shown in Table 1.5.

Table 1.5. Blood test results.

WCC	33 x 10⁹/L	Na^+	131mmol/L
Neutrophils	1.2 x 10⁹/L	K^+	3.1mmol/L
Lymphocytes	30 x 10⁹/L	Creatinine	110µmol/L
Platelets	100 x 10⁹/L	Urea	6mmol/L
CRP	100mg/L	Phosphate (PO_4^{3-})	1.4mmol/L
Procalcitonin (PCT)	0.3ng/ml	Ferritin	6000µg/L

What is the most appropriate treatment for the likely underlying cause?

a   Tazocin®.
b   Tocilizumab plus steroids.
c   Anakinra.
d   Noradrenaline infusion.
e   Intravenous (IV) fluids and rasburicase.

● Question 11

A patient has been on continuous renal replacement therapy (CRRT) for 4 days for AKI secondary to sepsis with citrate anticoagulation. Urine output has been around 20ml/hr for the past 12 hours. The charge nurse is concerned that the arterial blood gases (ABGs) look abnormal but there has been no change in the calcium infusion rate throughout the day.

Blood test results this morning are shown in Table 1.6.

Table 1.6. Blood test results.

pH	7.48	Na^+	146mmol/L
HCO_3^-	32mmol/L	K^+	4.5mmol/L
BE	+10mmol/L	Creatinine	110μmol/L
Ionised Ca^{2+}	1.3mmol/L	Urea	6.2mmol/L
		Total Ca^{2+}	2.6mmol/L

What is the best next step in the management of this patient's CRRT?

a   Reduce the blood flow rate on the CRRT.
b   Stop CRRT.
c   Increase the calcium infusion rate.
d   Continue to run CRRT but switch to heparin anticoagulation.
e   Reduce the citrate rate and run the patient off the standard dialysate to blood flow rate ratio.

● Question 12

A 35-year-old woman presents to the ED with acute-onset severe chest pain radiating into the back. A CT angiogram shows an aortic dissection from the left subclavian artery extending down into the abdominal aorta to the bifurcation of the aorta.

Clinical examination is as follows:

A: Maintaining own airway.
B: RR 24/min, O_2 sats 99% on 15L non-rebreathe mask (NRB), clear chest on auscultation.

C: BP 140/90mmHg, HR 101/min, CRT 3 seconds.
D: Alert and orientated, no focal neurological deficit. Ongoing pain despite morphine.
E: Abdomen soft, non-tender. Urinary catheter recently inserted, with minimal residual urine.

What is the immediate management priority?

a   Nicardipine infusion.
b   Endovascular stent grafting.
c   Urgent transfer to theatre for operative repair.
d   Labetalol infusion.
e   Glyceryl trinitrate (GTN) infusion.

● Question 13

A 22-year-old man is admitted to the ICU following a motorcycle crash without a helmet resulting in a significant traumatic brain injury (TBI) with diffuse axonal injury, a traumatic subarachnoid bleed and intraparenchymal bleeding consistent with a contusional injury. His GCS was 6 at the scene so he was intubated. Other injuries include left-sided rib fractures (2nd to 5th ribs with associated lung contusion) and a small splenic laceration (for conservative management). The neurosurgeons have placed an intracranial pressure (ICP) monitoring bolt.

You are called to review this patient because his ICP has been 25mmHg for the last 15 minutes.

On examination:

A: Intubated.
B: O_2 sats 97% on an FiO_2 of 0.4, PaO_2 10.5kPa, $PaCO_2$ 4.9kPa on ABG, PCV with a PEEP of 5cmH$_2$O.
C: BP 100/60mmHg (mean arterial pressure [MAP] 73mmHg), HR 75/min, sinus rhythm.
D: Pupils equal and reactive, propofol 4mg/kg/hr, alfentanil 0.5µg/kg/min, Bispectral Index (BIS) 25.
E: Temperature 36.8°C. Glucose 5.5mmol/L. His neck is in alignment, 30° bed tilt with nothing tight around his neck.

What is the next best step in the management of this patient's ICP?

a   3ml/kg of 3% hypertonic saline.
b   Start vasopressors aiming for a cerebral perfusion pressure (CPP) of 65mmHg.
c   Contact neurosurgeons for an urgent review.
d   Bolus sedation and increase maintenance rate.
e   Increase minute ventilation (MV) on the ventilator, aiming for a PaCO$_2$ of 4–4.5kPa.

● Question 14

A 45-year-old army sergeant presents to the hospital with a 4-day history of shortness of breath and haemoptysis. He is normally fit and well, and the only thing of note on his general practitioner (GP) community file is a record of recurrent courses of antibiotics for axillary boils. Swabs from his axilla have shown he is colonised with methicillin-resistant *Staphylococcus aureus* (MRSA). Whilst on a recent holiday to Thailand he went swimming in a lake and noticed there were multiple rats around the shoreline. On arrival in the ED, he is found to have a PaO$_2$ of 6kPa on a NRB mask so he is admitted to the ICU for intubation. Immediately following intubation, he requires a noradrenaline infusion to regain cardiovascular stability. Blood tests show a WCC of 6 x 10^9/L and CRP of 350mg/L. His creatinine is 150μmol/L, urea 7mmol/L, with unremarkable LFTs and coagulation tests, but a creatine kinase (CK) of 7000 IU/L. CT chest performed post-intubation shows dense right upper lobe consolidation with bilateral infiltrates and small pleural effusions. There are multiple cavitating areas within both lung fields.

What is the most appropriate antibiotic choice in this patient?

a   Augmentin and clarithromycin.
b   Clindamycin, linezolid and rifampicin.
c   Septrin™ (sulfamethoxazole and trimethoprim).
d   Benzylpenicillin and clindamycin.
e   Benzylpenicillin, doxycycline and ceftriaxone.

SBA Paper 1: Questions

● Question 15

An 18-year-old male presents with an acute asthma exacerbation. They have had 30 minutes of back-to-back salbutamol nebulisers with ipratropium and prednisolone 40mg orally. They look tired and have a silent chest on auscultation. Their ABG shows a PaO_2 of 10kPa on 6L nebuliser and a $PaCO_2$ of 5.5kPa. They are unable to do a peak flow measurement.

Which of the following is the next best step in the management of their asthma?

a   250mg IV aminophylline.
b   IV salbutamol infusion 5µg/min.
c   2g IV magnesium sulphate ($MgSO_4$) over 20 minutes.
d   Immediate intubation and ventilation.
e   Ketamine 1mg/kg IV bolus.

● Question 16

A 45-year-old lady presents to the ED having been found unconscious at home. She has recently had a bereavement and her family are concerned she may have taken a month's supply of her propranolol medication. She was last seen well around 4 hours ago.

Her initial observations are:

A: Maintaining own airway.
B: RR 15/min, O_2 sats 98% on 15L NRB.
C: HR 45/min, BP 80/40mmHg.
D: GCS 13 (E-3, M-6, V-4).

An ECG taken at triage 15 minutes ago shows a sinus tachycardia with a QRS of 140ms and prolonged PR interval. You are called to review her. On arrival she becomes less responsive:

A: Maintaining her airway.
B: O_2 sats 95% on 15L NRB.
C: HR 140/min, BP 65/40mmHg and ECG now shows ventricular tachycardia (VT).
D: GCS is 9 (E-2, M-5, V-2).

What is the best treatment option?

a   10mg glucagon IV.
b   1 unit/kg Actrapid® bolus then 1 unit/kg/hr infusion.
c   100ml 8.4% sodium bicarbonate.
d   Adrenaline infusion titrated to blood pressure.
e   Urgent intubation and ventilation.

● Question 17

A 72-year-old lady is admitted to the ICU having been urgently transferred from another unit with a suspicion of thrombotic thrombocytopenic purpura (TTP) for consideration of therapeutic plasma exchange. She presented to her local hospital with new confusion and a purpuric rash. Her medical history includes well-controlled systemic lupus erythematosus.

Her blood test results of note are shown in Table 1.7.

Table 1.7. Blood test results.

Hb	82g/L	Creatinine (Cr)	150µmol/L
Reticulocyte count	3%	Baseline Cr	80µmol/L
Mean corpuscular volume (MCV)	92fl	Bilirubin	45µmol/L
Platelets	3×10^9/L	Troponin	150ng/L
ADAMTS13	Result pending		

What is the management priority?

a   Therapeutic plasma exchange.
b   Platelet transfusion.
c   Plasma infusion.
d   Oral prednisolone.
e   Rituximab.

SBA Paper 1: Questions

 Question 18

A 60-year-old obese lady with a history of reflux, 40-pack-year smoking history and type 2 DM is being ventilated on the ICU for acute respiratory distress syndrome (ARDS) secondary to acute pancreatitis. She briefly required prone ventilation for severe acute hypoxia during her admission 2 weeks ago but has made steady progress and is now on an FiO_2 of 0.3 with a PaO_2 of 10kPa, PEEP of 7cmH_2O and PS of 5cmH_2O.

On review she is alert and appropriate on sedation hold, with a strong spontaneous cough and good peripheral power. You decide to commence a spontaneous breathing trial (SBT), which shows a Rapid Shallow Breathing Index (RSBI) of 40 breaths/min/L at 30 minutes. You then go on to assess with the cuff down and there is no audible leak.

What is the next most appropriate course of action?

a   Continue ventilator weaning and try again in 2 days.
b   Work the patient up for a tracheostomy.
c   Re-sedate and perform a laryngoscopy to assess the airway.
d   Continue to a trial of extubation.
e   Give a dose of methylprednisolone and extubate in 2 hours.

 Question 19

You are asked to review a 45-year-old lady in the ED who has presented with an acute asthma exacerbation. Despite an hour of full medical treatment including magnesium, she is still very wheezy. She states that she has had asthma for the last 10 years and the number of exacerbations requiring steroids has increased year on year. She has never required ICU admission for her asthma. Following review, she is admitted to the ICU for CPAP and ongoing asthma management. Over the course of the next 24 hours her chest slowly improves. On admission it is noted that her renal function is impaired which is new, and she complains of new skin lesions on her arms, as well as pain and numbness in her right hand and left foot. Due to the new multisystem nature of her presentation, you request extended blood tests.

Blood test results are shown in Table 1.8.

Table 1.8. Blood test results.

Hb	120×10^9/L	Creatinine	220μmol/L
WCC	14×10^9/L	Urea	12mmol/L
Neutrophils	8×10^9/L	MPO-ANCA	Positive
Lymphocytes	4×10^9/L	PR3-ANCA	Negative
Eosinophils	1.5×10^9/L	Rheumatoid factor	Weakly positive
Platelets	150×10^9/L	Immunophoresis	Mildly elevated IgE, otherwise normal
		Complement levels	Normal

CXR shows bilateral patchy infiltrates.

What diagnosis is most likely in this context?

a   Asthma.
b   Granulomatosis with polyangiitis.
c   Sarcoidosis.
d   Eosinophilic granulomatosis with polyangiitis.
e   Idiopathic acute eosinophilic pneumonia.

● Question 20

A 36-year-old man presents to the ED having fallen into a bonfire and sustained full-thickness burns to his torso (front and back) and upper arms. His estimated total body surface area (TBSA) burns is 30%. Fluid resuscitation has been initiated, and he is admitted to the ICU for ongoing management.

You are called to see him 30 minutes after admission to the ICU (around 4 hours post-burn) because he is feeling short of breath and his chest feels 'really tight'.

Examination reveals:

A: Patent, no airway swelling or burns seen.
B: Speaking in single-word sentences, SpO$_2$ 90% on an FiO$_2$ of 0.9 via high-flow nasal oxygen (HFNO), RR 40/min, poor air entry globally with fine

crepitations, no wheeze, CXR shows a clear chest, PaO_2 9kPa and $PaCO_2$ 6.5kPa on ABG.
C: BP 80/60mmHg, HR 120/min, sinus rhythm, CRT 4 seconds, raised JVP, urine output for the last hour is 20ml.
D: Alert and orientated, but very distressed.
E: Burns on chest and back as previously described.

Which of the following will treat the cause of his acute deterioration?

a   Intubation and ventilation.
b   CPAP.
c   Chest wall escharotomy.
d   IV fluid challenge.
e   Salbutamol and ipratropium nebuliser.

● **Question 21**
Which one of the following clinical scenarios would **not** meet the criteria for ARDS?

a O_2 sats of 90% on an FiO_2 of 0.5, 40L/min HFNO in a patient who is 4 days into admission with a positive swab for influenza A. CXR shows bilateral infiltrates.
b   Patient with a diagnosis of pancreatitis 3 days prior with O_2 sats of 92% on a NRB mask in a resource-poor setting. USS of the lung shows B-lines throughout both lung fields.
c   Patient intubated after a polytrauma laparotomy who has received a major haemorrhage pack, an FiO_2 of 0.8, PEEP of $8cmH_2O$, PaO_2 10kPa. Post-op CXR shows a left-sided haemopneumothorax with significant loss of volume on that side.
d   Patient who is day 11 on the ICU following a diagnosis of COVID-19. New deterioration in oxygenation, requiring CPAP with a PEEP of $10cmH_2O$, an FiO_2 of 0.7 with a PaO_2 of 8kPa.
e   Patient with right lower lobe (RLL) pneumonia diagnosed 3 days ago, has deteriorated requiring intubation. Now on an FiO_2 of 0.5 with a PaO_2 of 10kPa. Post-intubation CXR shows the presence of new left-sided infiltrates and worsening of the right side.

Question 22
A patient is admitted to your unit with a pacemaker. There is a medical student who asks you what the four different letters of the pacemaker mean. What is the correct answer?

a   Chamber sensed, Response to sensed event, Chamber paced, Rate modulation.
b   Chamber sensed, Chamber paced, Rate modulation, Response to sensed event.
c   Chamber paced, Chamber sensed, Response to sensed event, Rate modulation.
d   Chamber paced, Rate modulation, Chamber sensed, Response to sensed event.
e   Chamber paced, Chamber sensed, Rate modulation, Response to sensed event.

Question 23
You are looking after a 45-year-old patient who has taken 80g of paracetamol in a deliberate overdose 12 hours ago. They have received fluid resuscitation. Which one of the following factors would form part of a trigger for referral for liver transplantation?

a   Patient's age.
b   INR of 6.1.
c   Creatinine 250μmol/L.
d   Bilirubin 305μmol/L.
e   pH 7.27.

Question 24
Which of the following drugs is **least** likely to cause acute interstitial nephritis (AIN)?

a   Ibuprofen.
b   Penicillin V.
c   Omeprazole.
d   Simvastatin.
e   Co-amoxiclav.

SBA Paper 1: Questions

● **Question 25**

In a pregnant mother with known pre-eclampsia and a history of migraines and hypothyroidism, which of the following would lead to a diagnosis of pre-eclampsia with severe features?

a   Hyperreflexia.
b   Systolic blood pressure (SBP) of 165mmHg.
c   Headache.
d   Urinary protein creatinine (PCR) of 65mg/mol.
e   Platelet count of 110×10^9/L.

● **Question 26**

You admit a 16-year-old boy to the ICU with urosepsis. He is adamant that he will not have any lines inserted to enable management of his hypotension. He understands the risks of not having the lines in; he just really does not want a central line and arterial line inserted. His parents have given consent for the lines to be inserted. He currently only has one pink peripheral 20G intravenous cannula and is on 30mg/hr of metaraminol. With regards to consent in this patient which of the following is true?

a   One parent can consent to treatment (to overrule his decision).
b   Both parents need to consent to treatment (to overrule his decision).
c   As he has not consented, lines cannot be inserted.
d   The case needs court referral for a decision to be made.
e   Urgent discussion with the hospital legal team is needed, prior to a treatment decision.

● **Question 27**

With regard to head and neck injuries, which one of the following is true?

a   Bony C-spine injury is common after hanging.
b   An injury to zone 1 of the neck could result in a pneumothorax.
c   Hypotension and bradycardia after a C-spine injury could represent spinal shock.
d   A RTC at 50mph is an indication for neck imaging.
e   Retrograde amnesia is not an indication for a CT of the head.

Question 28

A polytrauma patient is on the ICU. They have multiple rib fractures with an associated haemopneumothorax and a chest drain *in situ*. They also have a splenic laceration which is being conservatively managed and left-sided femoral shaft, tibia and fibula fractures. You are asked to review this patient because he has worsening left lower leg pain despite a morphine patient-controlled analgesia (PCA) infusion. You are concerned about compartment syndrome. Which of the following is true regarding the identification and management of compartment syndrome?

a   Pain is typically only on active movement of the compartment.
b   Perfusion is only compromised once compartment pressures equal MAP.
c   The presence of a dorsalis pedis pulse rules out the diagnosis.
d   Fasciotomy is only considered when the compartment pressure is about diastolic pressure.
e   Irreversible ischaemia of the compartment happens within 4 to 8 hours.

Question 29

With regards to calcium homeostasis and abnormalities which of the following is correct?

a   Parathyroid hormone (PTH) increases the absorption of Ca^{2+} from the gut via the action of 1,25 vitamin D.
b   Hypercalcaemia is present in primary, secondary and tertiary hyperparathyroidism.
c   Hypercalcaemia causes a prolonged QTc.
d   Prednisolone is useful in all causes of hypercalcaemia.
e   Calcium gluconate contains more elemental calcium than calcium chloride.

Question 30

Which one of the following would **not** be a consideration for admission to the ICU in a patient with a diagnosis of diabetic ketoacidosis (DKA)?

a   Blood ketone level of 6.5mmol/L.
b   K⁺ on admission of 3.4mmol/L.
c   Bicarbonate on venous blood gas of 6mmol/L.
d   Pregnant patient.
e   SBP 85mmHg.

● Question 31

You come onto a day shift on your ICU which has 14 physical bed spaces. There are currently four level 3 patients and eight level 2 patients. According to United Kingdom (UK) Guidelines for the Provision of Intensive Care Services (GPICS), what is the correct minimum safe staffing for the current levels of bed occupancy?

a   Eight registered nurses plus nurse in charge.
b   Ten registered nurses.
c   Two ICU consultants and two resident junior intensive care staff (doctors or advanced critical care practitioners [ACCPs]).
d   One ICU consultant and one resident junior intensive care staff (doctor or ACCP).
e   Eight registered nurses plus two senior nurses.

● Question 32

Which term best describes the distribution of the data in this graph (Figure 1.1)?

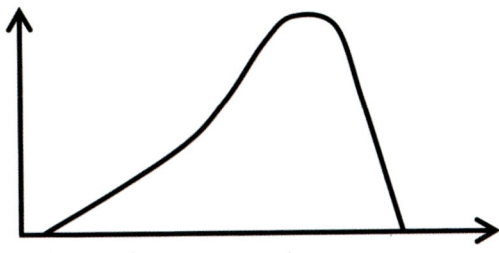

Figure 1.1. Distribution of data curve.

a   Negatively skewed distribution.
b   Gaussian distribution.
c   Bimodal distribution.
d   Positively skewed distribution.
e   Normal distribution.

● Question 33
Which of the following would be the correct daily requirement for a 60kg patient on the ICU?

a   120mmol K^+.
b   30mmol PO_4^{3-}.
c   30g protein.
d   120g fat.
e   60mmol Mg^{2+}.

● Question 34
You are asked to review a patient in the ED who has been admitted with sepsis. The patient tells you that she had chemotherapy 10 years ago for Hodgkin's lymphoma and has been told she must avoid oxygen therapy. Which chemotherapy agent is likely to have been given to the patient in the past?

a   Cyclophosphamide.
b   Methotrexate.
c   Vincristine.
d   Bleomycin.
e   Doxorubicin.

● Question 35
Which one of the following interventions should **not** be used for reducing the incidence of ventilator-associated pneumonia (VAP)?

a   Subglottic suction.
b   Daily sedation holds.
c   Selective digestive decontamination (SDD).
d   Toothbrushing with chlorhexidine toothpaste.
e   30° elevation of the head.

SBA Paper 1: Questions

● Question 36
With regard to intra-aortic balloon pumps (IABPs), which of the following is true?

a   The tip should lie 1–2cm distal to the right subclavian artery.
b   Deflation occurs at the peak of the T-wave.
c   A patient can safely sit upright with an IABP *in situ*.
d   Inflation of the IABP decreases aortic diastolic pressure.
e   Late deflation results in increased myocardial oxygen consumption.

● Question 37
Which of the following is true regarding nephrotic syndrome?

a   Characterised by a triad of proteinuria, hypertension and peripheral oedema.
b   The main cause in children is minimal change disease.
c   It can cause a reduced serum level of triglycerides and cholesterol.
d   An increased risk of bleeding is often seen.
e   Diagnosis is via urinary protein levels greater than 1.5g/24 hours.

● Question 38
Regarding the Gell and Coombs classification of hypersensitivity, which one of the following is **INCORRECT**?

a   Anaphylaxis is IgE-mediated.
b   Serum sickness is an example of type III hypersensitivity.
c   Goodpasture syndrome is an example of type IV hypersensitivity.
d   Type III hypersensitivity is caused by antigen-antibody complex deposition.
e   Type IV hypersensitivity is cell-mediated and has a delayed response.

Question 39

You are working on the cardiac ICU when you are urgently asked to review a patient who is 6 hours post-aortic valve replacement (AVR). He is still intubated and ventilated. The monitor shows a rhythm of ventricular fibrillation (VF) and no output on the arterial line. There is a defibrillator opposite the patient's bedspace. What is the most important next immediate step in management?

a   Start CPR.
b   Immediate resternotomy.
c   Increase FiO_2 to 1.0 and set PEEP to 0 on the ventilator.
d   Direct current (DC) shock up to three sequential attempts.
e   Amiodarone 300mg IV.

Question 40

You are asked to review a patient who requires transfer to a neurosurgical tertiary centre for management of a subarachnoid haemorrhage (SAH). On assessment they are opening their eyes to voice, have confused speech and are localising to pain. There is no obvious focal neurology. Which one of the following most accurately describes the grade of their SAH?

a   World Federation of Neurosurgical Societies (WFNS) grade IV.
b   Hess and Hunt grade V.
c   WFNS grade III.
d   Fisher grade III.
e   Fisher grade IV.

Question 41

Which one of the following is correct regarding multiple sclerosis (MS)?

a   Isolated sensory demyelination is seen.
b   In an acute attack, symptoms develop over minutes.
c   It is more common in men than women.
d   Investigative findings include oligoclonal bands in the cerebrospinal fluid (CSF) and white matter lesions in T2 magnetic resonance imaging (MRI) sequences.
e   Primary progressive MS has the best prognosis.

SBA Paper 1: Questions

Question 42
With regard to the presentation and treatment of tetanus, which one of the following is **not** true?

a   Treatments include magnesium and labetalol.
b   Motor symptoms only are seen in affected patients.
c   Tetanus toxin blocks inhibitory neurones.
d   Benzodiazepines are the mainstay of treatment for the muscle spasms.
e   Toxin reaches the anterior horn cells of the spinal cord via retrograde axonal transport.

Question 43
Regarding blast injury, which one of the following is correct?

a   Tertiary blast injury consists predominantly of long bone fractures and head injuries.
b   Primary blast injury is associated with the highest survival rates.
c   Blast lung is a type of secondary blast injury.
d   Primary blast injury affects solid organs more than air-filled organs.
e   Burns are regarded as secondary blast injuries.

Question 44
With regard to rescue therapies in the management of variceal bleeding, which one of the following is most accurate?

a   When using balloon tamponade methods, the gastric and oesophageal balloons should both be inflated.
b   Balloon tamponade methods can safely be left inflated for up to 36 hours.
c   A transjugular intrahepatic portosystemic shunt (TIPS) creates a connection between the portal vein and hepatic vein.
d   A self-expanding metal stent (e.g. Danis stent) is inserted without endoscopy.
e   A Sengstaken-Blakemore tube has an oesophageal suction port.

Question 45
With regards to renal tubular acidosis (RTA), which of the following is correct?

a   Alkali therapy is indicated in all types of RTA.
b   Type 1 RTA is due to a decrease in proximal tubule HCO_3^- reabsorption.
c   Types 1 and 2 are both associated with hyperkalaemia.
d   Type 1 RTA is associated with an increased risk of renal stones.
e   RTA results in a raised anion gap metabolic acidosis.

Question 46
With regards to drowning, which of the following statements is correct?

a   It is the leading cause of unnatural death in the UK.
b   There is a clinically significant difference between drowning in salt or fresh water.
c   Drowning victims may develop pulmonary oedema up to 12 hours after the drowning event.
d   There is no difference in the Advanced Life Support (ALS) management in a patient who has drowned.
e   Prophylactic IV antibiotics should be given routinely.

Question 47
In which of the following conditions is IV immunoglobulin (IVIg) **not** indicated?

a   Guillain-Barré syndrome (GBS).
b   Toxic epidermal necrolysis (TEN).
c   Haemophagocytic lymphohistiocytosis (HLH).
d   Toxic shock syndrome (TSS).
e   Myasthenia gravis (MG).

Question 48
Regarding the treatment of human immunodeficiency virus (HIV), which of the following is correct?

a   Monotherapy is standard.
b   Reverse transcriptase inhibitors are the mainstay of HIV treatment.
c   Integrase strand transfer inhibitors have the least favourable side-effect profile.
d   Non-nucleoside reverse transcriptase inhibitors (NRTIs) are active against HIV-1 and -2.
e   Anti-retroviral therapy (ART) is only started once the CD4 count is below 300 cells/mm^3.

Question 49
Which of the following results from an ascitic tap would lead you to a diagnosis of spontaneous bacterial peritonitis (SBP)?

a   Neutrophil count of 260/mm^3.
b   Red cell count of 900/mm^3.
c   Serum-ascites albumin gradient of 13g/L.
d   Ascitic WCC 260/mm^3.
e   Ascitic glucose 2.2mmol/L.

Question 50
High-dose euglycaemic insulin therapy is indicated in overdose of which of the following agents?

a   Paracetamol.
b   Ethylene glycol.
c   Digoxin.
d   Verapamil.
e   Sertraline.

Answer overview: Paper 1

Question:		Question:	
1	b	26	e
2	c	27	b
3	a	28	e
4	b	29	a
5	d	30	c
6	c	31	e
7	b	32	a
8	c	33	b
9	c	34	d
10	b	35	d
11	b	36	e
12	d	37	b
13	b	38	c
14	b	39	d
15	c	40	a
16	c	41	d
17	a	42	b
18	c	43	a
19	d	44	c
20	c	45	d
21	c	46	c
22	c	47	b
23	e	48	b
24	d	49	a
25	b	50	d

1 SBA Paper 1: Answers

 Answer 1: b

This history and biochemistry are consistent with a significant paracetamol overdose.

All of the options are reasonable, but the question is what the next treatment priority is. His glucose of 0.9mmol/L is life-threatening and, therefore, would be the treatment priority, although in reality it is likely that many of these treatments would be instituted in parallel in the emergency clinical setting.

 Answer 2: c

This lady has varicella zoster-induced acute respiratory distress syndrome (ARDS) (within 1 week of a known insult, bilateral opacities on chest imaging, and no evidence that this is heart failure, $PaO_2:FiO_2$ [P:F] <40kPa).

There is no indication in this question that any of the second-line ARDS treatments have been started. She has now deteriorated (P:F ratio 12kPa) and has severe ARDS based on the revised Berlin criteria (2024)(Table 1.9).

Table 1.9. Berlin criteria.

Intubated ARDS (Berlin 2024)	PaO_2: FiO_2 (mmHg)	PaO_2: FiO_2 (kPa)
Mild	P:F = 200< to ≤300mmHg	P:F = 26.7< to ≤40kPa
Moderate	P:F = 100< to ≤200mmHg	P:F = 13.3< to ≤26.7kPa
Severe	P:F = ≤100mmHg	P:F = ≤13.3kPa

Currently, of the interventions with evidence in ARDS, only two have evidence that is strongly in favour: tidal volume (Vt) ≤6ml/kg ideal body weight with a plateau pressure ≤30cmH$_2$O and prone positioning for ≥12 hours per days when P:F ≤20kPa.

Evidence is weakly in favour for: conservative fluid management, higher positive end-expiratory pressure (PEEP) (if P:F ≤27kPA), neuromuscular blockade infusion (if P:F ≤20kPa), extracorporeal membrane oxygenation (ECMO) (if meets criteria).

Evidence is against use in ARDS due to associated worse outcomes: salbutamol (BALTI-2, 2012) and high-frequency oscillation ventilation (HFOV) (OSCILLATE 2013 and OSCAR 2013).

References

1. The Faculty of Intensive Care Medicine (FICM). Guidelines on the management of acute respiratory distress syndrome, 2018. Available at: https://ficm.ac.uk/sites/ficm/files/documents/2021-10/Guidelines_on_the_Management_of_Acute_Respiratory_Distress_Syndrome.pdf.
2. Raghavendran K, Napolitano LM. Definition of ALI/ARDS. *Crit Care Clin* 2011; 27(3): 429–37.
3. Matthay MA, Arabi Y, Arroliga AC, et al. A new global definition of acute respiratory distress syndrome. *Am J Respir Crit Care Med* 2024; 209(1): 37–47.

● Answer 3: a

The history is consistent with cardiogenic shock, likely in this case due to viral myocarditis (lack of evidence of ischaemic disease and alcohol history, LV not dilated). Each of the inotropes suggested come with benefits and unwanted side effects. Direct beta-agonists such as dobutamine will further increase the heart rate, and given this patient is already significantly tachycardic this could lead to an acute further deterioration in cardiac function. Adrenaline would also worsen tachycardia and oxygen demand in an already critical heart. Milrinone will provide inotropy with limited increase in heart rate, but will cause vasodilatation, and she is already on a high dose of noradrenaline. Starting milrinone with a bolus may result in a catastrophic decrease in blood pressure (BP); therefore, starting milrinone as an infusion only is the best option. Vasopressin may well be needed once the milrinone is started but will not provide any inotropy on its own and so would not be the single best answer here.

The SCAI SHOCK stages classification provides an indication of the severity of cardiogenic shock from any aetiology. It is used across North America and some of Europe and has been validated for use in the UK population for prediction of circulatory aetiology death in patients after out-of-hospital cardiac arrest. It is graded A–E and can contribute to mortality risk prediction in patients with cardiogenic shock:

- **A**t risk: haemodynamically stable with no signs/symptoms of cardiogenic shock but is at risk of developing it (i.e. large MI, decompensated heart failure).
- **B**eginning: a patient with haemodynamic instability without hypoperfusion.
- **C**lassic: a patient with clinical evidence of hypoperfusion (i.e. lactate >2mmol/L) requiring pharmacological or mechanical support.
- **D**eteriorating: clinical evidence of hypoperfusion that is failing to improve or continuing to deteriorate despite an escalation in treatment.
- **E**xtremis: a patient with refractory shock or with impending/actual cardiovascular collapse.

References

1. Ostrowski P, Ahmadnia E, Price S, *et al.* Cardiovascular drugs. In: Waldmann C, Rhodes A, Soni N, Handy J, Eds. *Oxford desk reference: critical care*, 2nd ed. Oxford: Oxford University Press; 2019: chapter 12: pp. 178–204.
2. Naidu SS, Baran DA, Jentzer JC, *et al.* SCAI SHOCK Stage Classification expert consensus update: a review and incorporation of validation studies: This statement was endorsed by the American College of Cardiology (ACC), American College of Emergency Physicians (ACEP), American Heart Association (AHA), European Society of Cardiology (ESC) Association for Acute Cardiovascular Care (ACVC), International Society for Heart and Lung Transplantation (ISHLT), Society of Critical Care Medicine (SCCM), and Society of Thoracic Surgeons (STS) in December 2021. *J Soc Cardiovasc Angiogr Interv* 2022; 1(1): 100008.
3. Watson SA, Mohanan S, Abdrazak M, *et al.* Validation of the CREST model and comparison with SCAI shock classification for the prediction of circulatory death in resuscitated out-of-hospital cardiac arrest. *Eur Heart J Acute Cardiovasc Care* 2024; 13(8): 605–14.

Answer 4: b

Acute tubular necrosis (ATN) is the cause of acute kidney injury (AKI) in around 45% of hospitalised patients (pre-renal is around 21%).

It is renal injury that results in effacement and loss of proximal tubule brush border, some tubule cell loss and tubule casts.

Causes include: renal ischaemia, sepsis, nephrotoxins such as vancomycin, aminoglycosides, contrast media and mannitol.

The differences between pre-renal AKI and ATN are summarised in Table 1.10.

Table 1.10. Differences between pre-renal AKI and ATN.

	Pre-renal AKI	ATN
Urinalysis	Normal, no cells	Muddy brown granular, epithelial cell casts, tubule casts
$FENa^+$ – fractional excretion of Na^+	<1% (Na^+ retention)	>2%
Urine Na^+	<20mEq/L	>40mEq/L
Response to fluid	Creatinine normalises	No improvement in creatinine with fluid or increases in urine output
Urine osmolality	>500mOsmol/kg	<450mOsmol/kg
Urine output	Low	Low/normal

Management of ATN is via management of fluid balance, continuous renal replacement therapy (CRRT) if needed, supportive care and removal of the cause.

STOP-AKI is a useful pneumonic for the immediate management of AKI from any cause:

- **S** — **S**epsis: identify the source and treat if sepsis is suspected (early antibiotics, cultures, antimicrobial stewardship).

SBA Paper 1: Answers

- **T** — **T**oxins/drugs: medications review — withhold nephrotoxic drugs, e.g. non-steroidal anti-inflammatory drugs (NSAIDs), aminoglycosides. Withhold angiotensin-converting enzyme (ACE) inhibitors and angiotensin II receptor antagonists (ARA-IIs) and angiotensin II receptor blockers (ARBs). Withdraw herbal medicines. Stop all drugs that could lead to hypotension (e.g. diuretics/other antihypertensives) if safe to do so.
- **O** — **O**ptimise: assess volume status and optimise blood pressure/volume status with fluids and/or vasopressors. Avoid fluid overload. Exclude urinary obstruction (e.g. bladder USS scan, urinary system imaging).
- **P** — **P**revent harm: prevent volume depletion, identify the cause of AKI (consider rarer causes; urinary dipstick/intrinsic renal screen if positive for urinary blood and protein, urinary system imaging). Avoid nephrotoxic drugs. Adjust medication doses. There should be early referral for those patients who do not respond favourably to initial therapy (e.g. renal, urology, ICU). Monitor and treat promptly any complications, for example, pulmonary oedema/fluid overload, worsening acidosis (pH <7.25), hyperkalaemia (K$^+$ >5.5mmol/L), uraemic encephalopathy/pericarditis, anuria. If there is severe AKI (AKI-3) or AKI on chronic kidney disease (CKD) or if the cause of AKI is unknown or intrinsic renal disease (e.g. multi-system disease: myeloma, vasculitis) discuss urgently with a renal specialist.

References

1. www.uptodate.com. Etiology and diagnosis of prerenal disease and acute tubular necrosis in acute kidney injury in adults. UpToDate, 2024. Available at: https://www.uptodate.com/contents/etiology-and-diagnosis-of-prerenal-disease-and-acute-tubular-necrosis-in-acute-kidney-injury-in-adults.
2. International Society of Nephrology (ISN). Acute Kidney Injury Toolkit, 2024. Available at: https://www.theisn.org/initiatives/toolkits/acute-kidney-injury-aki-toolkit/#managing-patients.

● Answer 5: d

There are several conditions in pregnancy that can present with abnormal liver function.

There are those that are unrelated to pregnancy such as gallstone disease, which would potentially present with abdominal pain, tenderness at Murphy's point and an obstructed jaundice picture on bloods.

Those specific to pregnancy include:

- Hyperemesis gravidarum: persistent vomiting in early pregnancy, no hypertension (HTN), if hospitalised can get mildly elevated alanine transaminase (ALT) and aspartate aminotransferase (AST) (ALT>AST), bilirubin is normal.
- HELLP (haemolysis, elevated liver enzymes and low platelets): upper abdominal pain, nausea and vomiting, malaise, HTN in 85% of cases (systolic blood pressure [SBP] ≥140mmHg or a diastolic blood pressure [DBP] ≥90mmHg, onset in second half of pregnancy and into postpartum period. AST over two times upper limit, thrombocytopaenia platelets (Plt) <100 x 10^9/L, lactate dehydrogenase (LDH) >600 IU/L, raised bilirubin, elevated urinary protein:creatinine ratio (PCR) and uric acid.
- Pre-eclampsia with severe features: always HTN (SBP ≥160mmHg or DBP ≥110mmHg on two occasions at least 4 hours apart while the patient is on bed rest), onset second half of pregnancy. Impaired hepatic function: transaminases over two times the upper limit of normal. Plt <100 x 10^9/L, raised creatinine, urinary PCR and uric acid. New-onset cerebral or visual disturbances. Pulmonary oedema.
- Intrahepatic cholestasis of pregnancy: pruritus is a cardinal sign which starts in the palms and soles, and is worse at night. No HTN. Onset second trimester onwards. Mild elevation of transaminases (less than 2x), elevated serum bile acid, elevated bilirubin.
- Acute fatty liver of pregnancy (AFLP): non-specific signs (nausea and vomiting, abdominal pain, malaise), sometimes signs of acute liver failure (ALF). Occasionally HTN. Onset in third trimester. Transaminases elevated up to around 500 IU/L. Elevated WCC, creatinine, uric acid, ammonia, prolonged prothrombin time (PT) and activated partial thromboplastin time (APTT), low platelets, low glucose, low fibrinogen.

The clinical picture presented here is one of acute liver failure (ALF), and the only one of the options that results in this is acute fatty liver of pregnancy (AFLP).

References

1. Verma D, Saab AM, Saab S, El-Kabany M. A systematic approach to pregnancy-specific liver disorders. *Gastroenterol & Hepatol* 2021; 17(7): 322–9.

● Answer 6: c

In order to enable speech there needs to be airflow through the vocal cords. Aside from speech, restoring normal upper airway physiology has several other physiological and rehabilitation benefits, namely:

- Ability to generate PEEP from the upper airway.
- Creation of subglottic pressure to strengthen swallow and reduce the aspiration risk.
- Promotion of better cord closure resulting in a more effective cough and better airway protection.
- Improved laryngopharyngeal sensation and awareness of secretions and the need to swallow.
- Improved sense of taste and smell.

There are several ways by which airflow can be restored, and this can be done prior to or alongside ventilatory weaning; however, one must first establish that there is no limitation to airflow (such as significant airway oedema, anatomical abnormalities). If the patient is still requiring ventilatory support (as in this case) there are two options for vocalisation:

1. One-way inline valve (OWV, e.g. Passy-Muir valve) with the cuff down. This allows maintenance of inspiratory pressures, and the patient then generates PEEP via expiration through their own airway as the valve does not allow air to flow back through. The ventilator settings may need adjusting to compensate for the lack of expiratory airflow.
2. Above cuff vocalisation (ACV). This requires a tracheostomy tube with a subglottic suction port. The cuff remains inflated and so enables vocalisation earlier on by injection of air through the suction port. This also requires an intact upper airway.

Other options include:

- Leak speech: deflation of the cuff with ventilation which usually requires an increase in PEEP and doesn't prevent aspiration of secretions; the resulting voice may not be consistent.
- Voice-enabling specialist tracheostomy tubes.

Options for vocalisation once significant ventilatory support is no longer needed include: periods of cuff down (with external CPAP if needed) and insertion of a fenestrated tube (where a non-fenestrated liner can be inserted if ventilation is needed, for example, those needing overnight support).

In this question both inline and ACV are potential options, but this patient is not on high levels of ventilatory support and does not have a tracheostomy that has a subglottic suction port so, therefore, an inline OWV is the best answer.

References

1. Wallace S, McGowan S, Sutt A-L. Benefits and options for voice restoration in mechanically ventilated intensive care unit patients with a tracheostomy. *J Intensive Care Soc* 2022; p.175114372211131.

● Answer 7: b

This clinical scenario unfortunately represents a typical 'code red' trauma call. Code red calls have a specific set of criteria for triggering but are typically phoned ahead when the prehospital team feel that the patient may have suffered catastrophic bleeding.

The mechanism of injury is a very significant one and there is likely to be injuries to multiple areas. Haemorrhagic shock is a possibility; however, there is a strong clinical suspicion that this patient has suffered a significant C-spine injury. Up to 45% of spinal cord injuries are a result of road traffic collisions (RTCs).

This patient has the hallmarks of neurogenic shock (hypotension associated with an acute spinal cord injury [SCI] above the level of T6). In such cases, loss

SBA Paper 1: Answers

of sympathetic outflow below the level of the injury results in vasodilation and hypotension (usually trauma patients are very peripherally cold; in this case the patient is peripherally warm but centrally cold). The loss of sympathetic input to the heart results in bradycardia. Any vagal stimulus (such as intubation) may result in unopposed vagal input to the heart with severe bradycardia or even asystole seen. In addition, there may be urinary retention or priapism (again because of unopposed parasympathetic activity).

Other signs of a significant high SCI are respiratory arrest on arrival of the paramedics, and a lack of triggering spontaneous breaths on the ventilator.

References
1. Gillon S, Wright C, Knott C, *et al.* Injury: trauma and environmental. In: Gillon S, Wright C, Knott C, *et al*, Eds. *Revision notes in intensive care medicine*. Oxford: Oxford University Press; 2016: chapter 8: pp. 297–326.

Answer 8: c

This patient has acute severe pancreatitis, a known late complication of which is pancreatic fluid collections (PFCs). These are not an early complication and they usually take at least 4 weeks to form. They are divided into: walled-off PFCs with little or no necrosis (pancreatic pseudocyst); walled-off PFCs with necrosis; and walled-off pancreatic necrosis. These patients may have a prolonged clinical course with complications such as infection and intolerance of oral intake commonly seen. Drainage is not recommended for any pancreatic collection until it is walled off and matured; the CT abdomen shows a well-defined walled-off fluid collection amenable to drainage. For most patients with a symptomatic pancreatic pseudocyst abutting the stomach or duodenum, endoscopic ultrasound (EUS)-guided transmural drainage is preferred to surgery or percutaneous drainage because transmural drainage is effective for resolving walled-off PFCs but has a lower morbidity than surgery and no need for external drains.

The patient is not presenting as overtly septic so antibiotics may not be indicated as a treatment, but they may be given for procedural cover. As the patient is becoming symptomatic (no longer absorbing feed), drainage of the pseudocyst is indicated and appropriate.

References

1. www.uptodate.com. Approach to walled-off pancreatic fluid collections in adults. UpToDate, 2024. Available at: https://www.uptodate.com/contents/approach-to-walled-off-pancreatic-fluid-collections-in-adults.

● Answer 9: c

Oesophageal varices are a common complication of liver cirrhosis secondary to portal hypertension. The prevalence of varices increases with the severity of liver disease, with 76% of patients with Child-Pugh C disease having varices. Despite preventative therapies, around half of patients with cirrhosis will have an acute variceal bleed, and each of these episodes is associated with up to 20% mortality.

Management of a patient with an acute variceal bleed should focus on resuscitation and specific treatments. Regarding resuscitation, a Hb of 70–90g/L should be the target with the patient transfused only if below 70g/L. The use of TEG®/ROTEM® is advocated (if available) to guide product replacement as standard clotting tests are not always a true representation of coagulopathy in this patient group.

Treatment should include administration of a vasoactive agent to reduce portal pressure; terlipressin (2mg 6-hourly QDS) until the bleeding is controlled; octreotide or somatostatin can all be used. Prophylactic antibiotics should be considered as per local antibiotic guidance. Endoscopy should be undertaken as soon as possible and as allowed by the patient's haemodynamic status; guidance typically suggests this should be within 12 hours of presentation.

Terlipressin would be contraindicated in this situation, as there is suggestion of myocardial ischaemia, which terlipressin may worsen. Octreotide (50µg IV bolus followed by 25–250µg/hr infusion for 3–5 days) or somatostatin both reduce portal venous pressure without the risk of myocardial, gut or peripheral ischaemia and are suitable alternatives.

If bleeding continues despite blood products and octreotide, then intubation and placement of a Sengstaken-Blakemore tube may be necessary should access to endoscopy not be imminently available. In this situation the transfer to another hospital for an urgent scope may well take longer than arranging the endoscopy in house.

References

1. Edelson J, Basso JE, Rockey DC. Updated strategies in the management of acute variceal haemorrhage. *Curr Opin Gastroenterol* 2021; 37(3): 167–72.
2. www.uptodate.com. Methods to achieve hemostasis in patients with acute variceal hemorrhage. UpToDate, 2025. Available at: https://www.uptodate.com/contents/methods-to-achieve-hemostasis-in-patients-with-acute-variceal-hemorrhage.

Answer 10: b

There are a number of possible differentials in this case, including cytokine release syndrome (CRS) secondary to the CAR T-cell therapy, haemophagocytic lymphohistiocytosis (HLH) and sepsis. Given the recent CAR T-cell therapy, moderate increase in C-reactive protein (CRP) but low procalcitonin (PCT), CRS is more likely than sepsis. There is a high degree of crossover between HLH and CRS with many similar features seen on blood tests. However, hepatosplenomegaly, lymphadenopathy or haemophagocytosis are absent in CRS and would be seen with HLH. As we have no information on these signs, in this case HLH would fit as a diagnosis; however, clinical findings that occur after immune therapy should be considered as CRS not HLH.

CRS typically begins within 1–14 days after CAR T-cell therapy and can continue for up to 3 weeks. The symptoms range from mild fevers up to a severe systemic inflammatory response syndrome (SIRS)-type response. Leucocytosis may be present, as may leukopenia, neutropenia or thrombocytopaenia. Inflammatory markers such as CRP and ferritin are elevated, but PCT may not be and may help to differentiate from bacterial infection.

There is an American Society for Transplantation and Cellular Therapy (ASTCT) grading system for CAR T CRS:

- Grade 1: temperature ≥38°C, no hypotension or hypoxia.
- Grade 2: temperature ≥38°C plus hypotension that does not require vasopressors or hypoxia that requires less than 6L/min oxygen.

- Grade 3: temperature ≥38°C plus hypotension that requires one vasopressor and hypoxia requiring more than 6L/min (that is not attributable to any other cause).
- Grade 4: temperature ≥38°C plus hypotension that requires multiple vasopressors (excluding vasopressin) and hypoxia requiring CPAP, non-invasive ventilation (NIV) or invasive ventilation.

Management of CRS is dependent on the severity. Mild (grade 1) disease can be managed supportively. In severe CRS (grade 3–4 and some grade 2), the treatment is tocilizumab plus glucocorticoids as dual therapy resulting in more rapid and complete control of CRS compared to single-agent treatment. However, glucocorticoid use may deplete the CAR T-cells, so individualised decisions to use a single agent may be made. Patients with CRS may need between one and four doses of tocilizumab before an improvement is seen.

References

1. www.uptodate.com. Cytokine release syndrome (CRS). UpToDate, 2024. Available at: https://www.uptodate.com/contents/cytokine-release-syndrome-crs.
2. Lee DW, Santomasso BD, Locke FL, et al. ASTCT consensus grading for cytokine release syndrome and neurologic toxicity associated with immune effector cells. *Biol Blood Marrow Transplant* 2019; 25(4: 625–38.
3. Maakaron J, Penza S, El Boghdadly Z, et al. Procalcitonin as a potential biomarker for differentiating bacterial infectious fevers from cytokine release syndrome. *Blood* 2018; 132(Supplement 1): 4216.

Answer 11: b

Citrate anticoagulation is recommended by KDIGO (Kidney Disease: Improving Global Outcomes) as the first-line anticoagulation in CRRT. It provides good circuit anticoagulation and prolonged filter life (previously subtherapeutic heparin doses given concerns regarding bleeding effects have been cited as a reason for filter clotting) and reduces complications, therapy interruptions and costs compared to heparin.

Citrate is a weak organic acid used in CRRT primarily as trisodium citrate (other citrate complexes exist and there will be specific local protocols available). It works by complexing with free ionised calcium to form citrate calcium complexes. Calcium is a required cofactor for most of the enzymes in the coagulation cascade, so by removing free calcium, citrate acts as an effective anticoagulant. In CRRT, the citrate is introduced as the blood is removed from the patient (pre-filter) aiming for a concentration of around 3mmol/L (assessed by blood gas and aiming for a circuit ionised calcium level of around 0.2–0.35mmol/L). These citrate calcium complexes are then either cleared by the haemofilter (up to around 60% of complexes) or returned to the patient where they are metabolised in the liver, muscle or kidney (entering the Krebs cycle) with a half-life under normal conditions of around 5 minutes.

There are two acid-base complications that can occur with citrate:

- Citrate overload is relatively common, benign and straightforward to manage. If the patient is receiving too much citrate but their ability to metabolise the complexes is unimpaired, then the combination of citrate being metabolised to bicarbonate and the increase in SID (strong ion difference) from the Na^+ contained within the citrate leads to a metabolic alkalosis. This could be due to incorrect citrate dosing, the ultrafiltrate rate being too low in CVVH or an insufficient dialysate rate in CVVHD. However, more commonly it is a sign of reduced filter efficiency (due to clogging) causing low clearance. Along with signs of reducing biochemical clearance an increased bicarbonate level occurs on the blood gas. The total to ionised calcium ratio (T:I) is normal and there is no decrease in systemic ionised calcium levels. This can be corrected with a filter change, assuming no other factors relating to calcium delivery and metabolism have changed.
- Citrate accumulation/toxicity is a more concerning complication. If the patient's ability to metabolise citrate complexes is overwhelmed, the complexes remain in the blood. This can be due to very large doses of citrate with a normal metabolic threshold, or normal doses with a reduced metabolic threshold. The predominant cause of reduced metabolism of citrate is severe circulatory shock; decreased oxygen delivery to cells decreases Krebs cycle activity and therefore citrate metabolism. In addition, patients with acute or acute-on-chronic liver failure will have some reduction in their ability to metabolise citrate (but in isolation this can be managed with a reduced citrate protocol). There are also medications that can decrease citrate metabolism such as metformin, paracetamol and propofol. Citrate toxicity typically

occurs when there are multiple factors causing a reduction in citrate metabolism present. There is no way of directly measuring blood citrate levels, so accumulation is suggested by surrogate markers; limited metabolism means the complexed calcium is not released causing a systemic ionised hypocalcaemia (but increased total calcium) and, therefore, there will need to be increases in the calcium dosage given with the CRRT. The accumulated complexes lead to an increased anion and strong ion gap causing a metabolic acidosis, and there is likely to be rising lactate alongside this. The most specific marker is an elevation of the T:I ratio with a typical cut-off value being >2.5. The increase in bound calcium is measured in the total calcium levels and a reduction in the ionised calcium occurs as it is not being released from the citrate complex. Management of citrate accumulation depends on how unstable the patient is. If the patient is reasonably stable, the citrate load may be rapidly decreased. This can be achieved by decreasing the blood flow rate (reducing the number of citrate complexes formed), increasing the dialysate (CVVHD) or filtration (CVVH) rate to increase removal via the machine or decreasing the amount of citrate given. If the patient is unstable or does not improve despite the above measures, then the citrate should be replaced for an alternative anticoagulant (typically heparin).

In this clinical scenario, the patient has a biochemical picture pointing towards citrate overload. This patient has acceptable renal function, and a urine output that will likely be over 400ml in 24 hours, so a trial off CRRT would seem the best choice in this scenario.

References

1. Schneider AG, Journois D, Rimmelé T. Complications of regional citrate anticoagulation: accumulation or overload? *Crit Care* 2017; 21(1): 281.
2. Kidney Disease: Improving Global Outcomes (KDIGO). KDIGO clinical practice guideline for acute kidney injury, 2012. Available at: https://kdigo.org/wp-content/uploads/2016/10/KDIGO-2012-AKI-Guideline-English.pdf.

● Answer 12: d

The management of acute aortic dissection depends on the anatomical origin according to the Stanford and De Bakey classifications:

- Stanford type A: the tear originates in the ascending aorta. If this extends distal to the arch, this is a DeBakey type I; if it is contained within the ascending aorta, then this is a DeBakey type II. The management is surgical.
- Stanford type B: the tear originates distal to the left subclavian artery. If the tear involves the aorta only between the left subclavian and the coeliac artery, this is a DeBakey type IIIa; if it extends beyond the coeliac artery, then this is a DeBakey type IIIb. Management is based on whether they are complicated or uncomplicated.

Uncomplicated dissections: the mainstay of management is BP control. Regular monitoring of BP means that an arterial line may be indicated. First line is antihypertensive and anti-impulse therapy aiming for a SBP of <120mmHg and a HR of <60/min. To this end, IV beta-blockers such as labetalol or esmolol are preferred. It is thought that reducing the force of myocardial contraction slows aortic expansion and reduces the risk of rupture. Short-acting IV therapy is chosen for rapid reduction in BP and HR with transition onto oral medication occurring at a later stage once the patient can take oral medications. If the patient is unable to tolerate beta-blockers, diltiazem or verapamil (IV for rapid control then oral) can be used. If BP is elevated following maximal beta blockade (with HR <60/min), a vasodilator such as a calcium channel blocker (nicardipine for IV rapid reduction or enteral amlodipine) can be added in. Subsequent management would be with agents such as GTN or ACE inhibitors. If the patient presents hypotensive, then they should be resuscitated aiming for a systolic BP of around 100mmHg.

Complicated dissections are those associated with end-organ malperfusion or rapid expansion with impending or frank rupture (this represents around a third of patients with Type B dissection). In addition to BP management as for uncomplicated dissections, these patients should be referred for consideration of endovascular or surgical intervention. If the patient has uncontrolled pain, persistent hypertension despite over three classes of antihypertensives at maximum dose or propagation of the dissection flap, they can also be considered for intervention.

References

1. Isselbacher EM, Preventza O, Black JH, *et al*. 2022 ACC/AHA guideline for the diagnosis and management of aortic disease: a report of the American Heart Association/American College of Cardiology Joint Committee on Clinical Practice Guidelines. *Circulation* 2022; 146(24): e334–482.
2. www.uptodate.com. Management of acute type B aortic dissection. UpToDate, 2024. Available at: https://www.uptodate.com/contents/management-of-acute-type-b-aortic-dissection.

Answer 13: b

The Brain Trauma Foundation (BTF) guidelines detail the evidence level for each monitoring and management intervention in patients with TBI.

They advise keeping cerebral perfusion pressure (CPP) at 60–70mmHg (level IIb), intracranial pressure (ICP) below 20mmHg and management of ICP if it goes above 22mmHg. There is no evidence in support of therapeutic hypothermia, aggressive hyperventilation or burst suppression with barbiturates and they caution against excessive propofol use due to associated morbidity.

Hyperosmolar therapy has no evidence to support its use; however, the BTF states that it is a useful adjunct and may be used in these patients. When comparing mannitol to hypertonic saline, saline trends towards better ICP lowering but with no effect on long-term mortality.

When considering the options presented, the best response is to optimise BP and therefore CPP, as all the other factors are either within range, or the next step in management. Contact with the neurosurgical team is warranted, but will not immediately impact on the raised ICP.

References

1. Carney N, Totten AM, O'Reilly C, *et al*. Guidelines for the management of severe traumatic brain injury, 4th ed. *Neurosurgery* 2017; 80(1): 6–15.

SBA Paper 1: Answers

● Answer 14: b

Panton-Valentine leukocidin (PVL) is a toxin that causes destruction of white blood cells and may be expressed by *Staphylococcus aureus* strains with a specific genetic code. PVL can be expressed by methicillin-sensitive *Staphylococcus aureus* (MSSA) or methicillin-resistant *Staphylococcus aureus* (MRSA). PVL-*Staphylococcus aureus* (SA) predominantly causes skin and soft tissue infection which are often recurrent or difficult to treat. It is spread by skin-to-skin contact and risk factors for colonisation include frequent close contact with others in environments such as gyms, prisons and army barracks. Whilst it mainly results in superficial infections it can become invasive and cause necrotising pneumonias (associated with haemorrhage), necrotising fasciitis, and osteomyelitis in some cases. It should be suspected in patients with severe pneumonia and leukopenia +/- haemoptysis. Sputum samples require specific genetic testing and may take some time to yield results, but local laboratories will differentiate between MSSA and MRSA rapidly. If PVL infection is suspected, empiric treatment with linezolid, clindamycin (for switching off toxin production) and rifampicin — this covers MRSA and MSSA — should be instituted. Antibiotics can then be rationalised once sensitivities are known.

This patient is clearly profoundly unwell and has a haemorrhagic, necrotising pneumonia (based on the history and the imaging). There are several causative bacteria for haemorrhagic pneumonia aside from PVL-SA, such as: *Stenotrophomonas*, Group A *Streptococcus*, *Chlamydia* and leptospirosis. This gentleman has clues in his history that favour the diagnosis of PVL infection — recurrent skin infection not responding to antibiotics, a job that means he is likely to live in close quarters with others and a swab showing he is MRSA-positive. There is also the possible recent exposure to rat urine (via fresh water) which raises the possibility of leptospirosis.

The choice of initial antibiotics should provide MRSA cover given the presence of necrotising pneumonia with recent proven MRSA infection; the second option is the only one to do so. The first option would be appropriate for a standard community-acquired pneumonia (CAP), co-trimoxazole would treat *Stenotrophomonas*, benzylpenicillin would cover Group A *Streptococcus* and the final option is suitable for treatment of leptospirosis.

References

1. British Thoracic Society. CAP guideline Working Group 2014/15. Summary of recommendation: BTS guideline for the management of CAP in adults, 2009, annotated 2015. Available at: https://www.brit-thoracic.org.uk/document-library/guidelines/pneumonia-adults/annotated-bts-cap-guideline-summary-of-recommendations/.
2. PVL subgroup of the Steering Group on Healthcare-Associated Infection. Guidance on the diagnosis and management of PVL-associated *Staphylococcus aureus* infections (PVL-SA) in England, 2nd ed, 2008. Available at: https://assets.publishing.service.gov.uk/media/5a749fb7e5274a44083b82c1/Guidance_on_the_diagnosis_and_management_of_PVL_associated_SA_infections_in_England_2_Ed.pdf.

Answer 15: c

The British Thoracic Society (BTS) has clear guidance on the assessment and management of asthma in adults. The BTS classifies asthma severity as:

- Moderate acute asthma: increased symptoms, peak expiratory flow (PEF) 50–75% best or predicted, no features of severe asthma.
- Acute severe asthma: PEF 33–50%. RR ≥25/min, HR ≥110/min, unable to complete sentences in a single breath.
- Life-threatening asthma: clinical signs include decreased GCS, exhaustion, arrhythmias, hypotension, cyanosis, silent chest, poor respiratory effort. Measurements include PEF <33% best or predicted, O_2 sats <92%, PaO_2 <8kPa, 'normal' $PaCO_2$ 4.6–6kPa (as opposed to low in acute severe).
- Near fatal asthma: $PaCO_2$ >6kPa or need for mechanical ventilation, with high inflation pressures.

Treatment of asthma in adults is as follows:

- For moderate exacerbations: start with salbutamol via a spacer, and repeat if needed.
- For severe: first line is 5mg nebulised salbutamol (O_2 driven) repeated every 10–15 minutes, with ipratropium bromide 0.5mg added every 4–6 hours if there is a poor response to salbutamol. Prednisolone 40–50mg oral for 5 days. Consider IV $MgSO_4$ 1.2–2g if there is a poor response to initial therapy.
- Life-threatening: salbutamol, ipratropium bromide and steroids as per severe. Oxygen therapy should aim for O_2 sats of 94–98%. If there is no improvement or deterioration despite treatment, then the next line is

SBA Paper 1: Answers

IV MgSO$_4$ 1.2–2g over 20 minutes. IV salbutamol should be reserved for those patients in whom inhaled therapy is not reliable and, if used, lactate should be regularly measured. IV aminophylline should only be used after consultation with senior medical staff and is not likely to result in any additional bronchodilation.

- Near fatal: in addition to all the above, intubation and ventilation may be needed, with care given to ventilator settings (see page 124, Paper 2, Q7, for more details). ECMO referral should be considered.
- Additional treatments: there is no place for routine antibiotics and they should be given only if there is clear evidence of bacterial infection. Heliox is not recommended for use outside of a clinical trial setting. Ketamine has no evidence base in this patient group currently but may be used as an adjunct to other treatments in life-threatening/near fatal asthma.

Critical care should be involved if the patient has near fatal asthma or acute severe/life-threatening asthma that is failing to respond to therapy, as evidenced by: worsening peak flows, worsening oxygenation, hypercapnia, becoming more acidotic on ABG, tiring/exhaustion, altered conscious level and respiratory arrest.

References

1. British Thoracic Society (BTS)/Scottish Intercollegiate Guidelines Network (SIGN). BTS/SIGN British guideline on the management of asthma — a national clinical guideline, SIGN 158, 2024. Available at: https://www.sign.ac.uk/media/2269/sign-158-2024-update-final.pdf.

Answer 16: c

Propranolol is highly toxic in overdose. Toxicity in overdose arises from Na$^+$ channel blockade and beta-adrenergic blockade. Propranolol is lipid-soluble and penetrates the central nervous system (CNS) causing convulsions/coma. Peak plasma concentrations occur 1–2 hours after ingestion and its half-life is 3–6 hours.

Features of overdose are cardiovascular (CVS) collapse, CNS depression and seizures. ECG changes include QRS widening, bradycardias, heart blocks, ventricular tachycardia (VT)/ventricular fibrillation (VF). Significant hypotension is often encountered.

Management is as follows:

- A+B: keep the airway clear; early tracheal intubation may be of benefit in severe poisoning.
- C: treat hypotension with fluid resuscitation, early assessment of myocardial contractility (if available) and urgent ECG to guide specific treatments. If the QRS is prolonged, QRS ≥160ms or in arrest, treat with 100mmols of sodium bicarbonate (100ml of 8.4%). If QRS is 120–160ms, treat with 50mmols of sodium bicarbonate (50ml of 8.4%). Monitoring of QRS and serum pH (aiming for 7.5–7.55) is recommended. In patients with severe impairment of myocardial contractility, the first-line therapy is high-dose insulin treatment (1 unit/kg bolus then 1 unit/kg/hr); glucagon 5–10mg IV followed by an infusion can be used in those not improving. If the patient is symptomatically bradycardic, then atropine is indicated, followed by dobutamine, isoprenaline or pacing in unresponsive or hypotensive patients.
- D: treatment of seizures is with benzodiazepines, although this carries a risk of precipitating VT so ensure that the patient has received sodium bicarbonate first. Blood sugars should be checked regularly due to the risk of hypoglycaemia.

References

1. www.toxbase.org. TOXBASE — the primary clinical toxicology database of the National Poisons Information Service. Poisons-index-A-Z/p-products/propranolol. Available at: https://www.toxbase.org.

Answer 17: a

Thrombotic thrombocytopenic purpura (TTP) presents as thrombocytopaenia and a thrombotic microangiopathy (TMA). There may also be renal impairment, low-grade fever and neurological symptoms.

TTP is caused by deficiency of ADAMTS13, typically activity levels of under 20%. ADAMTS13 is a protease which cleaves von Willebrand factor (vWF); if not cleaved adequately, larger fragments of vWF remain which can result in excessive platelet activation. Severe deficiency, coupled with an inflammatory/prothrombotic stimulus, results in clots forming in areas of high sheer stress (e.g. small arterioles and capillaries). Immune TTP (as opposed to hereditary) is either autoimmune or acquired and is due to an autoantibody against ADAMTS13. ADAMTS13 activity can be reduced in sepsis, cardiac surgery, pancreatitis, liver disease and pregnancy, but not to a level associated with TTP (typically activity of around 20–60%).

Most patients are treated on the grounds of clinical suspicion alone as it can take up to a week in some centres to obtain the results of the ADAMTS13 level, and without prompt treatment the condition is almost invariably fatal. The PLASMIC score is a 7-tier system (Table 1.11) and is used to determine the likelihood of TTP and guide treatment of TTP prior to ADAMTS13 levels being known. A score of 0–4 indicates a low probability of TTP, whereas a high score of 5–7 would warrant treatment due to a high probability of TTP with severe ADAMTS13 deficiency.

Table 1.11. PLASMIC score.

PLASMIC Score: Category	Score
1. Platelet count <30 x 10^9/L	1
2. Haemolysis (indirect bilirubin >2mg/dL (34.2µmol/L) or reticulocyte count >2.5% or undetectable haptoglobin)	1
3. Active cancer	1
4. Previous transplantation	1
5. Mean corpuscular volume (MCV) <90fL	1
6. International Normalised Ratio (INR) <1.5	1
7. Creatinine <2.0mg/dL (177µmol/L)	1

TTP treatment consists of urgent therapeutic plasma exchange (TPE) for all patients (to replenish ADAMTS13 levels). Plasma infusion can be used as a temporising measure in hospitals where TPE is not available prior to transfer to a specialist centre. Platelets are avoided for insertion of lines as this propagates clot formation; the exception to this is the presence of significant active bleeding. Other treatment depends on the presence or absence of high-risk features (such as neurological abnormalities, decreased GCS, elevated troponin, signs of critical illness). Prednisolone is used for routine presentation and high-dose methylprednisolone for high-risk patients. Rituximab is only used once severe ADAMTS13 deficiency is confirmed (activity under 10%). If patients present with severe features of TTP, caplacizumab may be used (this blocks the interaction of vWF with platelets, preventing further clots or clot extension, but does not reduce autoantibodies). This has been shown in the HERCULES and TITAN trials which led to faster normalisation of the platelet count and shorter hospitalisation. Caplacizumab can be used instead of TPE in patients who refuse blood products, have a severe allergic reaction to plasma or have had a rapid platelet response to initial treatment meaning that TPE is deferred.

References
1. www.uptodate.com. Immune TTP: Initial treatment. UpToDate, 2025. Available at: https://www.uptodate.com/contents/immune-ttp-initial-treatment.

● Answer 18: c

Part of the assessment of suitability for extubation should be an assessment of the likelihood of post-extubation stridor. In some patients who have only been intubated for a short period of time, the likelihood is low and so no formal testing needs to be done. There are several risk factors for post-extubation stridor which, if present, should trigger a cuff leak test to be performed. These are: prolonged intubation (definitions vary from a few days to >6 days), age >80 years, large endotracheal tube (ETT), high APACHE II score, GCS <8, traumatic intubation, female and history of asthma. In these patients, a cuff leak test (deflating the cuff and listening for an air leak) can reduce the rates of reintubation and post-extubation stridor (as if the leak is absent, you should not proceed with extubation).

The most likely cause of this picture is laryngeal injury or oedema. Visualisation of the airway is important to determine the cause — oedema is likely to improve with time and steroid treatment, but it is important to check for other causes. If there is evidence of laryngeal oedema on laryngoscopy, then administration of steroids reduces the incidence of post-extubation stridor with multidose regimes having slightly better outcomes than single doses.

Tracheostomy would not be indicated at this stage as other criteria support the likelihood of successful extubation, but it may be a later consideration should the upper airway concerns persist. Equally, waiting for a period of time and trying again is not incorrect, but this approach does not seek to identify or address the underlying cause of the issue.

The Rapid Shallow Breathing Index (RSBI) is a tool used to assess weaning of mechanical ventilation on the ICU. The RSBI is defined as the ratio of respiratory frequency (rate per minute) to tidal volume (Vt, ml), where RSBI = f/Vt. A patient with a high RSBI will often not tolerate extubation. A patient with a RSBI <65 breaths/min/L will have a relatively low RR compared to Vt and is therefore more likely to successfully extubate. A patient with a RBSI <105 breaths/min/L will have an 80% chance of being successfully extubated, whereas a RSBI >105 breaths/min/L virtually guarantees extubation failure.

References
1. www.uptodate.com. Extubation management in the adult intensive care unit. UpToDate, 2025. Available at: https://www.uptodate.com/contents/extubation-management-in-the-adult-intensive-care-unit.
2. McConville JF, Kress, JP. Weaning patients from the ventilator. *N Engl J Med* 2012; 367(23): 2233–9.

Answer 19: d

The multisystem involvement in this case suggests an alternative diagnosis to acute exacerbation of asthma. Wheeze may be a presentation in several pathologies. This lady had a relatively long history of asthma and now presents with renal, skin and peripheral nerve involvement, which raises the possibility of a vasculitic cause.

The Chapel Hill Consensus Conference (CHCC) nomenclature for vasculitis is a widely used classification system for vasculitides which divides vasculitis into: large vessel, medium vessel, small vessel, variable vessel, single organ, associated with systemic disease and associated with probable pathology. In this case, the involvement of the kidneys and the peripheral nervous system suggests small-vessel vasculitis. Small-vessel vasculitis is divided into antineutrophilic cytoplasmic antibody (ANCA)-associated and immune complex-associated vasculitis.

ANCA-associated vasculitis (AAV) is a necrotising vasculitis that does not have deposition of immune complexes as a predominate feature. The variants of AAV are microscopic polyangiitis, granulomatosis with polyangiitis and eosinophilic granulomatosis with polyangiitis.

Eosinophilic granulomatosis with polyangiitis (EGPA) is also known as allergic granulomatosis and is a multisystem disease typically presenting with chronic rhinosinusitis, asthma and peripheral blood eosinophilia. The lungs are the most commonly involved organ, and asthma associated with the disease can precede the vasculitic phase by up to 10 years. The asthma is often poorly controlled, requiring multiple courses of oral steroids, which partially suppresses or slows the progression to the vasculitic phase. As it is a multisystem disease, the following may also be found in these patients: skin granulomas (normally during the vasculitic phase), heart involvement (heart failure, pericarditis or rhythm disturbance), thromboembolic disease, peripheral neuropathy (typically mononeuritis multiplex), renal impairment, eosinophilic gastroenteritis, myalgia and lymphadenopathy. Blood tests will reveal a peripheral eosinophilia (potentially ≥10% total WCC), positive ANCA — in most patients myeloperoxidase-specific ANCA (MPO-ANCA), and may also show positive rheumatoid factor or antinuclear antibody (ANA), elevation of IgE levels, hypergammaglobulinaemia and a normochromic normocytic anaemia. Chest imaging during the vasculitic phase is likely to show abnormalities, namely patchy bilateral opacities with or without effusions.

References

1. Chetcuti S, Jones RB, Varley J. Heritable connective tissue diseases, vasculitides, and the anaesthetist. *BJA Educ* 2016; 16(9): 316–22.
2. www.uptodate.com. Clinical features and diagnosis of eosinophilic granulomatosis with polyangiitis (EGPA). UpToDate, 2025. Available at: https://www.uptodate.com/contents/clinical-features-and-diagnosis-of-eosinophilic-granulomatosis-with-polyangiitis-egpa.

● Answer 20: c

Full-thickness burns result in the development of a tough non-distensible eschar. If the burns are circumferential around a limb, the chest or abdomen, this can lead to ischaemia in the limbs and respiratory/haemodynamic compromise in the chest/abdomen. The treatment to save the limb or to relieve respiratory or haemodynamic compromise is an escharotomy. An escharotomy is an emergency surgical procedure where incisions are made through the burnt skin, but unlike fasciotomies they do not breach the fascial layer. Full-thickness burns are dry, leathery, insensate and not painful and therefore the incision through the eschar will not be painful. However, the escharotomy may need to be extended into less burnt, sensate tissue for which local anaesthetic should be used along with sedation or general anaesthesia dependent on the clinical status of the patient.

Given the distribution of the burns in this case, the most likely cause of his shortness of breath is constriction of the chest wall, and escharotomies (with analgesia/sedation) would be the treatment that would improve his respiratory state. Intubation and ventilation would be unlikely to significantly improve his oxygenation alone but may still be necessary in due course or to aid the procedure.

References

1. Zhang L, Labib A, Hughes PG. Escharotomy. StatPearls [Internet]; 2023. Available at: https://www.ncbi.nlm.nih.gov/books/NBK482120/.
2. Escharotomy. In: *Zollinger's atlas of surgical operations*, 10th ed. Ellison EC, Zollinger RM, Jr., Eds. McGraw Hill Medical; 2024. Available at: https://accesssurgery.mhmedical.com/content.aspx?bookId=1755&sectionId=119131457.
3. www.uptodate.com. Emergency care of moderate and severe thermal burns in adults. UpToDate, 2025. Available at: https://www.uptodate.com/contents/emergency-care-of-moderate-and-severe-thermal-burns-in-adults.

● Answer 21: c

In January 2024, a new global definition of acute respiratory distress syndrome (ARDS) was released. This was developed after a series of consensus meetings of 32 critical care ARDS experts between 2021 and 2022. This definition added to the Berlin definition of ARDS and included new elements to the diagnosis. There are now three broad groups with slightly differing definitions: non-intubated ARDS, intubated ARDS, and ARDS in resource-limited settings.

The first new element was the inclusion of high-flow nasal oxygen (with a minimum flow rate of 30L/min) into the non-intubated category (in addition to CPAP/NIV with PEEP of at least 5cmH$_2$O). The second element was how hypoxia was identified — in addition to a P:F ratio of <300mmHg (40kPa), an SpO$_2$:FiO$_2$ of ≤315 (if the SpO$_2$ is ≤97%) can be used within all three of the ARDS groups. Therefore, the severity groupings now have SpO$_2$:FiO$_2$ ranges (in addition to the original P:F ratios, as stated in the original Berlin criteria) which are: mild ≤315, moderate ≤235, severe ≤148. The third new element was the addition of USS to the acceptable imaging modalities, for assessing bilateral lung involvement — as shown by 'bilateral B-lines and/or consolidation on USS not fully explained by effusions, atelectasis or nodules/masses'. The final new element was the addition of the resource-limited category, and in these patients, diagnosis is made on the SpO$_2$:FiO$_2$ ratio without reference to PEEP, oxygen flow rate or specific respiratory support devices.

There has also been a minor change to the wording with regards to timing — it still states within 1 week of the estimated onset of a predisposing factor but now adds new or worsening respiratory symptoms, allowing new significant deteriorations to be taken as day 1 with regard to the ARDS diagnosis.

They all meet the new criteria aside from answer c which does not as there is unilateral pathology and the criteria require bilateral involvement as stated above.

References
1. Matthay MA, Arabi Y, Arroliga AC, et al. A new global definition of acute respiratory distress syndrome. *Am J Respir Crit Care Med* 2024; 209(1): 37–47.

Answer 22: c
The modes of a pacemaker available depend on which wires are *in situ*, and utilise a five-letter code to describe function:

- Chamber paced (0 = none, A = atrium, V = ventricle, D = dual [A&V]).
- Chamber sensed (0, A, V, D).
- Response to sensing (0 = none, I = inhibited, T = triggered, D = dual [T&I]).

SBA Paper 1: Answers

- Rate modulation (0 or no letter = none, R = rate modulation).
- Multi-site pacing (0 or no letter = none, A, V or D).

VVI is the most commonly used pacing mode, i.e. ventricular pacing, ventricular sensing, and inhibition in response to sensing (so if an intrinsic beat is sensed there is no output from the pacemaker). AAI is used if there is an intact AV node.

References

1. Gall NP. Pacemakers and defibrillators. In: Davey A, Diba A, Eds. *Ward's anaesthetic equipment,* 6th ed. London: Saunders, Elsevier; 2012: chapter 25: pp. 465–74.
2. National Institute for Health and Care Excellence (NICE), guideline TA88. Dual-chamber pacemakers for symptomatic bradycardia due to sick sinus syndrome and/or atrioventricular block. Appendix D: Pacemaker nomenclature, 2014. Available at: https://www.nice.org.uk/guidance/ta88/resources/dualchamber-pacemakers-for-symptomatic-bradycardia-due-to-sick-sinus-syndrome-andor-atrioventricular-block-pdf-2294825703109.

Answer 23: e

Acute liver failure (ALF) is significant acute liver injury in patients with a previously healthy liver. It is categorised based on the time between the onset of jaundice to the development of encephalopathy and there are several different classification systems that divide ALF into hyperacute, acute and subacute or fulminant, sub-fulminant and late onset depending on different time scales.

ALF has a mortality of over 40% within the first 3 weeks of illness and orthotopic liver transplantation is an intervention that significantly reduces this mortality rate (survival of 84% if transplanted within 3.5 days of listing). Assessment of patients with ALF to determine if they would have a better outcome with a liver transplant in the UK and many other countries is performed using the King's College Criteria (KCC). Transplant-free survival differs dependent on the aetiology of the liver failure, with paracetamol-induced and hepatitis A-induced ALF having the highest transplant-free survival rates. Due to the difference with paracetamol-induced ALF outcomes, there are a different set of criteria for these patients compared to non-paracetamol-induced ALF.

Criteria for transplant in patients with paracetamol-induced injury are:

- pH <7.3 or all three of the following:
    - INR >6.5/PT >100 seconds;
    - creatinine >300µmol/L;
    - West Haven grade III/IV encephalopathy.

In 2002, Bernal *et al* proposed a modification to the KCC to increase sensitivity which includes the addition of a lactate of >3.5mmol/L after early resuscitation (4 hours) plus a pH <7.3 or a lactate >3.0mmol/L after fluid resuscitation 12 hours into the admission.

Criteria for transplantation in non-paracetamol-induced injury are as follows:

- PT >100 secs/INR >6.5 or any three of the following:
    - age <10 or >40;
    - aetiology — non-A/B viral hepatitis;
    - drug-induced;
    - time from jaundice to encephalopathy >7 days;
    - serum bilirubin >300µmol/L.

References
1. Renner E. How to decide when to list a patient with acute liver failure for liver transplantation? Clichy or King's College criteria, or something else? *J Hepatol* 2007; 46 (4): 554–7.
2. Bernal W, Donaldson N, Wyncoll D, Wendon J. Blood lactate as an early predictor of outcome in paracetamol-induced acute liver failure: a cohort study. *Lancet* 2002; 359(9306): 558–63.

● Answer 24: d

Acute interstitial nephritis (AIN) is an intrarenal lesion which causes a decline in renal function due to inflammatory infiltrates in the kidney interstitium. It may present with the signs and symptoms of acute kidney injury (AKI) or it can be asymptomatic. Around 50% of patients will be oliguric and, depending on the underlying cause, they may have other symptoms such as fever, eosinophilia and haematuria. Almost all patients will have a rise in their creatinine, which if the AIN is caused by medication will correlate with the initiation of the drug in question. Patients have a characteristic urine sediment including white blood cell casts and both red and white blood cells. In 70–75%, the cause is medication, with antibiotics being responsible for up to 50% of these cases. Beta-lactam antibiotics, particularly methicillin, are the highest risk for causing AIN. Although almost any drug can potentially cause AIN, a number are frequently cited as the precipitant including NSAIDs, penicillins, cephalosporins, rifampicin, Septrin™, diuretics (loop and thiazide), proton pump inhibitors (PPIs) and allopurinol. Other causes include systemic disease such as sarcoid, Sjögren's disease, systemic lupus erythematosus (SLE) (10–20%), infection (4–10%) and tubulointerstitial nephritis and uveitis (TINU)(<5%).

Management of these patients focuses on supportive treatment for the AKI, and cessation of medication in those which are caused by drug treatment. Treatment of the underlying cause in those not related to medications forms the mainstay of management. Recovery of renal function is variable with up to 40% of patients having persistent elevation of their creatinine, and around 10% of patients remaining dialysis-dependent.

References

1. www.uptodate.com. Treatment of acute interstitial nephritis. UpToDate, 2025. Available at: https://www.uptodate.com/contents/treatment-of-acute-interstitial-nephritis.
2. www.uptodate.com. Clinical manifestations and diagnosis of acute interstitial nephritis. UpToDate, 2025. Available at: https://www.uptodate.com/contents/clinical-manifestations-and-diagnosis-of-acute-interstitial-nephritis.

Answer 25: b

Pre-eclampsia is defined by the International Society for the Study of Hypertension in Pregnancy as new onset of hypertension (one or both of: systolic BP [SBP] ≥140mmHg, diastolic BP [DBP] ≥90mmHg) along with one or more of the following features at or after 20 weeks' gestation:

- Proteinuria: >1+ on urine dip, urine protein-creatinine ratio (PCR) ≥30mg/mmol, urine albumin-creatinine ratio (ACR) ≥8mg/mmol, AKI (creatinine ≥90µmol/L).

- Liver derangement: transaminases twice the upper limit of normal range or ALT ≥70 IU/L.
- Neurological complications: eclamptic seizures, severe headaches, clonus, blindness, confusion, stroke, visual disturbances.
- Haematological derangement: platelets <150 x 10^9/L, disseminated intravascular coagulation (DIC), haemolysis.
- Uteroplacental dysfunction.

Pre-eclampsia is a condition with the potential for significant clinical deterioration. In the presence of the following signs and symptoms, it would be described as pre-eclampsia with severe features:

- SBP ≥160mmHg, DBP ≥110mmHg, platelets ≤100 x 10^9/L, impaired liver function (transaminases twice normal and severe persistent right upper quadrant pain, or epigastric pain without alternative diagnosis), renal impairment (doubling of creatinine in the absence of other renal disease), pulmonary oedema, new-onset headache unresponsive to medication without alternative diagnosis, visual disturbance.
- HELLP (haemolysis, elevated liver enzymes and low platelets) syndrome would be characterised as pre-eclampsia with severe features and women may be critically unwell on presentation and may end up admitted to the ICU after major obstetric haemorrhage.

References
1. Goddard J, Wee MYK, Vinayakarao L. Update on hypertensive disorders in pregnancy. *BJA Educ* 2020; 20(12): 411–6.

● Answer 26: e
When a child is deemed 'incompetent' to make a decision (namely when they are too young to have capacity to consent), then consent may be given by the following people: either biological parents provided they are married; the father can sign if the parents are not married and he is named on the birth certificate; and other family members or guardians if they have been invested with parental authority by the court. If parents disagree over consent and this cannot be resolved with discussion, the case may be referred to the court for a ruling in the minor's best interests.

SBA Paper 1: Answers

As a child gets older, they will reach an age where they have the capacity to consent for treatment themselves; this age varies with each child and is assessed by the treating doctor. They are deemed to have Gillick competency if they have capacity to consent. Consent in these cases is analogous to the 'door and key' concept where consent is considered as a key that opens the door to treatment, and in the case of a child who is immature and incompetent, the parents hold the key to that door. As a child matures, they reach a point where they own their own key. Only one key is needed to open the door and once open it cannot be closed by another keyholder, so a parent cannot veto the consent of a competent minor and vice versa.

In the situation where a competent minor is refusing treatment (Gillick competent under 16 or ages 16 to 17 years old), if the refusal in treatment would in all probability lead to the death of the child or severe permanent injury then this refusal can be overruled by the parents. The General Medical Council (GMC) states that the law on parents overriding young people's competent refusal is complex, and you should seek urgent legal advice if you think treatment is in the best interests of a competent young person who refuses it. In this situation, as the patient with capacity has refused treatment but the parents have consented, urgent discussion with the hospital's legal team is the best course of action whilst continuing discussions with the child to explore the reasonings around their refusal. Mediation to establish an acceptable common ground solution is the best approach in such situations, as forcing a treatment on a child may result in significant psychological damage and loss of confidence in healthcare providers.

References
1. McCombe K, Bogod DG. Consent and capacity: issues for paediatric anaesthesia. *BJA Educ* 2020; 20(11): 377–81.

Answer 27: b

Hanging is sadly not an uncommon presentation to the ICU, but it is an uncommon cause of bony injury unless there has been a drop from a significant height onto a knot located over bony areas of the neck.

With traumatic spinal injury, the level of the injury dictates the resulting alteration in physiology. Patients who suffer fractures above the C3 level are likely to be apnoeic, whereas lower lesions may result in delayed phrenic nerve paralysis due to cord oedema. Airway compromise may occur as a result of associated facial trauma or retropharyngeal bleeding and oedema.

Spinal shock is the acute flaccid weakness that occurs post-spinal injury. Neurogenic shock results from damage to the sympathetic chain and results in hypotension and bradycardia (due to unopposed parasympathetic nervous system outflow above the level of the lesion).

Canadian C-spine rules provide guidance on the requirement for imaging post-injury. If high-risk criteria present, i.e. age >65 years, paraesthesia in the extremities or a dangerous mechanism (fall 1m/5 steps, axial loading to the head, RTC >62mph, ejection RTC, bike collision with static object), then the patient should undergo imaging of the C spine via X-ray or CT scanning.

If none of the above risks are present, then assessment for low-risk factors should take place along with a clinical examination of the neck. If the patient is unable to rotate their neck 45° to either side, imaging is indicated.

By definition, penetrating neck injuries always reach the level of the platysma and are divided into three zones based on anatomy:

- Zone 1 is the most inferior, bordered by the thoracic inlet and cricoid, and contains the trachea, oesophagus and lung so an injury to this area could conceivably result in a pneumothorax.
- Zone 2 extends from the cricoid to the angle of the mandible and contains the carotids, larynx and pharynx.
- Zone 3 covers the area from the mandible to the base of the skull and contains cranial nerves and the sympathetic chain.

References
1. Stiell IG, Wells GA, Vandemheen KL, *et al*. The Canadian C-spine rule for radiography in alert and stable trauma patients. *JAMA* 2001; 286(15): 1841–8.
2. Nowicki J, Stew B, Ooi E. Penetrating neck injuries: a guide to evaluation and management. *Ann Roy Coll Surg Engl* 2018; 100(1): 6–11.

Answer 28: e

Compartment syndrome most commonly occurs in the calf and the forearm. It is caused by any intrinsic or extrinsic pressure that leads to an increase in the compartment pressure, and is most commonly seen secondary to trauma.

Normal compartment pressure is 0–8mmHg. Perfusion becomes compromised within a compartment when the pressure is within 10–30mmHg of diastolic pressure (DBP – compartment pressure = delta pressure). Muscle oxygenation becomes impaired when the compartment pressure reaches MAP.

Nerve conduction is reduced with a compartment pressure of 30mmHg or delta pressure of 30mmHg. Ischaemia starts as delta pressure reaches zero. Damage tends to be reversible if increased pressure is resolved within 4 hours, with irreversible ischaemia occurring between 4 and 8 hours.

Symptoms of compartment syndrome include pain on passive movement, loss of pulses in the compartment area (so distal pulses may still be present if the artery doesn't pass through or near the affected compartment), tense tissues on palpation and reported pain out of proportion to the extent of injury seen.

If compartment syndrome is suspected, serial measurements of compartment pressures should be taken as trends are often more informative than isolated measurements. Directly inserted needles or indwelling catheters can be transduced to provide readings; an arterial transducer attached to an 18g needle placed within the compartment will suffice in an urgent setting.

A delta pressure of 30mmHg is used as a trigger for fasciotomy, which should be performed within 4 hours to save the extremity. If compartment syndrome is already established, a fasciotomy is unlikely to be of benefit and performing one more than 6 hours after onset results in an increased infection and amputation rate for no benefit, as the muscle is already dead.

References

1. www.uptodate.com. Acute compartment syndrome of the extremities. UpToDate, 2025. Available at: https://www.uptodate.com/contents/acute-compartment-syndrome-of-the-extremities.

Answer 29: a

Calcium and phosphate homeostasis is maintained by three hormones: parathyroid hormone, vitamin D and calcitonin.

Parathyroid hormone (PTH) is released from the four parathyroid glands (chief cells) and causes an increase in calcium (Ca^{2+}) and decrease in phosphate (PO_4^{3-}). It acts directly on the bone and indirectly on the kidney and gut by causing an increase in the production of 1,25 vitamin D.

Vitamin D is produced in the skin and undergoes metabolism in the liver followed by the kidney to 1,25 vitamin D. It causes an increase in calcium and phosphate via actions on the kidney, gut and bones.

Calcitonin is produced by parafollicular C-cells in the thyroid. Its production is triggered by a Ca^{2+} level >2.4mmol/L and it acts to decrease Ca^{2+} and PO_4^{3-}.

Hypercalcaemia can be caused by primary and tertiary hyperparathyroidism, malignancy, excess vitamin D, and several drugs. Patients are often described as suffering symptoms of 'stones, bones and psychic groans' and are often confused and dehydrated. ECG changes include shortening of the QTc interval and J waves in severe cases. Treatment is via rehydration, IV bisphosphonates, prednisolone (only in myeloma, sarcoid and increased vitamin D) and furosemide in some cases where fluid replenishment has taken place.

Calcium gluconate 10% contains 93mg Ca^{2+} per 10ml whereas calcium chloride 10% contains 273mg Ca^{2+} per 10ml (three times as much Ca^{2+} as calcium gluconate).

SBA Paper 1: Answers

References

1. Webster N, Strachan D. Metabolic disorders: electrolyte disorders. In: Waldmann C, Rhodes A, Soni N, Handy J, Eds. *Oxford desk reference: critical care*, 2nd ed. Oxford: Oxford University Press; 2019: chapter 25: pp. 452–6.
2. Power I, Kam P, Cousins MJ, Siddall PJ. Endocrine physiology. In: Power I, Kam P, Eds. *Principles of physiology for the anaesthetist*, 2nd ed. London: Hodder Arnold; 2008: chapter 11: pp. 323–54.

Answer 30: c

Diabetic ketoacidosis (DKA) is diagnosed when all three of the following are present:

- A blood glucose of over 11mmol/L (or a known diagnosis of diabetes).
- Ketone (capillary or blood) concentration of >3mmol/L or significant ketonuria (2+ or more on urine dip).
- Acidosis defined as bicarbonate concentration of <15mmol/L and or venous pH <7.3.

Note that the wording of hyperglycaemia or a known diagnosis of diabetes is such to allow inclusion of patients with euglycaemic DKA within the definition.

There are a number of indications for senior review and consideration of admission to critical care in patients with DKA. These include age 18–25 years or the elderly, pregnancy, evidence of heart or renal failure, additional serious comorbidities and the presence of severe DKA.

Severe DKA is defined by the presence of: blood ketone levels >6mmol/L, venous bicarbonate <5mmol/L, venous pH <7.0, hypokalaemia on admission (<3.5mmol/L), GCS <12, oxygen saturations below 92% on room air, SBP <90mmHg, HR of >100/min or <60/min and anion gap above 16 (anion gap = $([Na^+] + [K^+]) - ([Cl^-] + [HCO_3^-])$).

References

1. Joint British Diabetes Societies for Inpatient Care. The management of diabetic ketoacidosis in adults, March 2023. Available at: https://abcd.care/sites/default/files/site_uploads/JBDS_Guidelines_Current/JBDS_02_DKA_Guideline_with_QR_code_March_2023.pdf.

● Answer 31: e

The document 'Guidelines for the Provision of Intensive Care Services' was written by the Faculty of Intensive Care Medicine and the Intensive Care Society in 2022 and guides many aspects of intensive care provision, including recommendations on minimum safe staffing levels.

Medical staffing should consist of a daytime consultant to patient ratio of between 1:8 and 1:12, with the caveat that this will be dependent on several factors including the seniority and competency of junior staff on shift as well as the complexity of the patients. The resident doctor ratio should not normally exceed 1:8. Staff that work on the resident rota (doctors or ACCPs) must either have or have access to a practitioner with advanced airway skills. Nursing ratios recommended are a minimum of 1:1 for level 3 patients and a minimum of 1:2 for level 2 patients. In addition, there must be a supernumerary senior registered nurse to coordinate (nurse in charge). ICUs with greater than 10 beds must have additional supernumerary senior nursing staff, in addition to a nurse in charge, to enable delivery of safe care (+1 for 11–20 beds, +2 for 21–30 beds, etc.). In addition to numbers, a minimum of 50% of the registered nursing staff must be in possession of a post-registration academic programme in critical care nursing.

References
1. The Faculty of Intensive Care Medicine. Guidelines for the provision of intensive care services, Version 2.1, 2022. Available at: https://www.ficm.ac.uk/sites/ficm/files/documents/2022-07/GPICS%20V2.1%20%282%29.pdf.

● Answer 32: a

Distribution of data is dictated by the relationship between the mean, median and mode of the data. In Gaussian distribution or normal distribution there is a bell-shaped curve where the mean median and mode all have the same value. Most large data sets will form a normal distribution, or the data can be mathematically converted to one as this is what allows comparison between data sets with regard to the standard deviation.

In a positively skewed distribution, the curve is asymmetrical with most of the data clustered towards the left (the opposite of the above graph), and the mode < median < mean (the mean is closest to the tail of the data). An example of data with a positive skew is BP measurements across a

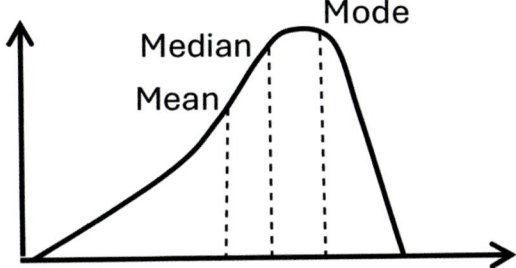

Figure 1.2. Negatively skewed distribution.

population. Figure 1.2 is a negatively skewed distribution, with the mean closest to the tail of the data on the left. Negative skews are less common, but an example would be the age of death. In a bimodal distribution there are two modes at two separate peaks and the dip in the middle is the antimode. An example of a bimodal distribution is the heights of a population with one mode for men and one for women.

References
1. Spoors C, Kiff K. Statistics for the anaesthetist. In: Spoors C, Kiff K, Eds. *Training in anaesthesia: the essential curriculum*. Oxford: Oxford University Press; 2010: chapter 24: pp. 561–72.

● Answer 33: b

Adult basal nutritional requirements per 24 hours in critical care are shown in Table 1.12.

Table 1.12. Adult basal nutritional requirements per 24 hours in critical care.

Na^+, Cl^-	1–2mmol/kg
K^+	0.8–1.2mmol/kg
Ca^{2+}, Mg^{2+}	0.1mmol/kg
PO_4^{3-}	0.2–0.5mmol/kg
Energy	25kcal/kg
Carbohydrate	2g/kg
Protein	0.8–2g/kg
Fat	1g/kg

This table describes basal requirements only and, depending on the patient's pathology, may be subject to some variation. The American Society for Parenteral and Enteral Nutrition (ASPEN) 2016 guidelines (updated in 2021) refer to several specific areas where this may be the case:

- Patients on CRRT should receive increased protein (very low-quality evidence).
- Patient with an open abdomen should receive additional protein.
- Patients with burns should receive higher amounts of protein up to 1.5–2g/kg/day.
- Indirect calorimetry should be used to guide energy need where available (expert consensus evidence).
- Patients with sepsis should receive trophic feeding (10–20kcal/hr) during the initial phase of their illness, building up to full feed as tolerated over 24–48 hours.

References
1. Chowdhury R, Lobaz S. Nutrition in critical care. *BJA Educ* 2019; 19(3): 90–5.
2. McClave SA, Taylor BE, Martindale RG, *et al*. Guidelines for the provision and assessment of nutrition support therapy in the adult critically ill patient: Society of Critical Care Medicine (SCCM) and American Society for Parenteral and Enteral Nutrition (ASPEN). *J Parenter Enteral Nutr* 2016; 40(2): 159–211.

Answer 34: d

Although detailed knowledge of chemotherapy agents is not necessary for an intensivist it is important to understand the side effects of the commonly used agents or significant side effects of less commonly used ones and which may affect management of critically ill patients.

One such example is bleomycin, which acts via interaction with the topoisomerase enzymes to damage DNA (other drugs with this mechanism of action include doxorubicin). Many of the chemotherapy agents can cause pulmonary toxicity but bleomycin has the potential for progression to life-threatening pulmonary fibrosis which may be triggered by exposure to high FiO_2 concentrations even for very short periods of time. In these patients oxygen therapy should be avoided if possible, and if the patient is hypoxic given at the lowest possible concentration of oxygen to achieve O_2

saturations of 88–92%. Clinical procedures mandating a high FiO_2 should be avoided where possible. The injury typically occurs in the first 6 months after treatment but the risk remains for the rest of the patient's life. Other agents that can cause pulmonary toxicity include alkylating agents such as cyclophosphamide, anti-metabolites such as methotrexate and azathioprine, plant alkaloids such as vincristine and etoposide and biological response modifiers such as interferon and the Bacillus Calmette-Guérin (BCG) vaccine.

References
1. Allan N, Siller C, Breen A. Anaesthetic implications of chemotherapy. *Contin Educ Anaesth Crit Care Pain* 2012; 12(2): 52–6.

Answer 35: d
Daily checklists for care are commonplace in intensive care practice. A large part of these checklists is to prevent hospital-acquired infections, notably ventilator-associated pneumonia (VAP). Different elements are included in these checklists and have different levels of supporting evidence. The following are regarded as essential in VAP prevention (levels of evidence in brackets):

- Avoidance of intubation and prevent reintubation (high), minimising sedation — avoiding benzodiazepines, protocols to minimise sedation such as daily sedation holds (moderate), maintenance and improvement of physical conditioning (moderate), elevation of the head of the bed to 30–45° (low), oral care with toothbrushing without chlorhexidine (moderate), early enteral nutrition (EN) vs. parenteral nutrition (PN) (high), change of ventilator circuit only if visibly soiled or malfunctioning (high).

Other actions that are considered as additional interventions include:

- Use selective oropharyngeal decontamination (SOD)/selective decontamination of the digestive tract (SDD) in countries with low prevalence of antibiotic-resistant organisms (high), ETT with subglottic suction drainage ports for patients expected to require >48 hours of ventilation (moderate), consideration of early tracheostomy (moderate), consideration of post-pyloric feeding for those with gastric intolerance or a high risk of aspiration (moderate).

There are also several interventions that all have moderate evidence, which are not recommended due to inconsistent reduction or no impact on VAP rates, mechanical ventilation, length of stay or mortality. These include:

- Oral care with chlorhexidine, use of probiotics, use of tapered ETT, automated cuff pressure device use, frequent cuff pressure measurement, kinetic beds, prone positioning, chlorhexidine bathing, stress ulcer prophylaxis, monitoring residual gastric volumes and early PN.

There have been a number of randomised controlled trials (RCTs) studying oral care with chlorhexidine and most showed no impact on VAP rates. A meta-analysis demonstrated an association between chlorhexidine oral care and higher mortality rates although this signal is uncertain, as other meta-analyses have not replicated this finding. Given the uncertainty regarding mortality coupled with the lack of evidence for benefit, it is no longer the standard of care.

References
1. Klompas M, Branson R, Cawcutt K, *et al.* Strategies to prevent ventilator-associated pneumonia, ventilator-associated events, and non-ventilator hospital-acquired pneumonia in acute-care hospitals: 2022 update. *Infect Control Hosp Epidemiol* 2022; 43(6): 687–713.

Answer 36: e

The intra-aortic balloon pump (IABP) was developed in the 1960s to provide circulatory support for patients in cardiogenic shock. It consists of a double-lumen balloon catheter that is attached to a console. The outer lumen is inflated with helium whilst the inner lumen provides a route for the guidewire to pass through during insertion via the femoral artery (it can also be inserted through the brachial or axillary arteries). Once inserted the patient must sit at 30° with their legs straight, as sitting upright may cause inward migration of the IABP balloon and potentially result in cerebral ischaemia.

The tip of the IABP should sit 2–3cm distal to the left subclavian artery, in line with the carina on a CXR. It contains 20–50ml of helium. Control of IABP inflation can be via the ECG trace, aortic pressure wave, pacing spikes or a

SBA Paper 1: Answers

pre-programmed rate for use during CPR. IABP inflation occurs at the onset of diastole marked by the dicrotic notch or the midpoint of the T wave and results in augmentation of the aortic diastolic pressure thus improving coronary artery blood flow. Deflation occurs at the onset of systole marked by the peak of the R wave.

Mistimed inflation and deflation of the IABP may cause significant clinical issues. If the balloon is inflated whilst the aortic valve (AV) is open (early inflation or late deflation), then an increase in oxygen demand and left ventricular (LV) wall stress may occur as the LV is emptying against the IABP. If the IABP is inflated too late, it is less effective in augmenting diastolic pressure; if it is deflated too early, it may result in poor function and retrograde coronary artery blood flow.

References
1. Ahmad I, John M. Cardiovascular therapy techniques: intra-aortic balloon counterpulsation pump. In: Waldmann C, Rhodes A, Soni N, Handy J, Eds. *Oxford desk reference: critical care*, 2nd ed. Oxford: Oxford University Press; 2019: chapter 2: pp. 61–3.

Answer 37: b

Nephrotic syndrome is characterised by the triad of proteinuria (>3.5g/24 hours), hypoalbuminemia (<35g/L) and peripheral oedema.

In children, the predominant cause of nephrotic syndrome is minimal change disease (MCD — no immune complex deposition, due to fusion of the podocyte cells) which accounts for 90% of cases in under 10-year-olds and 50% of cases over the age of 10.

In adults, nephrotic syndrome is caused by several conditions, namely: systemic diseases (30% — DM, amyloidosis, SLE, HIV); MCD (16%); focal segmental glomerulosclerosis (35% but over 50% in Afro-Caribbean populations); membranous nephropathy (24%); and drugs.

Clinically, patients have marked peripheral oedema, with hypercholesterolaemia, hypertriglyceridaemia and increased thromboembolic risk (both venous and arterial) often seen. The presence of AKI is not uncommon, and some patients may suffer protein malnutrition and infection (due to loss of IgG).

Treatment is with ACEis or ARBs, diuretics and Na^+ restriction, statins and aspirin or low-molecular-weight heparin (LMWH) for venous thromboembolism (VTE) prophylaxis depending on the albumin level.

Specific treatments for the underlying cause may be considered and in almost all cases involves the use of immunosuppressive agents. An exception is secondary focal segmental glomerulosclerosis (FSGS), where steroids are not recommended.

References
1. www.uptodate.com. Overview of the nephrotic syndrome and nephrotic range proteinuria. UpToDate, 2025. Available at: https://www.uptodate.com/contents/overview-of-the-nephrotic-syndrome-and-nephrotic-range-proteinuria.

Answer 38: c

The Gell and Coombs classification is traditionally used for hypersensitivity reactions, and describes four groups as below:

- Type I : IgE-mediated reactions, e.g. anaphylaxis. Occurs in minutes of exposure.
- Type II: autoantibody (IgG or IgM) reactions causing cytotoxicity, e.g. myasthenia gravis (MG), Goodpasture syndrome, immune thrombocytopaenia (ITP), transfusion reactions. Occurs in hours to days following exposure.
- Type III: antibody-antigen complex deposition, e.g. serum sickness, vasculitis, SLE, hypersensitivity pneumonitis. Occurs in hours to days to weeks following exposure.
- Type IV: cell-mediated delayed reactions (T cell-mediated), e.g. contact dermatitis, Stevens-Johnson syndrome (SJS), DRESS syndrome (drug rash with eosinophilia and systemic symptoms). These have a delayed onset and are usually seen 24–72 hours after contact.

References
1. Dispenza M. Classification of hypersensitivity reactions. *Allergy Asthma Proc* 2019; 40(6): 470–3.
2. Vaillant AAJ, Vashisht R, Zito PM. Immediate hypersensitivity reactions. StatPearls [Internet]; 2019. Available at: https://www.ncbi.nlm.nih.gov/books/NBK513315/.

SBA Paper 1: Answers

● Answer 39: d

Patients who suffer cardiac arrest after cardiac surgery have a better survival rate than the general population due to the high incidence of reversible causes for the arrest. In up to 50% of cases the cause is ventricular fibrillation (VF) with the majority of others being due to cardiac tamponade and bleeding, which can be successfully treated with prompt resuscitation and resternotomy.

The cardiac arrest algorithm for post-cardiac surgery patients differs from the standard in that CPR is not started immediately when a patient arrests. These patients will be in highly monitored environments and as such a change in rhythm and output will be picked up almost immediately. Therefore, you have up to 1 minute to either administer DC shocks (up to three stacked shocks) or optimise pacing in asystolic patients. In PEA, you would turn off pacing if present, to exclude underlying VF. There is no evidence of benefit for chest compressions in this patient cohort at this stage, and compressions may actually cause harm as a result of massive haemorrhage or damage to underlying structures.

A team approach in this setting is essential and whilst the first resuscitator is focusing on rhythm, the second person should increase the patient to 100% FiO_2 and if on a ventilator, switch the patient to a Waters circuit or bag/valve hand-ventilation system and verify correct ETT position. If there is no return of spontaneous circulation (ROSC) after that first minute of interventions, cardiopulmonary resuscitation (CPR) with a standard 2-minute cycle approach (chest compressions/ventilation) should be started. In patients with VF/VT, 300mg amiodarone IV is recommended and patients with a non-shockable rhythm should NOT receive adrenaline. The next step is to prepare for resternotomy and standard ALS cycles should be continued until resternotomy is performed.

References

1. Society of Thoracic Surgeons Task Force on Resuscitation After Cardiac Surgery: Dunning J, Levine A, Ley J, *et al*. The Society of Thoracic Surgeons expert consensus for the resuscitation of patients who arrest after cardiac surgery. *Ann Thorac Surg* 2017; 103(3): 1005–20.

● Answer 40: a

There are several grading systems available for the severity of subarachnoid haemorrhage (SAH), which can be used to plan treatment and predict outcome.

The World Federation of Neurological Societies (WFNS) score is frequently used and is based on the Glasgow Coma Scale (GCS) and the presence of any motor (M) deficits:

- Grade I: GCS 15, no motor deficit.
- Grade II: GCS 13–14, no motor deficit.
- Grade III: GCS 13–14 with motor deficit.
- Grade IV: GCS 7–12 with or without motor deficit.
- Grade V: GCS 3–6, with or without motor deficit.

The Hess and Hunt score is an alternative scoring system that was proposed in 1968 and is based on symptoms and examination:

- Grade 1: asymptomatic with mild headache and slight nuchal rigidity.
- Grade 2: moderate to severe headache, stiff neck, no neurological deficit except cranial nerve palsy.
- Grade 3: drowsy or confused, mild focal neurological deficit.
- Grade 4: stupor, moderate or severe hemiparesis.
- Grade 5: deep coma, decerebrate posturing.

Both of these scoring systems have a degree of subjectivity in their scoring, and demonstrate suboptimal sensitivity, specificity and predictive value.

The Fisher scale was devised in 1980 to provide an index of vasospasm risk (but not clinical outcome) and is scored based on the haemorrhage pattern seen on the initial CT head scan:

- Grade 1: no blood detected.
- Grade 2: diffuse thin layer of blood <1mm thick.
- Grade 3: localised clots and layers of blood 1mm or more thick.
- Grade 4: intracerebral or intraventricular clots with diffuse or no subarachnoid blood.

SBA Paper 1: Answers

References

1. www.uptodate.com. Subarachnoid hemorrhage grading scales. UpToDate, 2025. Available at: https://www.uptodate.com/contents/subarachnoid-hemorrhage-grading-scales.

Answer 41: d

Multiple sclerosis (MS) is the most common immune-mediated demyelinating disease. The precise mechanism that triggers the inflammatory demyelination and axonal degeneration seen in MS is unclear, but it is thought that genetic susceptibility and environmental factors are important factors. The strongest evidence of association is with prior Epstein-Barr virus (EBV) infection and smoking. MS is more common in women than men but carries a worse prognosis in males. The typical age of onset is between 15 and 50 years of age.

Several clinical subgroups of disease are recognised, namely:

- Clinically isolated syndrome (CIS): this is the initial presentation of MS in 80% of cases. A monophasic episode of focal or multifocal demyelination occurs over hours to days, lasts at least 24 hours and has no associated fever or infection. Typical examples include optic neuritis, Lhermitte's sign, internuclear ophthalmoplegia, sensory symptoms in limbs, and weakness in one area.
- Relapsing remitting multiple sclerosis (RRMS): this is the most common subtype of MS. Clearly defined attacks occur with complete or partial recovery and minimal disease progression between attacks. Diagnosis of RRMS requires more than one lesion to be disseminated in time and space, and can include a radiologically isolated lesion (RIS) consistent with MS that doesn't cause any associated symptoms.
- Secondary progressive: this is a progression of RRMS where remission is replaced by gradual decline with or without relapses. It usually occurs 10–15 years after the initial diagnosis of RRMS. Up to 80% of patients presenting with RRMS develop secondary progressive disease.
- Primary progressive: this has the worst prognosis and represents around 10–15% of patients with MS. A gradual decline in function with

or without acute episodes is seen. The mean age of onset is 40 years with males and females equally affected.

Diagnosis of MS is via MRI (where hyperintense white matter lesions which enhance with gadolinium on T2 sequences and older lesions are hypointense 'black holes' on T1 sequences are seen), the presence of oligoclonal bands (IgG) in cerebrospinal fluid (CSF) and abnormal evoked potential testing (visual, brainstem or somatosensory).

Treatment of MS focuses on acute relapse management (with steroids and treatment of any underlying trigger), use of disease-modifying treatments (β-interferon and glatiramer acetate) and symptomatic management.

References
1. Doshi A, Chataway J. Multiple sclerosis, a treatable disease. *Clin Med* 2016; 16(Suppl 6): s53–9.

● Answer 42: b

Clostridium tetani is an obligate anaerobe and therefore requires devitalised tissue or foreign bodies and an oxygen-poor environment to grow and produce the metalloprotease toxin 'tetanospasmin'. Once produced, tetanus toxin reaches the anterior horn cells of the spinal cord via retrograde axonal transport where it blocks inhibitory neurones and leads to an increase in discharge of excitatory neurones. This in turn leads to muscular spasms triggered by sensory stimulus and autonomic overactivity with tachycardia and sweating commonly seen.

Tetanus toxin causes destruction of the anterior horn cells. Recovery from infection is dependent upon horn cell regrowth and therefore takes a number of months. Several different patterns of disease are seen (including generalised, localised, cephalic and neonatal) and there are a number of differential diagnoses (strychnine poisoning, drug-induced dystonia, trismus due to dental infection, neuroleptic malignant syndrome and stiff person syndrome).

The treatment of tetanus is via halting toxin production with antibiotics (metronidazole and penicillin G, third-generation cephalosporin if a mixed

SBA Paper 1: Answers

infection), neutralisation of bound toxin with human tetanus immunoglobulin, active immunisation (as soon as the risk of tetanus infection is identified or suspected), control of muscular spasms with benzodiazepines, propofol and neuromuscular blocking drugs if required, and control of autonomic dysfunction with IV $MgSO_4$ infusion and labetalol (avoid beta-blockers due to unopposed alpha activation).

References
1. www.uptodate.com. Tetanus. UpToDate, 2025. Available at: https://www.uptodate.com/contents/tetanus.

Answer 43: a

Blast injuries are rare in civilian situations but can occur in major accidents or terrorist explosions, so some knowledge is important. Blast injury is categorised based on the chronology of the blast wave and its effects into:

- Primary injury: occurs due to the blast wave and causes damage at interfaces between tissues of different sound wave speeds (so more injurious to gas-filled organs such as the lungs, abdomen, intestines and ears). There is high mortality from primary blast injury, but survivors may initially present with minimal signs of injury and develop symptoms over time.
- Secondary blast injury: energised debris and weapon fragments that have been carried or displaced by the blast wind of the explosion may cause soft tissue and penetrating injuries. These represent the majority of injuries in survivors of an explosion and are also the most common cause of mortality. The force of the explosion can propel fragments many times faster than a bullet so a small external wound may overlay massive internal injury.
- Tertiary injury: occurs due to displacement of the patient by the blast winds impacting another object, or structural collapse of a building on to the patient. Typically, long bone fractures and head injuries are seen and structural collapse can lead to crush injury and compartment syndrome.
- Quaternary: all injuries sustained from an explosion that are not included in primary, secondary or tertiary but still directly resulting from the explosion are termed quaternary. Examples include burns

from fire and chemical agents, biological agent exposure, toxin exposure, environmental exposure and the psychological impact of the event.

References

1. Jorolemon MR, Lopez RA, Krywko DM. Blast Injuries. StatPearls [Internet]; 2019. Available at: https://www.ncbi.nlm.nih.gov/books/NBK430914/.

Answer 44: c

Several rescue therapies are available for the management of variceal bleeding. These are indicated if medical management with vasopressor therapy (terlipressin or octreotide), resuscitation with blood products and endoscopic management have not resulted in haemostasis.

A transjugular intrahepatic portosystemic shunt (TIPS) is performed via right internal jugular vein (IJV) access and places a stent between the hepatic vein and portal vein. It is important to ascertain RV function prior to TIPS as the procedure results in a large increase in RV preload. A systematic review in 2020 evaluating the role of early TIPS versus standard medical therapy in acute bleeding showed that early TIPS (as opposed to rescue) in high-risk patients (Child Pugh C) reduced the rates of treatment failure and improved 6-week survival with reducing rebleeding rates at 6 weeks and 1 year. This, however, has not yet been widely implemented into clinical practice.

Up to 20% of variceal bleeds can be refractory to initial therapy, and in these cases balloon tamponade devices can provide a rescue option. Examples include the Sengstaken-Blakemore tube (large gastric balloon, oesophageal balloon and gastric suction port), the Minnesota tube (as above with the addition of an oesophageal port) and the Linton-Nachlas tube (single gastric balloon). The tubes are inserted to around 50–55cm and then the gastric balloon is first partially, then fully, inflated once the position has been confirmed on CXR. Traction is then applied (a 500ml bag of fluid is often used as traction weight). The oesophageal balloon is only inflated if bleeding despite traction on the gastric balloon occurs. The gastric balloon can stay inflated for a maximum of 12 hours at a time and *in situ* for no more than 48 hours. The oesophageal balloon, if used, should be inflated to a pressure of 30–45mmHg and be deflated for 15 minutes every 4 hours.

SBA Paper 1: Answers

Another rescue therapy being increasingly used is the endoscopically-guided placement of a self-expanding metal stent (one of which is called a Danis stent). These have a lower short-term failure rate than balloon methods with regards to control of bleeding and also have the advantage of being safe to leave *in situ* for up to 14 days, allowing a longer time for a bridging plan to definitive management to be made.

References

1. Edelson J, Basso JE, Rockey DC. Updated strategies in the management of acute variceal haemorrhage. *Curr Opin Gastroenterol* 2021; 37(3): 167–72.
2. www.uptodate.com. Methods to achieve hemostasis in patients with acute variceal hemorrhage. UpToDate, 2025. Available at: https://www.uptodate.com/contents/methods-to-achieve-hemostasis-in-patients-with-acute-variceal-hemorrhage.

● Answer 45: d

Renal tubular acidosis (RTA) refers to a group of conditions that cause a hyperchloraemic metabolic acidosis with a normal anion gap. It is divided into hypokalaemic RTA (types 1 and 2) and hyperkalaemic RTA (type 4 and distal tubule Na^+ transport defects):

- Type 1 RTA is due to impaired acidification in the distal tubules from a combination of reduced proton pump activity and increased permeability of the luminal membrane to H^+. Plasma HCO_3^- can range from <10 to 20mmol/L. Hypocitraturia also occurs, resulting in increased free calcium and an elevated risk of renal stones. Causes include Sjögren's syndrome, hereditary spherocytosis, specific genetic abnormalities and amphotericin therapy.
- Type 2 RTA is due to impaired proximal HCO_3^- reabsorption (normally 85–90% of sodium bicarbonate is reabsorbed in the proximal tubule). Plasma HCO_3^- ranges between 12–18mmol/L. The most common cause in adults is monoclonal gammopathy and myeloma followed by genetic mutations and carbonic anhydrase inhibitor drugs (e.g. acetazolamide and methazolamide). If serum bicarbonate is below the patient's threshold for reclaiming, then bicarbonate will be reabsorbed and the urinary pH will be normal; however, if given alkali therapy, these patients have the potential to become profoundly hypokalaemic as they will not reabsorb excess bicarbonate resulting in reduced reabsorption of potassium.

- Type 4 RTA is due to hypoaldosteronism or resistance to aldosterone. These patients are hyperkalaemic and correction of hyperkalaemia will improve the acidosis (which is often mild with a plasma HCO_3^- of over 17mmol/L).

References
1. Mustaqeem R, Arif A. Renal tubular acidosis. StatPearls [Internet]; 2020. Available at: https://www.ncbi.nlm.nih.gov/books/NBK519044/.

Answer 46: c

Drowning is the second most common cause of unnatural death in the United Kingdom (UK) after road traffic collisions, and claims the lives of over 40 people per hour worldwide. It is estimated that over 90% of drownings are preventable. Drowning is defined as the process of experiencing respiratory compromise as a result of submersion or immersion in liquid. The commonly used terms around drowning are:

- Submersion (the airway is below the surface of the liquid).
- Immersion (liquid splashes over the airway).
- Non-fatal drowning (patient rescued such that the drowning process is interrupted).
- Fatal drowning (the patient dies).

Non-fatal downing is then categorised dependent on the severity of respiratory and neurological impairment encountered into mild (fully alert, breathing, involuntary distressed coughing), moderate (disorientated but conscious, difficulty in breathing) and severe (unconscious and not breathing).

On immersion, water hits the airway and often causes laryngospasm. This breaks once the patient is hypoxic causing aspiration of water into the lungs, worsening hypoxia, loss of consciousness and apnoea in seconds to minutes. Hypoxic cardiac arrest will follow this if the patient is not rescued. Water in the alveoli causes surfactant washout resulting in acute lung injury (ALI). Drowning patients are at increased risk of pulmonary oedema for up to 12 hours post-drowning. There is no significant difference in the pathology caused by salt or freshwater aspirations, and as little as 1–3ml/kg of water aspirated into the lungs can cause significant alteration in pulmonary gas exchange and decreased lung compliance.

Most bodies of water have insufficient bacterial colonisation to cause pneumonia in the immediate post-drowning period, so prophylactic antibiotics are not indicated, unless drowning has occurred in a liquid with a known high pathogen load.

There is a difference in initial life support provided to victims of drowning. If the patient has no or abnormal breathing after a witnessed drowning event, five rescue breaths should be given first (slow breaths at a higher pressure as surfactant may have been washed out), before proceeding with ALS if the patient has no pulse or continuing ventilation if there is a pulse but no respiratory effort.

References
1. Szpilman D, Morgan P. Management for the drowning patient. *Chest* 2021; 159(4): 1473–83.

Answer 47: b
IV immunoglobulins (IVIgs) are a blood product derived from the pooled plasma of between 1000 and 15,000 donations. As it is pooled from many donors, each unit is screened for HIV, hepatitis B and C, and processes are undertaken for viral inactivation and to reduce the risk of viral transmission. IVIg has a number of proposed mechanisms of action, including:

- Fab receptor binding: the Fab area of the antibody is the variable region responsible for antigen recognition which neutralises autoantibodies and pro-inflammatory cytokines. Due to the large pool of donors used to produce IVIg — and the varied immune exposures of these donors — many different antigens can be neutralised.
- Fc receptor binding: the Fc receptor is the other distinct region of the immunoglobulin and is constant across all immunoglobulins of a certain class (IgA, IgG, etc.). It is thought that the presence of high levels of Fc in IVIg leads to decreased production of autoantibodies as well as reducing the half-life of all IgGs (including auto-antibodies).

- Inhibitory effects on B cells: IVIg can induce apoptosis of B cells. Given that IgE is produced by activation of B cells, which leads to histamine and leukotriene release, IVIg may downregulate this response.

The indications for IVIg use in critical care can be categorised as follows:

- Neurological: Guillain-Barré syndrome (GBS), myasthenia gravis (MG), chronic inflammatory demyelinating polyneuropathy (CIDP) and acute disseminated encephalomyelitis.
- Infectious: toxic shock syndrome (TSS) and *C. difficile* infection. It is no longer recommended for necrotising fasciitis and there is equipoise for its use in Group A Streptococcal sepsis (used in the UK but the US).
- Rheumatological and haematological: haemophagocytic lymphohistiocytosis (HLH), vaccine-induced thrombocytopaenia and thrombosis (VITT), post-transfusion purpura and CAR-T syndrome.
- Dermatological: Stevens-Johnson syndrome (SJS) and toxic epidermal necrolysis (TEN) are no longer on the list of indications for IVIg in the UK. However, it may still be used but assessed on a case-by-case basis.

References
1. Sylvester J, Lobaz S, Boules E. The use of intravenous immunoglobulin in intensive care. *BJA Educ* 2024; 24(1): 31–7.

● Answer 48: b

Anti-retroviral therapy (ART) consists of a combination of a number of different groups of drugs used for the treatment of human immunodeficiency virus (HIV). There are two variants of HIV: HIV-1 and HIV-2. HIV-1 affects up to 95% of those with HIV and represents the more aggressive variant. HIV-2 is predominantly confined to West Africa and tends to develop more slowly, be less transmissible and very rarely results in critical illness.

ART is started as soon as a diagnosis of HIV has been made, as treatment reduces viral load (and thus the risk of onward transmission) and improves CD4 count. It is also thought that treatment improves the immune system's ability to control the virus and thus reduce the risk of ART failure. Combination therapy is standard with almost all initial regimes and contains

SBA Paper 1: Answers

reverse transcriptase inhibitors which stop the conversion of viral RNA to DNA. There are two groups of drug that affect this pathway: nucleoside reverse transcriptase inhibitors (NRTIs) which are active against both HIV-1 and -2, and non-nucleoside reverse transcriptase inhibitors (NNRTIs) which are only active against HIV-1. NRTIs are recognised as having the most side effects, causing mitochondrial toxicity leading to peripheral neuropathy, pancreatitis, lipoatrophy, lactic acidosis and renal injury amongst others. NNRTI and INSTIs (integrase strand transfer inhibitors) have relatively few adverse effects by comparison.

Protease inhibitors are relatively safe but may cause insulin resistance, hyperlipidaemia and sometimes hepatotoxicity.

References
1. www.uptodate.com. Overview of antiretroviral agents used to treat HIV. UpToDate, 2025. Available at: https://www.uptodate.com/contents/overview-of-antiretroviral-agents-used-to-treat-hiv.
2. Burtle D, Marsh S, Matin N. Update on the management of patients with HIV infection in anaesthesia and critical care. *BJA Educ* 2023; 23(7): 264–72.

● Answer 49: a

An ascitic tap is often performed in patients with known liver disease and ascites to rule out spontaneous bacterial peritonitis (SBP). In this situation it is ideal to take a sample of the ascitic fluid prior to starting antibiotics provided this does not delay the administration of the antibiotics.

In patients with SBP the ascitic fluid is likely to be a cloudy yellow colour, but it may be transparent yellow or blood-stained following a traumatic tap. If the tap is blood-stained, a correction factor is used to estimate the true WCC, where 1 WBC is subtracted per 750 RBCs and 1 neutrophil per 250 RBCs. There is not a specific cut-off for WCC with regards to SBP diagnosis, with the main criteria being neutrophils (or polymorphonuclear leukocytes [PMN]) ≥250cells/mm^3. This measure alone is sufficient for a diagnosis of SBP and antibiotics to be started. Fluid is also sent for culture with single-organism infection typical in SBP. Patients undergoing peritoneal dialysis (PD) use a different diagnostic threshold for SBP of a WCC of over 100 cells/mm^3 or a raised WCC (normal in PD patients is <8) with >50% neutrophils considered diagnostic of infection.

Although SBP is the most common cause of a raised ascitic WCC, other causes exist including secondary bacterial peritonitis (SecBP). Should ascitic culture grow multiple organisms, SecBP should be suspected.

Runyon's criteria may also be used for SecBP where the presence of two of the following confirms diagnosis: total protein >1g/dL, glucose <2.8mmol/L, LDH greater than the upper limit of normal for serum. If two of these are present, the patient should undergo further imaging to rule out intra-abdominal pathology (such as bowel perforation) as the underlying cause of peritonitis.

The serum ascites albumin gradient (SAAG) is ≥1.1g/dL in patients with portal hypertension. This does not help to identify the cause of portal hypertension; however, if the total protein is <2.5g/dL, this suggests cirrhosis and if the total protein is ≥2.5g/dL, a cardiac cause is more likely. The SAAG will also be elevated in patients with SBP.

References
1. Akriviadis EA, Runyon BA. Utility of an algorithm in differentiating spontaneous from secondary bacterial peritonitis. *Gastroenterol* 1990; 98(1): 127–33.
2. www.uptodate.com. Evaluation of adults with ascites. UpToDate, 2024. Available at: https://www.uptodate.com/contents/evaluation-of-adults-with-ascites.
3. www.uptodate.com. Clinical manifestations and diagnosis of peritonitis in peritoneal dialysis. UpToDate, 2024. Available at: https://www.uptodate.com/contents/clinical-manifestations-and-diagnosis-of-peritonitis-in-peritoneal-dialysis.

● Answer 50: d

Hyperinsulinaemic euglycaemic therapy (HIET) is emerging as a treatment for myocardial depression secondary to poisoning. The mechanism of action is not fully understood but it is thought to increase uptake of glucose and lactate into the cardiac muscle thus improving myocardial contractility without increasing oxygen demand and also increases concentration of calcium in the cytoplasm of myocardial cells.

HIET was originally used for the treatment of calcium channel blocker (CCB) and beta-blocker overdose. The non-dihydropyridine CCBs (such as verapamil and diltiazem) tend to cause greater myocardial depression than dihydropyridine CCBs (such as amlodipine), which predominantly cause vasodilation. In CCB overdose, insulin release is decreased as it is dependent on calcium uptake into beta cells of the islets of Langerhans and so is impaired and insulin resistance leading to hyperglycaemia is also seen. HIET helps to attenuate these effects.

The regime recommended by Toxbase is as follows:

- Correct hypokalaemia and ensure glucose is >10mmol/L prior to starting HIET.
- Bolus of 1 unit/kg short-acting insulin IV over 2–3 minutes.
- Start insulin infusion of 1 unit/kg/hr, titrate up by 2 units/kg/hr every 15 minutes until there is a satisfactory clinical response to a maximum of around 10 units/kg/hr.
- Run an infusion of 10% glucose 100ml/hr initially and titrate to blood glucose, measuring glucose levels every 10 minutes initially and following rate changes and every 30–60 minutes when on a stable rate.

HIET is cited as a possible treatment for refractory cases of amitriptyline poisoning but is not indicated in any of the other poisonings listed.

References

1. Hamzić J, Raos D, Radulović B. High-dose insulin euglycemic therapy. *Acta Clin Croat* 2022; 61(Suppl 1): 73–7.
2. www.toxbase.org. TOXBASE — the primary clinical toxicology database of the National Poisons Information Service. Information/antidote/high-dose-insulin-euglycaemic-therapy-adults-only. Available at: https://www.toxbase.org.
3. www.toxbase.org. TOXBASE — the primary clinical toxicology database of the National Poisons Information Service. Poisons-index-A-Z/d-products/diltiazem. Available at: https://www.toxbase.org.

2 SBA Paper 2: Questions

● Question 1

You are working in a district general hospital and are on a night shift. There is a paediatric arrest call in the emergency department (ED) that you attend as the resident critical care physician. There is also an anaesthetic registrar in attendance. The infant girl is 4 months old and is normally fit and well. Delivery was pre-term at 36 weeks secondary to maternal pre-eclampsia; all developmental milestones have been reached without delay and the infant has no current medical conditions. The mother reports recent coryzal symptoms and poor milk intake for several days. Tonight, the child has become lethargic and tachypnoeic, hence her mother has bought her to hospital. The ED team have put out an arrest call because the child is cyanosed and mottled, and looks peri-arrest.

On examination:

A: Grunting sounds, small amounts of air movement, no secretions.
B: Respiratory rate (RR) 80/min, shallow breaths, oxygen sats are 95% on a 15L non-rebreathe (NRB) mask, wheeze on auscultation with poor air entry globally, intercostal and sternal recession is noted.
C: Peripherally cool and mottled, capillary refill time (CRT) 5 seconds, heart rate (HR) 160/min, sinus rhythm. There has not been a wet nappy today.
D: Groaning when cannulated, with some attempt to withdraw from painful stimulus. Eyes only opening to pain.
E: Temperature 38.4°C, abdomen soft.

What is the most appropriate next step in the management of this child?

a   Immediate intubation and ventilation.
b   Fluid challenge.
c   Back-to-back salbutamol nebulisers.
d   Broad-spectrum antibiotics.
e   5x rescue breaths.

● Question 2

You asked to review a 66-year-old patient who has attended the ED, with shortness of breath (SOB) and a productive cough. The patient has recently bought a new dehumidifier for their home. The patient has diaphoresis and there is increased work of breathing.

A: Maintaining own airway.
B: Oxygen sats 95% on 15L NRB, RR 32/min, chest X-ray (CXR) — patchy bilateral lower zone consolidation.
C: Blood pressure (BP) 90/55mmHg, HR 98/min, sinus rhythm.
D: Alert and orientated.

You suspect a diagnosis of atypical community-acquired pneumonia (CAP) and start intravenous co-amoxiclav and clarithromycin. The patient remains hypotensive despite fluid resuscitation, and is admitted to the intensive care unit (ICU). A metaraminol infusion is commenced, along with omeprazole (gastric ulcer prophylaxis) and dalteparin (venous thromboembolism [VTE] prophylaxis) as part of the standard ICU admission bundle. You subsequently establish in the past medical history that the patient had a renal transplant secondary to reflux nephropathy several years ago and takes regular oral tacrolimus.

Which of the following medications may need stopping or altering, in view of the patient being on tacrolimus?

a   Co-amoxiclav.
b   Metaraminol.
c   Omeprazole.
d   Clarithromycin.
e   Dalteparin.

Question 3

You are reviewing a 44-year-old gentleman who has been in the ICU for the last 25 days. He was initially admitted with necrotising pancreatitis which has been complicated by infected pancreatic collections. A drain remains *in situ* for this, which is continuing to drain brown fluid. He had a tracheostomy sited on day 16 following several failed extubation attempts, due to a mixture of agitation and secretion load. He has recently finished a course of meropenem and anidulafungin and is not currently on any antimicrobials. He has had a persistent temperature for the last week but in the context of recent sterile blood cultures and a falling C-reactive protein (CRP) it was felt that stopping antibiotics was appropriate. Overnight, nursing staff report that he is pyrexial with very high temperatures and looks sweaty and uncomfortable. A full septic screen has been sent off and his current observations and bloods are as follows:

A: Tracheostomy *in situ*, cuff is inflated.
B: Ventilated: pressure support (PS)/continuous positive airway pressure (CPAP) mode (PS 10cmH$_2$O, CPAP 7.5cmH$_2$O), an FiO$_2$ of 0.4, RR 30/min. Crepitations at both lung bases on auscultation.
C: BP 100/60mmHg (on noradrenaline 0.1µg/kg/min), HR 95/min, sinus rhythm, warm peripherally, CRT 3 seconds.
D: Alert but unsettled. Not obeying commands consistently. Clonidine 3µg/kg/hr infusion.
E: Temperature 39.5°C, abdomen distended, soft, mildly tender in the left flank. Pancreatic drain draining brown fluid as before.

Blood test results are shown in Table 2.1.

Table 2.1. Blood test results.

	Today	Yesterday		Today	Yesterday
Hb	91g/L	102g/L	Na$^+$	133mmol/L	136mmol/L
WCC	10.4 x 10^9/L	9.5 x 10^9/L	K$^+$	3.8mmol/L	3.5mmol/L
Platelets	110 x 10^9/L	140 x 10^9/L	Creatinine	110µmol/L	80µmol/L
PT	12.2 seconds	11.5 seconds	Urea	8.5mmol/L	6.0mmol/L
APTT	35 seconds	34 seconds	AST	300 U/L	120 U/L
Fibrinogen	1.6g/L	3.2g/L	Albumin	30g/L	31g/L
CRP	60mg/L	30mg/L	Bilirubin	20µmol/L	18µmol/L
PCT	0.4ng/ml	-	Ferritin	5800µg/L	-

What additional test would be most likely to confirm the diagnosis?

a   Galactomannan.
b   Serum triglycerides.
c   CT abdomen.
d   Beta-D-glucan.
e   Full set of cultures.

● Question 4

You are called to the resuscitation department to assist with the care of a 65-year-old man, who has attended with a large gastrointestinal (GI) bleed. He has significant haematemesis, and the ED team have begun to administer a major haemorrhage pack. The patient takes regular apixaban for a previous pulmonary embolus (PE).

What is the most appropriate specific treatment for this gentleman?

a   Andexanet alfa.
b   Prothrombin factor concentrate.
c   Idarucizumab.
d   Tranexamic acid.
e   Phytomenadione.

● Question 5

You are the registrar on-call for the ICU on a night shift. Whilst you are in the ED reviewing a patient, you overhear a police officer in the department discussing a potential terrorist attack at a local night club. Five minutes later, the resuscitation team receive a pre-alert: there has been a massive explosion at a night club with multiple casualties. There are reported to be at least 30 patients with serious injuries. A major incident has been declared; the current status is 'standby'.

What is the most important next step?

a	Stay in the ED to help manage the incoming patient load.
b	Ring the ICU consultant and ask them to come in.
c	Go back to the ICU and start to identify which patients could be discharged.
d	Become the ICU bronze commander until the consultant arrives.
e	Consult your hospital's major incident protocol on what to do next.

● Question 6

You are called to assist with a patient in the ED, who has attended with headache and vomiting and subsequent collapse. Their Glasgow Coma Scale (GCS) at presentation is 4 (E-1, V-1, M-2). It is felt that the patient should be intubated for airway protection, to facilitate an urgent CT head. The patient is normally a fit and well 45-year-old man. The only additional history of note is from the patient's husband, who states that the patient needed an ICU stay after a previous routine operation (tonsillectomy) whilst a teenager. He also states that his husband's father has reported having a similar problem but cannot recall any detail.

The anaesthetic machine in the ED is equipped with a sevoflurane vaporiser on the back-bar, as well as a Waters circuit and a transport Hamilton ventilator.

What is the safest way to proceed in this case?

a	Ensure there is a new circuit on the anaesthetic machine. Anaesthetise with propofol, alfentanil and rocuronium.
b	Use a Waters circuit to pre-oxygenate, use the transport ventilator post-intubation. Anaesthetise with propofol, alfentanil and rocuronium.
c	Use the current anaesthetic machine as it currently is. Anaesthetise with propofol, alfentanil and rocuronium.
d	Ensure there is a new circuit on the anaesthetic machine. Anaesthetise with propofol, alfentanil and suxamethonium.
e	Use a Waters circuit to pre-oxygenate, use the transport ventilator post-intubation. Anaesthetise with propofol, alfentanil and suxamethonium.

Question 7

A 21-year-old asthmatic patient has been admitted to the ICU a few hours previously, as he was hypoxic and wheezy despite back-to-back nebulised salbutamol, 4-hourly ipratropium bromide, intravenous (IV) magnesium sulphate and an aminophylline infusion. He is currently on CPAP and appears to be struggling and dyspnoeic. A decision is made for intubation. He has an ideal body weight of 70kg.

What is the most appropriate invasive ventilation settings for this patient?

a   PCV — PHigh to aim Vt 490ml, PEEP of 10cmH$_2$O, RR 16/min. I:E 1:2.
b   VCV — Vt 420ml, PEEP of 5cmH$_2$O, RR 16/min. I:E 1:2.
c   Pressure-regulated volume-controlled (hybrid) mode — Vt 420ml, PEEP of 5cmH$_2$O, RR 10/min. I:E 1:2.
d   VCV — Vt 600ml, PEEP 0cmH$_2$O, RR 10/min. I:E 1:5.
e   Pressure-regulated volume-controlled (hybrid) mode — Vt 420ml, PEEP of 0cmH$_2$O, RR 10/min. I:E 1:5.

Question 8

You are undertaking a daily review of a 65-year-old man, who has been admitted with community-acquired pneumonia (CAP). During his stay the renal function has deteriorated, and he has now been anuric for over 12 hours, with a rising potassium. You make the decision to start him on continuous renal replacement therapy (CRRT). He is currently taking IV Tazocin® (piperacillin with tazobactam) 4.5g every 12 hours as his antimicrobial therapy. He is also on unfractionated heparin for treatment of an acute pulmonary embolus.

What medication changes need to be made, in the context of starting on CRRT?

a   Tazocin 4.5g 8-hourly. Switch to treatment dose dalteparin.
b   Tazocin dosing can remain the same. Remain on unfractionated heparin.
c   Tazocin dosing can remain the same. Switch to treatment dose dalteparin.
d   Tazocin 4.5g 8-hourly. Remain on unfractionated heparin.
e   Tazocin 4.5g 8-hourly. Switch to prophylactic dose dalteparin.

Question 9

You are asked to review a 35-year-old man on the infectious disease ward for consideration of CRRT. He was admitted with a fever having recently returned from a holiday in India 2 weeks ago. His liver and renal function are acutely deranged. His travel history is that he was visiting friends in Mumbai, staying in the city the whole time. He did eat some street food. It was the monsoon season hence he had walked through flood water, but otherwise there was no outdoor water exposure. He sustained several mosquito bites but had taken malaria prophylaxis. The man states that he started to feel feverish on the plane home, with a mild cough and generalised myalgia. This lasted a few days and then improved for around 5 days, before worsening again. His fever returned and he noticed his eyes were getting a bit yellow, so he came into hospital.

His blood test results are shown in Table 2.2.

Table 2.2. Blood test results.

Hb	130g/L	Na$^+$	129mmol/L
WCC	14 x 10^9/L	K$^+$	6.1mmol/L
Neutrophils	12 x 10^9/L	Creatinine	350μmol/L
Platelets	150 x 10^9/L	Urea	15.4mmol/L
PT	11 seconds (INR 1)	ALT	100 IU/L
		ALP	120 IU/L
		Bilirubin	300μmol/L

What is the most likely unifying diagnosis?

a   Leptospirosis.
b   Hepatitis A.
c   Malaria.
d   Hepatitis C.
e   Cholecystitis.

Question 10

You are called to see a 64-year-old patient on the haematology ward. The patient has had a recent diagnosis of Hodgkin's lymphoma. He has been started on induction chemotherapy that morning. Pre-treatment with allopurinol and IV hydration have been administered. Other medical comorbidities include ischaemic heart disease with a recent ECHO showing a left ventricle (LV) ejection fraction (EF) of 40%, diabetes mellitus (DM) and stage 3 chronic kidney disease (CKD).

You have been asked to review the patient, as despite ongoing IV fluid therapy, they have been oligo-anuric having passed only 10ml in the last 4 hours. An ECG has been done which shows a sinus tachycardia and peaked T waves, but a normal QRS and no ischaemic changes. The patient feels nauseous but has no pain or weakness.

Blood test results including a venous blood gas taken 1 hour ago are shown in Table 2.3.

Table 2.3. Blood test results.

Na$^+$	135mmol/L	AdjCa	1.8mmol/L	pH	7.29
K$^+$	6.3mmol/L	PO$_4^{3-}$	2.2mmol/L	pCO$_2$	4.5kPa
Urea	15mmol/L	Uric acid	600µmol/L	HCO$_3^-$	15mmol/L
Creatinine	250µmol/L			BE	−9mmol/L
Baseline Cr	135µmol/L			Cl$^-$	105mmol/L

What is the definitive treatment here?

a   Initiation of CRRT.
b   Insulin and dextrose.
c   Rasburicase.
d   Urinary alkalinisation with sodium bicarbonate.
e   Further aggressive fluid resuscitation.

Question 11

A 35-year-old woman attends the ED with a 2-day history of nausea and vomiting with development of weakness, initially in her arms and now in her legs as well. She mentions that she cut her leg whilst digging in her allotment and the wound became contaminated with soil. She has noticed that the cut now looks infected and is painful. Over the next 2 hours her weakness progresses, with a significant postural BP drop, tachycardia and worsening respiratory failure. She is admitted to the ICU for monitoring plus respiratory support as needed.

The lab has just rung the ICU to say that the blood cultures taken in the ED are growing a Gram-positive bacillus with full identification to follow.

What Is the most appropriate antimicrobial therapy for this patient?

a   Gentamicin.
b   Metronidazole and gentamicin.
c   Co-amoxiclav and clindamycin.
d   Benzylpenicillin.
e   Antibiotics are not indicated.

Question 12

You are asked to help with a patient who is having a seizure in the ED. The patient has had two self-terminating seizures and is now quite confused and agitated. The patient is a 55-year-old lady who has been on citalopram for depression for the last 6 months but is otherwise fit and well. She takes no other medications. Her wife states she has been a little muddled of late and started with fits today.

A blood gas shows a Na$^+$ of 111mmol/L so a bolus of 150ml of 2.7% hypertonic saline is given IV. You admit her to the ICU for sodium correction and management.

On examination:

A: Maintaining own airway.
B: O$_2$ sats 94% on room air, RR 20/min.

C: BP 135/80mmHg, HR 80/min, no peripheral oedema, normal skin turgor, CRT <2 secs.
D: GCS 14 (confusion).

Blood test results are shown in Table 2.4.

Table 2.4. Blood test results.

Hb	122 g/L	Na⁺	111mmol/L
WCC	12 x 10⁹/L	K⁺	4.5mmol/L
Platelets	350 x 10⁹/L	Urea	6.2mmol/L
Liver function tests	Normal	Creatinine	85µmol/L
Cortisol	Normal	Glucose	5.4mmol/L
Thyroid function	Normal	Urinary Na⁺	37mmol/L
Serum osmolality	240mOsmol/kg	Urine dipstick	Protein 1+, no WCC or blood
		Urine osmolality	300mOsmol/kg

What is the most likely diagnosis?

a   Syndrome of inappropriate anti-diuretic hormone (SIADH) secretion.
b   Diuretic abuse.
c   Nephrotic syndrome.
d   Water intoxication.
e   Addison's disease.

● **Question 13**

You are reviewing a 25-year-old patient who was admitted overnight to the ICU for treatment of pyelonephritis and vasopressor support. CT-KUB (kidneys, ureters and bladder) has shown a large obstructing ureteric stone which required emergency nephrostomy insertion. On speaking to the patient, she informs you she has had several renal stones in the past and has been told she has something wrong with her kidneys. She also sees a rheumatologist for Sjögren's syndrome.

Her blood test results including a venous blood gas are shown in Table 2.5.

Table 2.5. Blood test results.

Hb	122g/L	pH	7.25
WCC	18.5 x 10^9/L	pCO_2	4.5kPa
Platelets	230 x 10^9/L	HCO_3^-	9mmol/L
Na^+	136mmol/L	Lactate	2.1mmol/L
K^+	2.8mmol/L	Cl^-	120mmol/L
Creatinine	140μmol/L	Urinary pH	6.0
Urea	8.4mmol/L		
CRP	280mg/L		

What is the most likely cause of her acid-base derangement?

a   Sepsis.
b   Acute kidney injury (AKI).
c   Renal tubular acidosis type 2.
d   Diabetic ketoacidosis.
e   Renal tubular acidosis type 1.

● Question 14

An 18-year-old patient has been on the neuro ICU for 7 days following a severe traumatic brain injury (TBI). He has had several episodes of raised intracranial pressure (ICP), all of which resolved with medical management. He has now had an ICP of 40mmHg for 30 minutes. A CT head scan revealed a very tight-looking brain with early signs of cerebral herniation. On ABG, he has a $PaCO_2$ of 4.5kPa. His cerebral perfusion pressure (CPP) is 68mmHg. He is optimally sedated and paralysed with a Bispectral Index (BIS) of 25 and 1 twitch on a train of four (TOF) monitoring. He has received two doses of hypertonic saline.

Which one of the following is the next best step in his ICP management?

a   Insertion of an external ventricular drain (EVD).
b   He should be cooled to 34°C.
c   Increased CPP target to 70–80mmHg.
d   Increased sedation aiming for burst suppression.
e   Reduction in $PaCO_2$ to 4–4.5kPa whilst further urgent management options are considered.

● Question 15

A 52-year-old man who is normally fit and well is admitted to the ICU following a large spontaneous intracranial haemorrhage (ICH). His pupils are fixed and dilated and he is taking intermittent spontaneous breaths on the ventilator. After a discussion with the family a decision is made for withdrawal of life-sustaining treatment (WOLST) followed by organ donation after cardiac death (DCD). His liver, lungs, kidneys and pancreas (but not heart) have been accepted for donation by the transplant team.

He is moved into an anaesthetic room in theatres with his family for WOLST. His systolic BP is 100mmHg prior to WOLST and drops to 50mmHg 5 minutes after withdrawing support. The patient dies 45 minutes after WOLST. Death is confirmed and he is immediately transferred into theatre, where the transplant surgical team undertake organ retrieval.

Which organs would still be deemed viable for donation?

a   Kidneys, liver, pancreas and lungs.
b   Liver, pancreas and lungs.
c   Kidneys, pancreas and lungs.
d   Kidney and lungs.
e   Kidney, liver and lungs.

● Question 16

You are asked to prescribe CRRT for an ICU patient. The patient is a 64-year-old man with a history of alcoholic liver disease (ALD) who is 1 year abstinent and on the liver transplant list. He came into hospital with an acute variceal bleed requiring banding under general anaesthesia (GA) and was transferred to the ICU after this. He remains intubated and ventilated. His renal function has significantly deteriorated since admission and a diagnosis of hepatorenal syndrome–acute kidney injury (HRS-AKI) is suspected. There has been a decision to commence CRRT whilst work-up for a transjugular intrahepatic portosystemic shunt (TIPS) is performed. He is already on the maximum terlipressin dose. There is no ongoing variceal bleeding.

Blood test results of note are shown in Table 2.6.

Table 2.6. Blood test results.

Platelets	56 x 10^9/L	ALT	350 IU/L
PT	15 seconds	AST	400 U/L
APTT	30 seconds	Albumin	25g/L
Fibrinogen	2.2g/L		

What is the best type of anticoagulation for his CRRT?

a   Systemic anticoagulation with heparin.
b   Systemic anticoagulation with danaparoid.
c   Circuit anticoagulation with citrate.
d   Circuit anticoagulation with prostacyclin.
e   No anticoagulation.

● Question 17

A 55-year-old man is referred to the ICU from the neurology ward. He has been admitted with progressive ascending weakness over the last 24 hours. Prior to the weakness he had noticed numbness and pins and needles in his feet. He had his flu vaccine a week ago (as he is a healthcare worker) but otherwise has no medical problems.

You have been asked to review him because his oxygen requirements over the last 6 hours have increased from an FiO_2 of 0.3 to 0.5 via a Venturi mask. His RR is 26/minute and he states he is struggling to breathe.

What would be the most useful investigation to guide ongoing management?

a   Arterial blood gas.
b   Chest X-ray.
c   Lumbar puncture.
d   Serial vital capacity measurements.
e   Serial peak flow measurements.

● Question 18

A 22-year-old patient presents with fevers, confusion and altered behaviour. Aside from occasional cold sores and mild asthma he is normally fit and well. A CT head is undertaken which is normal, so a lumbar puncture (LP) is subsequently performed. His blood results show a WCC 14 x 10^9/L, CRP 45mg/L and glucose 6.5mmol/L.

Which LP results are most consistent with this history?

a   Clear fluid, protein 0.6g/L, glucose 3.5mmol/L, WCC 650 cells/µL with monocytes and lymphocytes predominant.
b   Clear fluid, protein 0.4g/L, glucose 3.5mmol/L, WCC 2 cells/µL.
c   Cloudy fluid, protein 0.15g/L, glucose 1.5mmol/L, WCC 200 cells/µL with a high proportion of monocytes.
d   Turbid fluid, protein 1.2g/L, glucose 2mmol/L, WCC 550 cells/µL with 90% polymorphonuclear leukocytes (PMNs or neutrophils).
e   Clear fluid, protein 1.3g/L, glucose 4mmol/L, WCC 550 cells/µL with 90% PMN.

● Question 19

A 45-year-old man presents to the ED with acute respiratory failure. He has recently had a viral infection and for the last few days has been coughing up green sputum and becoming increasingly short of breath (SOB). He has a background history of a few months of weakness, and at a neurology appointment last week he was diagnosed with motor neurone disease (MND). He is awaiting a further appointment to discuss treatment options and is being considered for riluzole.

SBA Paper 2: Questions

His observations are as follows:

A: Maintaining own airway.
B: O_2 sats 88% on 15L NRB mask, RR 35/min, PaO_2 7.6kPa, $PaCO_2$ 8.2kPa, HCO_3^- 24mmol/L and pH 7.28 on ABG, CXR consistent with right lower lobe pneumonia.
C: BP 90/40mmHg after 500ml fluid challenge, HR 110/min, warm peripherally, CRT 4 seconds.
D: Rousable to voice.

His wife has done some research and says they've had a conversation where he said he was not keen on the idea of long-term ventilation, but they have no advanced directives yet. The patient is not confused but finds conversation difficult due to his severe SOB. He has already received broad-spectrum antibiotics in the ED.

What is the best management option in this case?

a Immediate intubation and ventilation.
b Admit to the ICU for a trial of NIV to allow further discussions with the patient and his team.
c Best supportive ward care only.
d Start riluzole and admit to the ICU with no treatment limitations.
e Admit to the ICU with a ceiling of level 2 treatment.

● Question 20

You are asked to review a 35-year-old patient in the ED for consideration of admission to the ICU for management of malignant hypertension. The patient presented with severe headache and a BP of 250/125mmHg. Despite analgesia their BP is still above 240mmHg systolic, and the headache has only marginally improved. The patient had a parathyroidectomy 5 years ago and says several of his family members have needed operations on their thyroid and parathyroid glands. He states that for the last few weeks he has been intermittently having these headaches with palpitations and feeling hot and flushed. He says he does use cocaine socially and admits to taking some a few hours ago.

On examination:

A: Maintaining own airway.
B: O_2 sats 99% on room air, RR 22/min.
C: BP 245/120mmHg, HR 130/min, sinus rhythm, warm peripheries.
D: Alert and orientated.
E: Temperature 38.5°C, no rashes, sweaty.

What would be the best choice of agent for management of his hypertension?

a   IV lorazepam.
b   Labetalol infusion.
c   Hold off management until further investigations have been undertaken.
d   Doxazocin.
e   Atenolol.

● Question 21

Which antibiotic/s would be the best choice in a patient presenting with severe community-acquired pneumonia (CAP) with a CURB-65 score of 3 who has anaphylaxis to penicillin?

a   IV Tazocin®.
b   PO doxycycline.
c   PO clarithromycin.
d   IV cefuroxime and clarithromycin.
e   IV levofloxacin.

● Question 22

With regard to mechanical left ventricular assist devices (LVADs) which one of the following is correct?

a   LVAD pump inflow is from the left atrium (LA) and outflow goes to the left ventricle (LV).
b   A LVAD cannot be used as a destination treatment in patients with heart failure.
c   A peripheral pulse is present with all types of LVAD.
d   Bleeding is the most common device-related complication.
e   The LV ejection fraction (EF) must be <10% for consideration of LVAD insertion.

● Question 23
Which one of the following factors on admission to the ICU would carry the biggest risk for refeeding syndrome?

a   Negligible oral intake for 8 days.
b   K⁺ 3.4mmol/L.
c   BMI 16.4kg/m².
d   5% weight loss in the last month.
e   Evidence of moderate loss of muscle mass.

● Question 24
Which of the following does **not** form part of the Child-Pugh-Turcotte scoring system for chronic liver disease (CLD)?

a   Bilirubin.
b   Age.
c   INR.
d   Ascites.
e   Albumin.

● Question 25
Which of the following would be calculated by the formula [A/(A+B)] (Figure 2.1)?

		Actual outcome	
		+ve	-ve
Test outcome	+ve	A	B
	-ve	C	D

Figure 2.1. 2 x 2 table: actual outcome and test outcome.

a Sensitivity.
b Specificity.
c Positive predictive value (PPV).
d Odds ratio (OR).
e Negative predictive value (NPV).

● Question 26

A 25-year-old 70kg man presents to the ED after being hit with a firework. He has full-thickness burns to his anterior torso and both arms excluding his hands. He said that the injury occurred about an hour ago and he made his way straight to the hospital in his friend's car. You have calculated him as having 20% total body surface area (TBSA) burns using a Lund and Browder chart. What is the best fluid regime for this patient?

a 300ml/hr of 0.9% saline over the next 7 hours.
b 400ml/hr of 0.9% saline over the next 8 hours.
c 400ml/hr of Hartmann's solution over the next 7 hours.
d 300ml/hr of 0.9% saline over the next 11 hours.
e 400ml/hr of Hartmann's solution over the next 11 hours.

SBA Paper 2: Questions

● Question 27
Which of the following thromboelastography (TEG®) traces would be seen in a patient with an isolated platelet deficiency (Figure 2.2)?

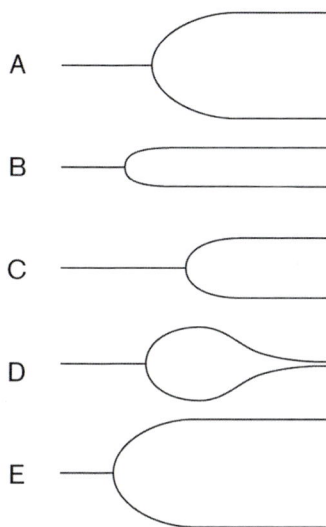

Figure 2.2. Thromboelastography (TEG®) traces.

● Question 28
Which element of a patient's ICU stay contributes the highest carbon footprint in the UK?

a   Energy.
b   Consumables.
c   Waste management.
d   Water.
e   Staff travel.

Question 29

You are asked to review an acutely hypoxic patient who has an established tracheostomy (patent upper airway). The nurses have applied oxygen to their face and tracheostomy stoma. They have removed the inner tube. The patient is making respiratory effort but is obviously distressed with O_2 saturations of 70%. What is the next best step?

a   Attempt to ventilate with a Waters circuit via the tracheostomy.
b   Pass a suction catheter down the tracheostomy to assess patency.
c   Deflate the cuff of the tracheostomy.
d   Remove the tracheostomy and ventilate via the stoma using a paediatric face mask.
e   Start CPR.

Question 30

Which of the following drugs can be safely used without dose adjustment in a patient with myasthenia gravis (MG)?

a   IV magnesium.
b   Atracurium.
c   Labetalol.
d   Clarithromycin.
e   Alfentanil.

Question 31

Which of the following antivirals would **not** be effective against one of the herpes viruses?

a   Foscarnet.
b   Cidofovir.
c   Oseltamivir.
d   Aciclovir.
e   Ganciclovir.

SBA Paper 2: Questions

Question 32
Which of the following ECG changes would you expect to see in a patient with a K⁺ of 1.5mmol/L?

a   Tented T waves.
b   Widened QRS.
c   Flattened P wave.
d   U wave.
e   Shortened QT interval.

Question 33
A patient with longstanding alcohol dependency presents with ataxia, confusion and ophthalmoplegia. Deficiency of which vitamin is likely to be responsible for this clinical picture?

a   Vitamin B12.
b   Thiamine.
c   Folate.
d   Vitamin D.
e   Vitamin K.

Question 34
You are reviewing a patient who is day 4 after an out-of-hospital cardiac arrest (OOHCA). On sedation hold they are extending bilaterally. During assessment at or after 72 hours post-OOHCA, which of the following is **not** a predictor of a poor outcome?

a   Bilaterally absent N20 SSEP wave.
b   Status myoclonus.
c   Neuron-specific enolase (NSE) >60μg/L at 48 or 72 hours.
d   Highly malignant EEG at >24 hours.
e   Isolated loss of pupillary reflexes.

Question 35
In which of the following conditions would a patient require irradiated blood products?

a   Non-Hodgkin lymphoma (NHL).
b   Allogeneic haematopoietic stem cell transplant.
c   HIV infection.
d   Renal transplant.
e   Pregnancy.

Question 36
Which of the following is correct regarding carbon monoxide (CO) poisoning?

a   It can be diagnosed on standard oximetry.
b   It has a lower affinity for haem than oxygen.
c   The half-life of carbon monoxide is around 90 minutes when breathing room air.
d   The mainstay of treatment is high-flow oxygen.
e   Carboxyhaemoglobin (COHb) levels above 15% are an indication for hyperbaric oxygen therapy.

Question 37
According to the MBRRACE-UK 2022 report, which of the following is correct regarding maternal mortality in the UK?

a   Haemorrhage is the most common cause of death.
b   Black women have four times the mortality rate of white women in pregnancy.
c   Causes of death are either direct or indirect.
d   In the last 10 years maternal mortality has consistently decreased.
e   COVID-19 did not increase maternal mortality rates.

SBA Paper 2: Questions

Question 38
Which of the following is true regarding intra-abdominal pressure (IAP) measurement?

a   Abdominal compartment syndrome (ACS) is defined as IAP >20mmHg with new organ dysfunction.
b   Normal IAP is <5mmHg in critically ill adults.
c   IAP should be measured using a rectal pressure monitor.
d   An IAP of 15mmHg is classified as grade II abdominal hypertension.
e   Surgical decompression is the first-line management of ACS.

Question 39
Regarding fire in the ICU, which one of the following is correct?

a   Fire requires the presence of oxygen, heat and an ignition source.
b   There should be evacuation equipment available for each ICU bed space (e.g. ski pad or sheet).
c   When administering oxygen via a cylinder, the mask should be attached to the patient, then to the cylinder, and then flow turned on.
d   Only senior nursing staff need to know fire evacuation procedures.
e   There should be a minimum of five air changes per hour in the ICU.

Question 40
You are intubating a patient in the ICU. The patient has received a modified rapid sequence induction (RSI) using ketamine and 1mg/kg of rocuronium. You are oxygenating the patient with a Waters circuit and supplemental nasal oxygen. The patient is positioned 30° head up. You are unable to intubate with a standard laryngoscope, so you try a video laryngoscope, which is also unsuccessful. Your registrar colleague then attempts and fails to intubate with cricoid pressure off. You declare a failed intubation. The patient is starting to desaturate (O_2 saturations currently 90%).

Which of the following would **not** be a next reasonable step?

a   Oxygenate and ventilate using a two-person technique with oropharyngeal adjunct (Guedel) and facemask.
b   Insertion of a supraglottic airway.
c   Get a front-of-neck access (FONA) airway set prepared.
d   Further attempt at intubation by the consultant.
e   Nasal intubation with a fibreoptic scope.

Question 41

Which of the following scoring systems has the best published performance AUROC (area under the receiver operating characteristic curve)?

a   ICNARC.
b   qSOFA.
c   APACHE III.
d   APACHE II.
e   SAPS II.

Question 42

A patient is admitted to the ICU on the devastating brain injury pathway. On day 3 of their admission, brainstem death testing (BSDT) is performed and confirms death. The family had previously mentioned organ donation, and the specialist nurse for organ donation is currently discussing this with the family, with a view to gaining consent. Which of the following actions would be deemed to be 'unlikely' or 'very unlikely' to be in the patient's best interests (after death before consent)?

a   Insertion of a central line.
b   Starting the patient on vasopressors.
c   Giving methylprednisolone.
d   Taking blood samples for organ donation purposes.
e   Sharing the medical notes with the organ donation team.

Question 43

Which of the following best describes the mechanism of action of ticagrelor?

a   Irreversibly acetylates COX-1.
b   P2Y12 ADP receptor antagonism.
c   GPIIb/IIIa receptor antagonism.
d   Adenylate cyclase stimulation.
e   Phosphodiesterase inhibition.

● Question 44

Which of the following interventions has the best evidence for prevention of cerebral vasospasm and delayed cerebral ischaemia in patients with aneurysmal subarachnoid haemorrhage (SAH)?

a   Regular IV magnesium.
b   Elevation of BP targets with symptomatic vasospasm.
c   Starting a statin.
d   Fluid resuscitation aiming for hypervolaemia.
e   Regular enteral nimodipine.

● Question 45

Which of the following antibiotics are **not** associated with an increased risk of *C. difficile* infection?

a   Clindamycin.
b   Tazocin®.
c   Fidaxomicin.
d   Meropenem.
e   Ciprofloxacin.

● Question 46

Which of the following drugs is most likely to cause prolongation of the QT interval and an increased risk of torsade de pointes?

a   Magnesium sulphate.
b   Metoclopramide.
c   Amiodarone.
d   Haloperidol.
e   Propofol.

Question 47

Which of the following is the most accurate statement regarding pulmonary hypertension (PH)?

a   It occurs most commonly secondary to lung disease.
b   It is defined as a mean pulmonary artery pressure (mPAP) >20mmHg at rest.
c   It is defined as mPAP >25mmHg at rest.
d   In pre-capillary PH, pulmonary artery wedge pressure (PAWP) is >15mmHg.
e   Vasoreactivity testing is indicated in all causes of PH.

Question 48

Which of the following best describes what is happening during phase 2 of this cardiac action potential (Figure 2.3)?

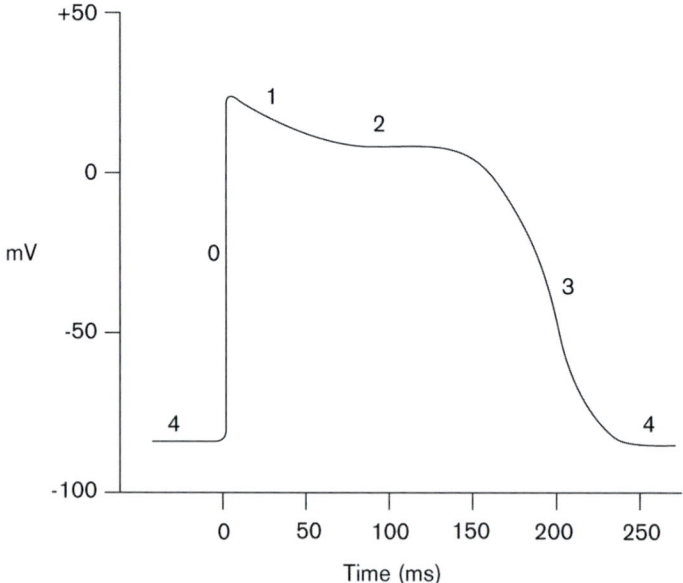

Figure 2.3. Cardiac muscle action potential curve.

a   Rapid Na⁺ influx into the cell.
b   Na⁺/K⁺ pump moves three Na⁺ ions out of the cell in exchange for two K⁺.
c   L-type Ca^{2+} channels open.
d   Na⁺ channels close and K⁺ channels open.
e   L-type Ca^{2+} channels close as K⁺ efflux continues.

● Question 49

Which of the following is best described as a lipopolysaccharide (LPS) toxin which stimulates release of tumour necrosis factor alpha (TNF-α) and interleukin 1, is associated with Gram-negative sepsis, does **not** stimulate an adaptive immune response and causes symptoms including fever, tachycardia and hypotension?

a   Type 1 exotoxin.
b   Type 2 exotoxin.
c   Type 3 exotoxin.
d   Endotoxin.
e   Cytotoxin.

● Question 50

Which of the following would be classified as a never event?

a   Transfusion-associated circulatory overload (TACO).
b   Intra-arterial insertion of a central venous catheter (CVC) line.
c   Accidental iatrogenic opiate overdose.
d   Oesophageal intubation.
e   Intra-arterial injection of propofol.

Answer overview: Paper 2

Question:		Question:	
1	b	26	c
2	d	27	b
3	b	28	a
4	a	29	b
5	c	30	e
6	b	31	c
7	e	32	d
8	d	33	b
9	a	34	e
10	a	35	b
11	d	36	d
12	a	37	b
13	e	38	a
14	e	39	b
15	d	40	e
16	c	41	c
17	d	42	c
18	a	43	b
19	b	44	e
20	d	45	c
21	e	46	d
22	d	47	b
23	a	48	c
24	b	49	d
25	c	50	e

2 SBA Paper 2: Answers

● Answer 1: b

The likely diagnosis is acute bronchiolitis. The child is extremely unwell and needs immediate resuscitation to prevent cardiac arrest. She is in severe respiratory distress but is currently maintaining adequate oxygen saturations. There is no immediate clinical indication for five rescue breaths; however, if the child deteriorates further this may become necessary. The immediate priority is resuscitation of the child. Intubation and ventilation may be indicated at some point, but this should be undertaken following optimisation of their cardiovascular status (if possible), to avoid further deterioration especially potentially during induction of anaesthesia. There is no strong evidence for the use of salbutamol in infants with bronchiolitis, and the National Institute for Heath and Care Excellence (NICE) does not recommend the use of antibiotics. It is likely given how unwell this child is that antibiotics would be given to cover sepsis; however, the primary concern here is resuscitation, so the single best answer here is a fluid bolus (10ml/kg) in the first instance.

References

1. National Institute for Heath and Care Excellence (NICE), guideline NG9. Bronchiolitis in children: diagnosis and management, 2021. Available at: www.nice.org.uk/guidance/ng9.

● Answer 2: d

Tacrolimus is an immunosuppressant drug with a relatively narrow therapeutic window. Tacrolimus is metabolised by cytochrome P450

(CYP450) enzymes in the liver, hence caution needs to be exercised when using any drugs that either induce or inhibit CYP450.

The British National Formulary (BNF) highlights that certain drugs can have serious interaction risks with tacrolimus; however, anything that affects the CYP450 enzyme pathway should be considered a risk:

- Drugs that increase tacrolimus blood concentration (risk of toxicity) include amiodarone, ciclosporin, macrolides (clarithromycin and erythromycin), diltiazem, verapamil, felodipine, nicardipine, azole antifungals (e.g. fluconazole, itraconazole, ketoconazole), and tigecycline.
- Drugs that decrease tacrolimus blood concentration (risk of inadequate immunosuppression and organ rejection) include: carbamazepine, phenobarbital, phenytoin, rifampicin, orlistat and St John's wort.

In addition, other interactions to consider include:

- Concurrent use of tacrolimus with medications known to have nephrotoxic or neurotoxic effects may increase the risk of these effects (e.g. aminoglycosides, vancomycin, NSAIDs [ibuprofen], aciclovir and amphotericin B) and should be used with caution or avoided.
- Not to drink grapefruit juice or eat grapefruit as this can increase tacrolimus levels.
- Potassium-sparing medications (e.g. amiloride, spironolactone) may exacerbate tacrolimus-induced hyperkalaemia and should be only initiated with regular monitoring of U&Es. Dalteparin may cause hyperkalaemia in combination with tacrolimus, but this would not require dose adjustment provided K^+ is monitored in the ICU. The risk of venous thromboembolism with no prophylaxis is higher than the hyperkalaemia risk in this situation. Trimethoprim and co-trimoxazole can also increase serum K^+.
- Avoid the use of live vaccines as immunosuppression may affect vaccine effectiveness.

It is important to liaise with critical care pharmacists and transplant teams.

SBA Paper 2: Answers

References

1. BNF. Tacrolimus interactions. Available at: https://bnf.nice.org.uk/interactions/tacrolimus/.
2. EMC. Tacrolimus contraindications. Available at: https://www.medicines.org.uk/emc/product/585/smpc.

Answer 3: b

Haemophagocytic lymphohistiocytosis (HLH) is a condition with significant morbidity and mortality that is caused by a loss of immune regulation, leading to an uncontrolled immune system response resulting in very high cytokine levels and immune-mediated organ damage. It can be primary (often seen in children due to genetic mutations) or secondary due to malignancy (typically haematological), infection or autoimmune causes.

Symptoms and signs include fever (often out of proportion to inflammatory markers), coagulopathy, liver dysfunction, hepatosplenomegaly, cytopaenias and haemophagocytosis of the bone marrow.

As the treatment for HLH involves immunosuppression, which would not be part of routine ICU treatment, early diagnosis is paramount including calculation of the H-score.

The H-score is based on diagnostic criteria published in 2014 and has been validated with good sensitivity and specificity. A cut-off score of 169 correlates with a diagnosis of HLH.

It has nine criteria with different score weightings (see Table 2.7 overleaf).

This clinical picture is consistent with likely HLH; to enable a full H-score one would need to measure triglycerides. If the triglycerides are raised this would result in a score above 169 and treatment would be indicated (e.g. high-dose steroids — dexamethasone or methylprednisolone, anakinra or etoposide).

Table 2.7. H-score diagnostic criteria.

HScore criteria	Extent	Value
1. Immunosuppression, e.g. HIV positive or receiving long-term immunosuppression therapy	No	0
	Yes	18
2. Fever	<38.4°C	0
	38.4–39.4°C	33
	>39.4°C	49
3. Organomegaly	None	0
	Liver or spleen	23
	Liver and spleen	38
4. Cytopaenia Hb ≤92g/L, WCC ≤5,000/mm^3, Plt ≤110,000/mm^3	0–1 lineages	0
	2 lineages	24
	3 lineages	34
5. Ferritin	<2000ng/ml	0
	2000–6000ng/ml	35
	>6000ng/ml	50
6. Triglycerides	<1.5mmol/L	0
	1.5–44mmol/L	44
	>4mmol/L	64
7. Fibrinogen	>2.5g/L	0
	≤2.5g/L	30
8. AST	<30 U/L	0
	≥30 U/L	19
9. Haemophagocytosis on BM aspirate	No	0
	Yes	35

SBA Paper 2: Answers

References

1. Al-Samkari H, Berliner N. Hemophagocytic lymphohistiocytosis. *Annu Rev Pathol: Mech Dis* 2018; 13(1): 27–49.
2. Fardet L, Galicier L, Lambotte O, *et al.* Development and validation of the HScore, a score for the diagnosis of reactive hemophagocytic syndrome. *Arthritis Rheumatol* 2014; 66(9): 2613–20.

Answer 4: a

The management of bleeding in a patient on direct oral anticoagulants (DOACs) can be divided into: 1) supportive; and 2) agent-specific management.

Management also depends on the severity of the bleeding. Minor superficial bleeding can often be managed with direct compression. Significant bleeding necessitates a multipronged approach.

Activated charcoal may be considered if a DOAC has been taken within 2 hours of the bleeding event. The DOAC should be stopped, and no further doses given until haemostasis is achieved. Tranexamic acid (TXA) (1g) IV should be given along with blood products, except in cases of GI bleeding where routine administration of TXA is not recommended. Early source control of any bleeding patient is a treatment priority. DOACs have variable renal clearance and in the case of dabigatran, which is highly renally cleared, management may include CRRT. Most DOACs tend to be eliminated from the body within five half-lives.

The use of four-factor prothrombin complex concentrate (PCC) products such as Octaplex® or Beriplex®, can be used for all DOACs but will not completely reverse bleeding.

Other specific agents:

- Idarucizumab is a dabigatran-specific Fab fragment. It completely binds to dabigatran and hence only one dose is indicated. It should not be given with PCC. The availability of this drug is currently a limiting factor.
- Andexanet alfa can be given for reversal of apixaban or rivaroxaban. It is a recombinant form of human factor Xa, which specifically binds to

these drugs. It needs to be given as an infusion that continues until all the drug is cleared.

References

1. www.uptodate.com. Management of bleeding in patients receiving direct oral anticoagulants. UpToDate, 2024. Available at: https://www.uptodate.com/contents/management-of-bleeding-in-patients-receiving-direct-oral-anticoagulants.
2. HALT-IT Trial Collaborators. Effects of a high-dose 24-h infusion of tranexamic acid on death and thromboembolic events in patients with acute gastrointestinal bleeding (HALT-IT): an international randomised, double-blind, placebo-controlled trial. *Lancet* 2020; 395(10241): 1927–36.

● Answer 5: c

All NHS providers in the UK are required by law, to prepare for major incidents and other large-scale emergencies. A health-related major incident is described as 'any occurrence presenting a serious threat to the health of the community'. It is likely to involve disruption of services and require the coordination of hospitals, ambulance services and primary care trusts.

There are different types of major incidents:

- Big bang (explosion/major road traffic collision (RTC).
- Cloud on the horizon (a significant chemical or nuclear release developing elsewhere but needing preparation by your hospital).
- Rising tide (epidemic or pandemic of infectious disease, or a capacity and/or staffing crisis, e.g. industrial action).
- Headline news (public or media alarm about an actual or potential situation).
- Internal incidents (utility or equipment failure, fire, hospital-acquired infections, violent crime).
- CBRN(e) (deliberate [criminal intent] release of chemical, biological, radioactive or nuclear materials or explosive device).
- HAZMAT (incident involving hazardous materials).

SBA Paper 2: Answers

There are different phases of major incidents:

- Major incident standby: incident has occurred but in the early stages, key personnel on major incident call-out list are contacted (likely to include an ICU consultant).
- Major incident declared: all personnel on call-out list are notified; they should retrieve their role incident action cards and proceed to their designated location.
- Major incident stand down: major incident stood down, transition into recovery phase.

With regards to the answers, there should already be an awareness of your hospital's major incident plan. If the consultant needs to attend as part of the hospital's major incident plan then they will be contacted by the major incident team. You may well want to ring the consultant for advice or ask them to come in for alternative reasons, but asking them to attend specifically for the major incident is not your role within the standby phase of a major incident. Although the current escalation phase is standby, there is a high likelihood of significant casualties. Therefore, the first stage to prioritise is preparation, the first step of which is freeing up resources. In relation to critical care capacity this will involve communicating with your team and identifying which patients could step down to the ward, and ensuring anything that needs to be done for these patients is undertaken to facilitate timely discharge.

References
1. Johnson C, Cosgrove JF. Hospital response to a major incident: initial considerations and longer-term effects. *BJA Educ* 2016; 16(10): 329–33.
2. CAB International. Health emergency preparedness and response. Sellwood C, Wapling A, Eds. CAB International; 2016: chapter 1 – Introduction: Why do we need to prepare? Available at: https://www.cabi.org/Uploads/CABI/OpenResources/44554/Chap1%20 9781780644554.pdf.

● Answer 6: b
This history is unclear and there could be many reasons why this patient went to the ICU post-op previously. In the context of his young age at the time of operation and also the routine nature of the procedure, two anaesthetic diagnoses to consider are malignant hyperpyrexia (MH) and suxamethonium apnoea. In addition, there is a family history of a similar presentation which would increase concerns around either one of these diagnoses.

Although a volatile anaesthetic is unlikely to have been used in the ED machine, this cannot be guaranteed, and hence the need to eliminate the potential trigger. Appropriate management guidance can be found within the *Association of Anaesthetists quick reference handbook* (MH protocol section). Placing activated charcoal filters on both limbs of the anaesthetic machine breathing circuit can be considered. A safe and viable alternative in the ED is to use the Waters circuit and transport ventilator, as there is an airway that needs to be urgently secured. This approach effectively removes the potential anaesthetic machine trigger. As for the choice of muscle relaxant, the safest option is to avoid suxamethonium completely, as this is a trigger of both conditions and use an appropriate dosage of rocuronium instead.

References

1. *The Association of Anaesthetists quick reference handbook*. Malignant hyperpyrexia. The Association of Anaesthetists; 2013: chapters 3–8. Available at: https://anaesthetists.org/Portals/0/PDFs/QRH/QRH_complete_June_2023.pdf?ver= 2023-06-23-141011-603.

● Answer 7: e

Ventilating asthmatic patients can be extremely difficult and should be considered once appropriate medical management has been instituted (in the context of a life-threatening asthma exacerbation). Ventilation should try and replicate what is happening in the lungs. Asthma is an inability to effectively expire air due to airway narrowing, whereas inspiration may only be partially limited. Therefore, the key ventilator strategies are to allow as long as possible for expiration, by having a slow respiratory rate (10–12 per minute) and prolonging the expiratory time — Inspiratory: Expiratory ratio (I:E), e.g. to 1:4 or 1:5. In addition, the choice of mode is important. Modern-day ventilators usually have a hybrid setting and this can be ideal, as it allows you to target the tidal volume (Vt) whilst limiting peak pressures. Set the Vt to the lower end of lung-protective ventilation, aiming for 5–7ml/kg of ideal body weight, with peak pressure between 30–35cmH$_2$O. With regards to the PEEP setting, this should be set as low as possible, and often the initial settings would be with a PEEP of zero (ZEEP) to promote expiratory flow. Later, PEEP can be individualised with measurement of intrinsic PEEP (PEEPi). In asthma, a significant issue is dynamic hyperinflation of the lungs, and management of this can become more problematic once the patient is intubated. Hyperinflation can be assessed by measuring the level of PEEPi on the ventilator (usually done using an expiratory hold manoeuvre. It often underestimates the true PEEPi). If present, this indicates the presence of hyperinflation and ideally should be kept below 12cmH$_2$O.

The plateau pressure (PPlat) should be measured using an inspiratory pause manoeuvre; this should be used to guide ventilation and be kept below 25cmH$_2$O. If it is consistently above this, then the RR should be reduced.

References
1. Tuxon D, Hew M. Acute severe asthma. In: Bersten AD, Handy JM, Eds. *Oh's intensive care manual*, 8th ed. London: Elsevier; 2018; chapter 35: pp. 449–56.

Answer 8: d

There are useful resources available for the management of medications in patients with renal failure or those on CRRT (the UK's *Renal drug handbook* is a popular resource). Whilst we often work in a multi-disciplinary team (MDT) with critical care pharmacists, it is important that we know how to alter some regularly used medications for patients with poor renal function or those on CRRT.

In the case of dalteparin, prophylactic dalteparin dosing does not need to be altered for any level of renal impairment, or if commencing CRRT. It is generally well tolerated. However, if a patient has an estimated glomerular filtration rate (eGFR) under 20ml/min or is on CRRT, the use of treatment dose dalteparin is not recommended as it is highly likely to accumulate with a risk of significant bleeding. Therefore, in this patient group it is recommended to use unfractionated heparin as this can be more easily monitored and adjusted.

Tazocin® is predominantly excreted unchanged in the urine (piperacillin 60–80%, tazobactam 80%) and is impacted by renal impairment. The dosing of Tazocin® is unchanged down to an eGFR of 20ml/min. However, below this eGFR, the Tazocin® dose should be decreased or the interval between administration increased, e.g. TDS to BD. In patients on CRRT, Tazocin® is dialysed and therefore the dose can be increased back up to normal, 4.5g every 8 hours (e.g. TDS or QDS depending on local policy).

References

1. Ashley C, Dunleavy A. *The renal drug handbook: the ultimate prescribing guide for renal practitioners*, 5th ed. Available at: https://medicinainterna.net.pe/sites/default/files/The_Renal_Drug_Handbook_The_Ultimate.pdf.

● Answer 9: a

This history suggests a diagnosis of leptospirosis. This is an infection caused by the pathogenic spirochete of the genus *Leptospira*. Mammals primarily act as the reservoir for *Leptospira*, but it can be caught from water if this is contaminated by the urine of infected mammals. *Leptospira* can survive for days to months in urine-contaminated soil and fresh water. Entry is via cuts or abrasions on the skin, mucous membranes or conjunctiva.

Illness follows a biphasic pattern. Initially there is an acute phase, which lasts a few days and symptoms include fever, myalgia and headache. Very rarely you can get a rapidly progressive pulmonary haemorrhage within this acute phase (though more common in the immune phase).

Most people with leptospirosis will only have the acute phase of illness. A minority of patients then go on to experience an immune phase which either overlaps the acute phase or more commonly is separated by a period of improvement. This phase lasts up to 30 days and is due to antibodies towards the *Leptospira* (no organisms are remaining in the blood). There can be multi-organ involvement, but most commonly you see systemic symptoms such as fever and headache from an aseptic meningitis.

Weil's disease or icteric leptospirosis occurs in around 5–10% of cases and is a rapidly progressive multisystem illness with mortality rates of 5–15%. These patients have very high bilirubin, with only mildly elevated transaminases, and liver failure is rare. They have renal failure with markedly elevated creatinine. Hyponatraemia and raised potassium are common. These patients may also suffer with pulmonary haemorrhage (in less than 5%) and myocarditis.

In hepatitis A infection, there is often a more marked elevation in transaminases and ALP. There is also a shorter progression from the initial symptoms of fever, nausea and vomiting and abdominal pain to significant jaundice within a few days to a week, without improvement between.

SBA Paper 2: Answers

References

1. www.uptodate.com. Leptospirosis: epidemiology, microbiology, clinical manifestations, and diagnosis. UpToDate, 2025. Available at: https://www.uptodate.com/contents/leptospirosis-epidemiology-microbiology-clinical-manifestations-and-diagnosis.

● Answer 10: a

This patient is suffering from tumour lysis syndrome (TLS). This is an oncological emergency that is a result of massive tumour cell breakdown, most commonly after the initiation of chemotherapy. This cell breakdown results in significant increases in serum potassium, phosphate (tumour cells can contain up to four times the amount of phosphate as normal cells) and nucleic acids — resulting in hyperuricaemia. The uric acid precipitates in the renal tubules resulting in AKI from a combination of renal vasoconstriction, decreased renal flow, oxidation and inflammation. Hyperphosphataemia with calcium phosphate deposition in the renal tubules can also cause AKI. The presence of high phosphate and high uric acid potentiates the risk of AKI, as uric acid precipitates more readily in the presence of calcium phosphate and vice versa. Laboratory findings may include hyperkalaemia, hyperphosphataemia, hypocalcaemia (caused by precipitation of calcium phosphate), hyperuricaemia, increased lactate dehydrogenase (LDH), and AKI. The Cairo-Bishop criteria defines TLS from laboratory parameters (Table 2.8).

Table 2.8. The Cairo-Bishop criteria.

Laboratory variable	Value	Change from baseline
Uric acid	≥476µmol/L (8mg/dL)	25% increase
K^+	≥6.0mmol/L	25% increase
PO_4^{3-}	≥2.1mmol/L (6.5mg/dL) for children or ≥1.45mmol/L (4.5mg/dL) for adults	25% increase
Ca^{2+}	≤1.75mmol/L (7mg/dL)	25% decrease

Two or more laboratory changes within 3 days before or 7 days after cytotoxic therapy defines laboratory TLS.

Clinical TLS according to the Cairo-Bishop criteria, is defined as laboratory TLS plus at least one clinical complication. TLS is graded 0 to 5 depending on the presence of three complications: creatinine rise (AKI), cardiac arrhythmia and seizure presence.

TLS is almost exclusively secondary to haematological malignancy but can occasionally occur with other bulky or rapid turnover cancers such as inflammatory breast cancer.

Patients undergoing chemotherapy, if assessed as being higher risk for TLS, will undergo prophylaxis. This consists of IV hydration (aiming for a urine output of around 2ml/kg, patients may need furosemide to assist), and a hypouricaemic agent such as allopurinol, rasburicase or febuxostat. Excess purine catabolism results in the production of hypoxanthine and xanthine, which are metabolised to uric acid via the enzymatic action of xanthine oxidase (XO). Urate oxidase metabolises uric acid to the more water-soluble allantoin.

Allopurinol is a hypoxanthine analogue that competitively inhibits XO, blocking metabolism of hypoxanthine and xanthine to uric acid. This decreases formation of uric acid and reduces the incidence of obstructive nephropathy. It is inexpensive and given orally. Allopurinol does not reduce the pre-existing uric acid amount, hence does not bring down serum uric acid levels if already high. Allopurinol can cause AKI by increasing levels of other purine precursors. It also has the potential to interact with many other drugs (including cyclophosphamide, methotrexate, ampicillin, amoxicillin, carbamazepine and diuretics). A dose reduction is required if the patient is on mercaptopurine or azathioprine. Hypersensitivity reactions can also rarely occur, e.g. vasculitis and Stevens-Johnson syndrome.

Rasburicase is a recombinant urate oxidase and lowers serum uric acid by promoting degradation to allantoin; it is useful if serum uric acid levels are already high. Rasburicase is superior to allopurinol in children and has been shown to reduce the need for renal replacement therapy (RRT). Rasburicase is not without side effects. It can cause haemolysis, haemoglobinuria and methaemoglobinaemia and interferes with serum uric acid measurement. It can also be a trigger for anaphylaxis. Rasburicase should not be given in those with glucose-6-phosphate deficiency (G6PD) (predisposition in patients of African American, Mediterranean or south east Asian descent). At-risk patients should undergo genetic testing and/or assays to determine their G6PD status.

Febuxostat is a selective XO inhibitor; it is not a purine base analogue like allopurinol. It inhibits both reduced and oxidised forms of XO and has minimal effects on other enzymes involved in purine and pyrimidine metabolism. Febuxostat is associated with fewer drug interactions and reactions, compared to allopurinol but is more expensive.

Aside from hydration and uric acid management, the focus of TLS treatment is the management of electrolyte complications. Hyperphosphataemia can be managed by limiting intake of phosphate, and the use of phosphate binders. In cases of severe TLS, the early use of RRT is indicated. Hypocalcaemia should only be treated if the patient is symptomatic, as calcium may bind to serum phosphate and precipitate in the renal tubules exacerbating renal injury. Patients with tetany or cardiac arrhythmias associated with the low calcium should be given a slow IV infusion of calcium gluconate or calcium chloride (see local guidelines).

Hyperkalaemia should be managed depending on severity as per UK Kidney Association (UKKA) guidelines or equivalent (see Figure 2.4). The definitive management of severe refractory hyperkalaemia is the institution of RRT. Insulin dextrose would temporarily bring down the potassium but is not the definitive management in this case.

References
1. www.uptodate.com. Tumor lysis syndrome: prevention and treatment. UpToDate, 2025. Available at: https://www.uptodate.com/contents/tumor-lysis-syndrome-prevention-and-treatment.
2. www.uptodate.com. Tumor lysis syndrome: pathogenesis, clinical manifestations, definition, etiology and risk factors. UpToDate, 2024. Available at: https://www.uptodate.com/contents/tumor-lysis-syndrome-pathogenesis-clinical-manifestations-definition-etiology-and-risk-factors.

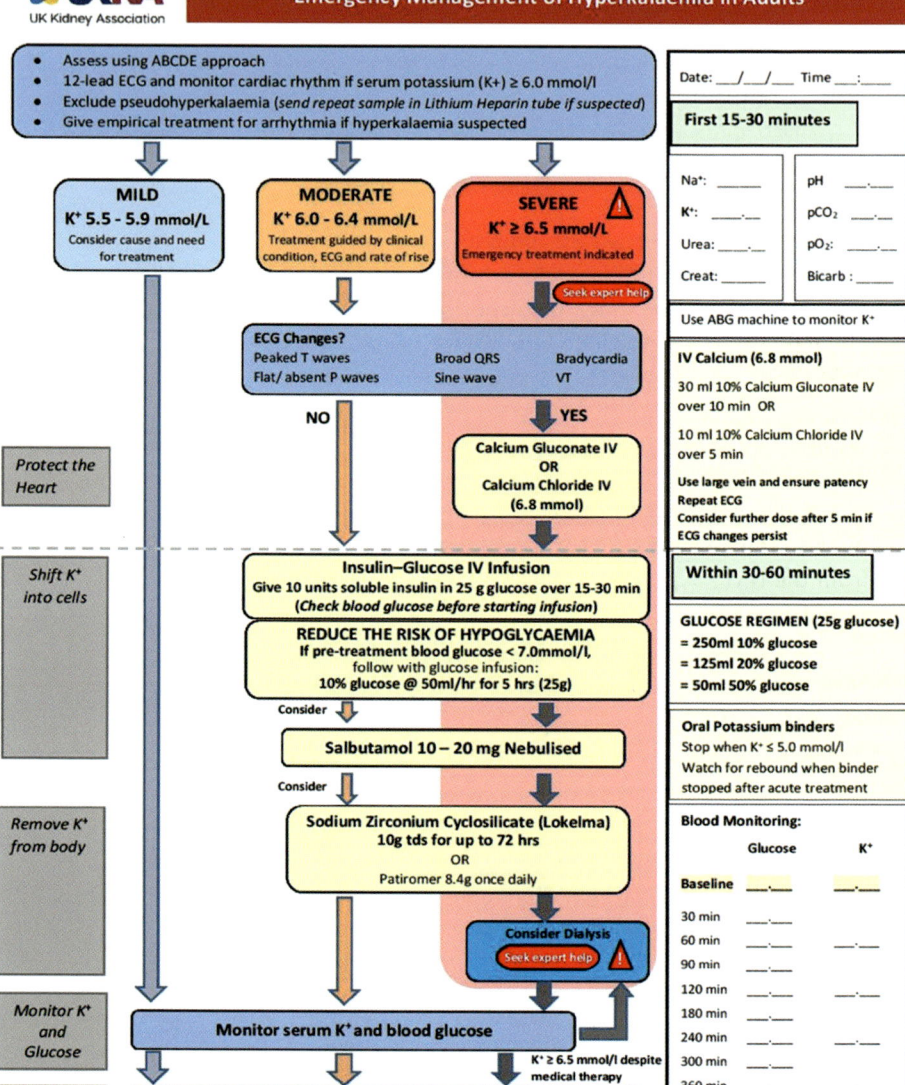

Figure 2.4. Emergency management of hyperkalaemia in adults. *Reproduced with permission from the UK Kidney Association.*

3. Coiffier B, Altman A, Pui CH, *et al.* Guidelines for the management of paediatric and adult tumor lysis syndrome: an evidence-based review. *J Clin Oncol* 2008; 26: 2767.
4. UK Kidney Association (UKKA). Clinical practice guidelines: treatment of acute hyperkalaemia in adults, 2023. Available at: https://ukkidney.org/sites/renal.org/files/FINAL%20VERSION%20-%20UKKA%20CLINICAL%20PRACTICE%20GUIDELINE%20-%20MANAGEMENT%20OF%20HYPERKALAEMIA%20IN%20ADULTS%20-%2020191223_0.pdf.

Answer 11: d

The patient history and microbiological findings strongly suggest a diagnosis of botulism.

Botulism is caused by a neurotoxin exotoxin produced by the Gram-positive anaerobic bacillus *Clostridium botulinum*. The toxins target presynaptic receptors of the neuromuscular junction (NMJ) in peripheral cholinergic nerves. This leads to an irreversible failure of acetylcholine (ACh) release from the NMJ, autonomic ganglia and parasympathetic nerve terminals and results in weakness and paralysis.

Several different botulism syndromes — including infant, food-borne, wound, iatrogenic, adult intestinal, inhaled — are recognised although only wound botulism requires antibiotic therapy.

Antibiotics effective against *Clostridium botulinum* include penicillin G, benzylpenicillin and metronidazole. Antibiotics that may potentiate NMJ blockade by any mechanism (i.e. aminoglycosides [e.g. gentamicin], tetracyclines, clindamycin and polymyxins) should be avoided.

Therefore, the most appropriate choice of antimicrobial therapy in this case is benzylpenicillin as this will cover wound infection without potentially worsening the botulism-induced NMJ blockade and weakness.

References

1. www.uptodate.com. Botulism. UpToDate, 2025. Available at: https://www.uptodate.com/contents/botulism.

Answer 12: a

This patient has low serum osmolality (240mOsmol/kg) suggesting either hypotonic hyponatraemia or 'true' hyponatraemia as the underlying cause. Other causes of hyponatraemia include pseudohyponatraemia (serum osmolality of 285–295mOsmol/kg) and translocational hyperosmolar hyponatraemia (serum >295mOsmol/kg) and require a different management approach.

In determining a cause for this patient's hypotonic hyponatraemia, measurement of urinary osmolality and urinary sodium, combined with the patient's history and assessment of their fluid volume status

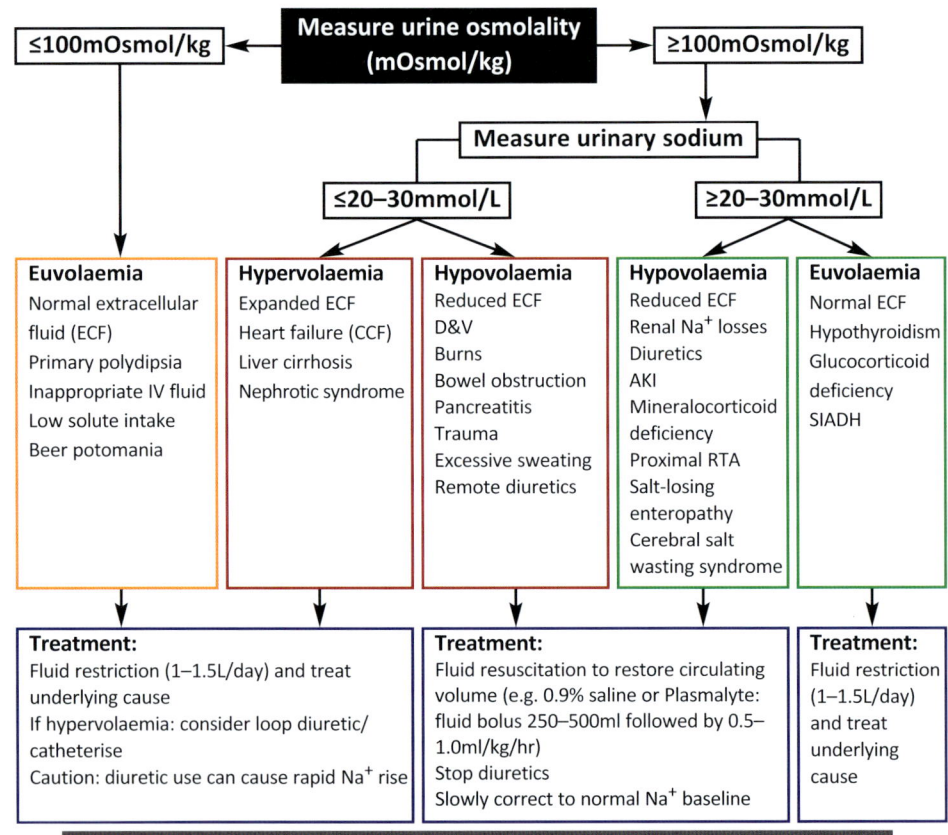

Figure 2.5. Algorithm for the management of hyponatraemia.

(hypo/euvolaemic/hyper), helps to narrow the differential diagnosis and ensure correct management. The algorithm on the facing page detailing causes of hyponatraemia and their management (modified from Spasovski 2014 ESICM) may be used as a guide (Figure 2.5).

This patient has a raised urine osmolality of 300mOsmol/kg and urinary sodium of 37mmol/L. Clinically she is euvolaemic and has had no recent diuretic use. She has normal cortisol and thyroid function. She has no renal impairment with normal K^+ and she is not Addisonian.

SIADH is a diagnosis of exclusion based on the presence of a number of essential and supplemental criteria and exclusion of other possible causes. The criteria are listed below. Ideally for the diagnosis to be made, all essential criteria should be present; if not, the presence of supplemental criteria increases the likelihood of SIADH.

Essential criteria:

- Effective serum osmolality <275mOsmol/kg.
- Urine osmolality >100mOsmol/kg at some level of decreased effective osmolality.
- Clinical euvolaemia.
- Urine sodium concentration >30mmol/L with normal dietary salt and water intake.
- Absence of adrenal, thyroid, pituitary or renal insufficiency.
- No recent use of diuretic agents.

Supplemental criteria:

- Serum uric acid <0.24mmol/L (<4mg/dL).
- Serum urea <3.6mmol/L (<21.6mg/dL).
- Urine specific gravity >1.003.
- Failure to correct hyponatraemia after 0.9% saline infusion.
- Fractional sodium excretion (FENa) >0.5%.
- Fractional urea excretion >55%.
- Fractional uric acid (urate) excretion >12%.
- Correction of hyponatraemia through fluid restriction.

There are many causes of SIADH including malignancies (e.g. lung carcinoma), pulmonary disorders (e.g. pneumonia, tuberculosis, asthma, ICU ventilation), neurological disorders (e.g. CNS infection, encephalitis, meningitis, SAH, GBS, MS, head trauma), drugs (e.g. antidepressants, SSRIs, tricyclics, MAOIs, venlafaxine, anticonvulsants, antipsychotics, anticancer drugs, opiates, MDMAs, nicotine, NSAIDs) and other causes (e.g. pain, stress, nausea, exercise, idiopathic, transient and hereditary).

Citalopram is a recognised cause of SIADH and the most likely cause in this case. This drug should be held and 1–1.5L/day oral fluid restriction started with close serum Na$^+$ monitoring.

References

1. Yaqoob M, McCafferty K. Water balance, fluids and electrolytes. In: Kumar P, Clark M, Eds. *Kumar and Clark's clinical medicine*, 10th ed. London: Elsevier; 2020: chapter 9: pp. 168–202.
2. www.uptodate.com. Pathophysiology and etiology of the syndrome of inappropriate antidiuretic hormone secretion (SIADH). UpToDate, 2024. Available at: https://www.uptodate.com/contents/pathophysiology-and-etiology-of-the-syndrome-of-inappropriate-antidiuretic-hormone-secretion-siadh.
3. Spasovski G, Vanholder R, Allolio B, *et al.* Clinical practice guideline on diagnosis and treatment of hyponatraemia. *Nephrol Dial Transplant* 2014; 29 Suppl 2: i1–39.
4. Differences between SIADH and cerebral salt wasting. Adapted from Sherlock M, O'Sullivan E, Agha A, *et al.* The incidence and pathophysiology of hyponatraemia after subarachnoid haemorrhage. *Clin Endocrinol* 2006; 64: 250–4.
5. Lobaz S, Merza Z, Sylvester J, Wyatt S. Management of hyponatraemia in adults guideline. Barnsley Hospital NHS Foundation Trust, 2024.

● Answer 13: e

The combination of a history of renal stones and the significant normal anion gap (hyperchloraemic) metabolic acidosis raises the possibility of renal tubular acidosis (RTA). For further information on the four different types of RTA please see page 79, Paper 1, Q45.

In this case, RTA type 1 (also known as distal RTA) is seen. This causes a failure of H$^+$ excretion in the distal tubules, which in turn means that the urine cannot be maximally acidified and the daily acid load cannot be excreted. It is characterised by a low serum bicarbonate (under 15mmol/L) with hypokalaemia that corrects with bicarbonate administration. It is also associated with hypocitraturia which results in increased calcium in the urine and a risk of nephrolithiasis.

 Answer 14: e

The Brain Trauma Foundation (BTF) has useful guidelines for monitoring and the management of patients with traumatic brain injury (TBI). This is a case of refractory high ICP despite first- and second-stage management. Decompressive craniectomy is a potential treatment option; however, evidence from clinical trials suggest that whilst a decrease in mortality may be seen with decompression, survivors have a significantly worse Glasgow Outcome Scale Extended score than survivors who were not decompressed. Therefore, decompression is not currently recommended by the BTF. In practice, decompression may still take pace in this setting should a multi-disciplinary team (MDT) discussion (including the patient's family) conclude that this is an acceptable treatment avenue in spite of the potential limitations.

Therapeutic hypothermia is not recommended (the Eurotherm 3235 trial showed worse neurological outcomes and increased mortality) and there is no evidence for burst suppression or higher cerebral perfusion pressure (CPP) targets in this scenario. Lowering of $PaCO_2$ targets should not be used routinely but may be used as a short-term measure to help reduce ICP until a definitive treatment is agreed upon; BTF guidance states that 'hyperventilation is recommended as a temporizing measure for the reduction of elevated intracranial pressure (ICP). Hyperventilation should be avoided during the first 24 hours after injury when cerebral blood flow (CBF) is often critically reduced'.

References
1. Brain Trauma Foundation. Guidelines for the management of severe TBI, 4th ed, 2016. Available at: https://braintrauma.org/coma/guidelines/guidelines-for-the-management-of-severe-tbi-4th-ed.
2. Sahuquillo J, Dennis JA. Decompressive craniectomy for the treatment of high intracranial pressure in closed traumatic brain injury. *Cochrane Database Syst Rev* 2019; 12(12): CD003983.

Answer 15: d

In organ donation after cardiac death (DCD), warm ischaemic time (WIT) is the period of time between the systolic BP dropping below 50 (or O_2 sats below 70%) and the onset of cold perfusion. Cold perfusion occurs in theatre with rapid instillation of intra-arterial cold fluid and ice slush around the organs to be retrieved. Different organs have different WIT time limits for suitability for donation as below:

- Pancreas and liver — 30 minutes.
- Lungs — 60 minutes from onset of WIT to reinflation.
- Kidneys — dependent on transplant surgeon but normally up to 3 hours.

In the case in question, the WIT was longer than 30 minutes but less than 60 minutes meaning that the pancreas and liver could not be used for donation, but the kidneys and lungs were still suitable.

References

1. Organ donation after circulatory death report of a consensus meeting. Available at: https://nhsbtdbe.blob.core.windows.net/umbraco-assets-corp/1360/donation-after-circulatory-death-dcd_consensus_2010.pdf.
2. British Transplantation Society. UK guidelines on transplantation from deceased donors after circulatory death — British Transplantation Society, 2023. Available at: https://bts.org.uk/transplantation-from-deceased-donors-after-circulatory-death/#retrieval.

 ## Answer 16: c

The Kidney Disease: Improving Global Outcomes (KDIGO) group recommends the use of anticoagulation in RRT if there is no patient coagulation impairment or clotting risk (1B). Heparin is preferred for intermittent RRT (IHD) and citrate for continuous RRT (CRRT) (2A) and in those in whom systemic anticoagulation would result in a significant bleeding risk.

KDIGO guidance recommends citrate anticoagulation for CRRT unless there is a contraindication to citrate such as severely impaired liver function or shock with muscle hypoperfusion, as these are associated with a risk of citrate accumulation. In this case, although there is a potential bleeding risk and a degree of liver impairment, it would still be appropriate to use citrate and monitor closely for signs of citrate accumulation and toxicity, namely:

- Hypocalcaemia (decreased iCa^{2+}, normal total Ca^{2+} as bound to citrate) symptoms, e.g. long QT, tetany, hypotension, systemic hypocoagulability, etc.
- Metabolic alkalosis (due to HCO_3^- formation).
- High anion gap metabolic acidosis (HAGMA) due to citrate accumulation.
- Electrolyte disturbance including hypernatraemia (due to sodium load from sodium citrate), hypomagnesaemia and hypokalaemia.

For more information on complications of citrate use, please see page 42, Paper 1, Q11.

References

1. Kidney Disease: Improving Global Outcomes (KDIGO). KDIGO clinical practice guideline for acute kidney injury, 2012 Available at: https://kdigo.org/wp-content/uploads/2016/10/KDIGO-2012-AKI-Guideline-English.pdf.
2. Nickson C. Citrate toxicity. Life in the fast lane (LITFL); 2024. Available at: https://litfl.com/citrate-toxicity/.

Answer 17: d

This history fits with a diagnosis of Guillain-Barré syndrome (GBS). Several subtypes of GBS are recognised:

- AIDP: acute inflammatory demyelinating polyneuropathy — affects any myelinated nerve and is the most common variant representing 85–90% of cases.
- AMAN: acute motor axonal neuropathy — only motor nerves are affected.
- AMSAN: acute motor and sensory axonal neuropathy — AMAN with some sensory nerve involvement.
- Miller Fisher syndrome: ophthalmoplegia, ataxia and areflexia with or without limb weakness.
- Bickerstaff brainstem encephalitis: encephalopathy with ophthalmoplegia and ataxia.

- Pharyngeal-cervical-brachial weakness: weakness of oropharyngeal, neck and shoulder muscles associated with swallowing dysfunction.

GBS is 1.5x more common in males than females, with an increased incidence with increasing age; the aetiology of GBS is discussed further on page 340, Paper 4, Q30.

Around half of patients experience distal paraesthesia and numbness as the first feature, followed by progressive ascending flaccid weakness that may become flaccid paralysis. The cranial nerves are involved in around 45% of cases with the facial and glossopharyngeal nerves typically affected. Weakness peaks at 2–4 weeks after onset and plateaus at 4 weeks. Autonomic nervous system involvement occurs in 20% of GBS patients and sensory nerve involvement is usually mild.

Approximately 30 to 35% of patients require ventilatory support and 25% of patients will need invasive ventilation due to respiratory weakness. Vital capacity (VC) monitoring is an important bedside test to assess respiratory weakness and GBS progression; once VC is <20ml/kg, patients should be admitted to critical care and intubation considered if VC falls to <15ml/kg.

Nerve conduction studies can help to distinguish GBS from other causes of weakness, and the findings vary slightly depending on the type of GBS. Cerebral spinal fluid analysis will reveal a normal WCC with elevated protein levels in 80% of patients at 2 weeks post-symptom onset. Blood should be tested for anti-ganglioside antibodies such as anti-GM1 and anti-GQ1B.

Supportive management is vital, with assessment of impending respiratory failure and the need for ventilatory support as described above. Autonomic dysfunction management includes vasopressors for hypotension and labetalol or nicardipine for hypertension and tachycardia. Specific management includes either plasma exchange or IVIg. These interventions are equally effective as lone therapies but confer no benefit in combination. Treatment should ideally begin within 2 weeks of symptom onset. Steroids are not indicated in GBS as they have been shown to increase mortality.

References

1. www.uptodate.com. Guillain-Barré syndrome in adults: pathogenesis, clinical features, and diagnosis. UpToDate, 2025. Available at: https://www.uptodate.com/contents/guillain-barre-syndrome-in-adults-pathogenesis-clinical-features-and-diagnosis.
2. Nguyen TP, Taylor RS. Guillain-Barré syndrome. StatPearls [Internet]; 2023. Available at: https://www.ncbi.nlm.nih.gov/books/NBK532254/.

Answer 18: a

Healthy cerebrospinal fluid (CSF) is clear in appearance unless there has been a traumatic lumbar puncture (LP) tap. In viral meningitis the appearance of CSF tends to remain clear. In bacterial meningitis, CSF is often turbid due to the high white cell count (WCC) and presence of bacteria. In fungal and TB meningitis, it appears cloudy or turbid and contains fibrin webs.

The protein content of the CSF in health is 0.18–0.45g/L. In viral infection, CSF protein can be elevated but does not normally go above 1g/L. In fungal and TB infection, the protein level is low/normal (0.1–0.5g/L) and in bacterial CSF infection, it is elevated above >1g/L.

Glucose in the CSF in health is around 0.6 of the serum glucose, so assuming normoglycaemia, it is usually in the range of 2.5–3.5mmol/L. CNS viral infections do not tend to have any effect on the glucose except in rare infections like mumps. In fungal, TB and bacterial infections, the CSF glucose is low and often below 2.5mmol/L.

The WCC of normal CSF is under 3 WBCs/mm^3 (unless there has been a traumatic tap, in which case the WCC may be closer to serum levels). Viral infection causes an elevation in WCC but not typically above 1000 WBCs/mm^3 with the cell type predominantly monocytes with some elevation in polymorphonuclear leukocytes (PMNs or neutrophils). Bacterial infection causes a very high CSF WCC (>1000 WBCs/mm^3) with over 90% PMN. Fungal and TB infections cause a moderately elevated WCC with predominantly monocytes.

If you have had a traumatic tap, you can estimate the CSF WCC by subtracting 1 WCC for every 500–1500 RBCs or use an online calculator (see second reference).

Therefore, the answer in this case is a — viral — as the case history is consistent with herpes simplex virus (HSV) encephalitis. In CNS infection, any delay in performing LP should not delay antimicrobials.

Table 2.9 summarises the diagnostic features of CSF analysis in meningoencephalitis.

Table 2.9. Diagnostic features of CSF analysis in meningoencephalitis.

	Normal	Bacterial	Viral	Fungal	TB	SAH
Opening pressure (cmH$_2$O)	7–20	>30 high	Normal/high	Very high	High	Increased (60% of cases)
Appearance	Clear, colourless	Turbid	Clear	Fibrin web	Turbid	Bloody/xantho-chromic or clear
Protein (g/L)	<0.45	High >1	Normal	High 0–2.5	High 1–5	Increased
Glucose (mmol/L)	⅔ serum glucose	Decreased	Normal	Low/normal	Very low	Normal
Glucose CSF: serum ratio	50–66%	Low <50%	Normal	Low/normal	Very low <30%	Normal
Gram stain	Negative	Positive	Negative	Negative	Negative or weakly positive	Negative
Cell count (per mm^3)	<5	>1000	<500	100–500	50–1500	May see an increase with bleeding
WCC differential	Lymphocytes	Predominantly neutrophils	Lymphocytes	Lymphocytes	Lymphocytes	May see an increase with bleeding

References

1. www.uptodate.com. Cerebrospinal fluid: physiology, composition, and findings in disease states. UpToDate, 2024. Available at: https://www.uptodate.com/contents/cerebrospinal-fluid-physiology-composition-and-findings-in-disease-states.
2. https://reference.medscape.com/calculator/642/csf-wbc-correction-in-blood-contaminated-csf#.

● Answer 19: b

Patients with motor neurone disease (MND) who are intubated for respiratory complications have a high likelihood of requiring long-term ventilatory support either via a tracheostomy or non-invasive ventilation (NIV). A study of 24 MND patients admitted to the ICU for ventilatory support from 2002 found that 16 of 17 patients surviving to ICU discharge required long-term ventilatory support.

Therefore, proceeding to intubation and ventilation in this case (particularly in the context of the history provided by his wife) should only be considered following detailed MDT and patient discussion. If there is an option that can allow time for further discussions whilst keeping the patient safe such as NIV, this may be the preferred course of action in the first instance.

References

1. Bradley MD, Orrell R, Clarke J, *et al.* Outcome of ventilatory support for acute respiratory failure in motor neurone disease. *J Neurol, Neurosurg Psychiatry* 2002; 72: 752–6.

● Answer 20: d

Phaeochromocytomas are rare tumours which secrete the catecholamines adrenaline, noradrenaline or dopamine. They may secrete catecholamines intermittently or continuously so patients can present with 'hyperadrenergic spells' typically consisting of palpitations, sweating, headache and tremors. However, the classic triad of headache, sweating and tachycardia is relatively unusual and most patients present with sustained or paroxysmal hypertension (85–95%) and headache (90%). Some patients are asymptomatic, with the tumour being picked up incidentally as part of other investigations.

Most tumours are sporadic with around 40% being familial, such as multiple endocrine neoplasia type 2 (MEN2) which is implied within the stem of the question for this patient. MEN2a includes the risk of medullary carcinoma of the thyroid, phaeochromocytoma and parathyroid adenoma/hyperplasia.

The mainstay of treatment is surgical resection of the tumour. However, before surgery can be performed medical management is essential to prevent an intra-operative phaeochromocytoma crisis (hypertension/ hypotension, temperature >40°C, altered GCS, organ dysfunction). Hypotension may also occur perioperatively as patients are often significantly hypovolaemic due to chronic vasoconstriction. Medical therapy is initially with α-blockade with doxazosin for 7–10 days pre-op to allow reversal of hypovolaemia. It is important to start α-blockade prior to β-blockade to avoid unopposed α-action causing worsening vasoconstriction and a hypertensive crisis.

In this case it is possible that cocaine use may have contributed to the hypertension, but it is unlikely to be the sole cause and benzodiazepines are unlikely to result in an improvement in symptoms. β-blockers such as labetalol (even though it provides some α-blockade) and atenolol can result in some unopposed α-action and therefore are contraindicated for initial treatment. This patient's BP needs controlling and results may take some time to come back, so waiting for results prior to treatment is not advisable. Therefore, starting doxazosin for hypertension management is the best answer here.

References

1. www.uptodate.com. Clinical presentation and diagnosis of pheochromocytoma. UpToDate, 2024. Available at: https://www.uptodate.com/contents/clinical-presentation-and-diagnosis-of-pheochromocytoma.
2. www.uptodate.com. Treatment of pheochromocytoma in adults. UpToDate, 2025. Available at: https://www.uptodate.com/contents/treatment-of-pheochromocytoma-in-adults.

Answer 21: e

The National Institute for Health and Care Excellence (NICE) in the UK has produced guidance on antibiotic therapy for community-acquired pneumonia (CAP). Treatment is based on the severity of pneumonia (using the CURB-65

SBA Paper 2: Answers

score) and the allergy status. For patients with moderate severity (CURB-65 score 2), the recommendations are: amoxicillin plus clarithromycin or erythromycin (in pregnancy) if atypical pathogens are suspected, or doxycycline or clarithromycin if the patient has a penicillin allergy.

For high-severity pneumonia (CURB-65 score 3 to 5), the recommendations are: Augmentin® IV/PO plus clarithromycin or erythromycin (in pregnancy), or levofloxacin PO/IV if the patient has a penicillin allergy.

The British Thoracic Society (BTS) guidelines on treatment of CAP have significant overlap with NICE recommendations but differ in suggesting use of a cephalosporin in place of Augmentin® in severe CAP. This patient has anaphylaxis to penicillin so avoidance of cephalosporins is advised due to the risk of immune cross-reactivity to the shared beta-lactam ring. Although this risk is low, it is well recognised and higher with first-generation cephalosporins such as cefuroxime, thought to be due to the similar R1 side chain in the structure, but negligible increased risk with second- or third-generation cephalosporins. Therefore, based on current guidance and recommendations, the correct answer here is levofloxacin.

References

1. National Institute for Health and Care Excellence (NICE), guideline NG138. Pneumonia (community-acquired): antimicrobial prescribing, 2019. Available at: https://www.nice.org.uk/guidance/ng138/resources/pneumonia-communityacquired-antimicrobial-prescribing-pdf-66141726069445.
2. British Thoracic Society. CAP Guideline Working Group 2014/15. Summary of recommendation: BTS guideline for the management of CAP in adults, 2009, annotated 2015. Available at: https://www.brit-thoracic.org.uk/document-library/guidelines/pneumonia-adults/annotated-bts-cap-guideline-summary-of-recommendations/.
3. Chaudhry SB, Veve MP, Wagner JL. Cephalosporins: a focus on side chains and β-lactam cross-reactivity. *Pharmacy* 2019; 7(3): 103.

● Answer 22: d

Left ventricular assist devices (LVADs) are inserted either percutaneously (in the case of the shorter-term devices) or surgically. There have been several generations of devices used to treat acute left ventricular failure, but they all take blood from the apex of the left ventricle and pump this blood into the aorta (most commonly the ascending aorta but sometimes the descending). Similar devices exist to support the right heart. Earlier generation devices were pulsatile, but now devices employ continuous flow using either axial flow or centrifugal pumps, meaning the patient will not have a peripheral pulse.

These devices are used for the management of heart failure in a small subset of patients when medical management has failed. The broad indications include:

- Bridge to transplantation.
- Bridge to decision-making relating to transplantation (e.g. in patients who are not eligible for transplantation but with optimisation may become so).
- Destination therapy (if the patient is not eligible for transplantation, devices can last up to 10 years).
- Bridge to recovery of ventricular function.

All the following characteristics must be present for consideration for LVAD insertion: class IV NYHA for 60–90 days, on maximal medical therapy, dependence on ionotropic agents, LVEF <25%, SBP ≤90mmHg or cardiac index ≤2L/min/m² with evidence of declining right ventricle or renal function.

Contraindications to LVAD insertion include right ventricular dysfunction (unless secondary to left heart failure as impaired function will lead to inadequate filling of the left side), neurological compromise as a result of heart failure (as improving cardiac output is unlikely to improve neurology), terminal comorbidity, active bleeding or coagulopathy that will prevent anticoagulation, and lack of social support to enable the patient to care for the LVAD.

Complications of LVAD insertion include bleeding (both immediately following insertion and later due to long-term anticoagulation), right heart failure, infection (most commonly *Staphylococcus aureus*), stroke (haemorrhagic or ischaemic) and arrhythmias.

SBA Paper 2: Answers

References
1. Vaidya Y, Riaz S, Dhamoon AS. Left ventricular assist devices (LVAD). StatPearls [Internet]; 2020. Available at: https://www.ncbi.nlm.nih.gov/books/NBK499841/.

● Answer 23: a

Refeeding syndrome is a condition characterised by metabolic and electrolyte disarray when feeding is reinstituted following a period of decreased or absent calorific intake. It can be triggered by any form of nutrition including an infusion of 5% dextrose. It is important to recognise patients at risk of refeeding as the condition is preventable with appropriate rates of calorie reintroduction.

Typically, chronic malnutrition leads to protein and fat catabolism for energy with total body phosphate depletion despite normal serum phosphate. Upon refeeding and the introduction of carbohydrate, glycaemia leads to an increase in insulin secretion and a decreased secretion of glucagon. Insulin stimulates an anabolic state stimulating glycogen, fat and protein synthesis. This process requires phosphate, magnesium and cofactors such as thiamine. Insulin stimulates the absorption of potassium into the cells through the Na^+/K^+-ATPase symporter, which also transports glucose, magnesium and phosphate into cells. Water then follows by osmosis. Intracellular uptake of glucose and depleted electrolytes results in a decrease of serum levels of phosphate, potassium and magnesium causing potentially fatal clinical complications including arrhythmias, heart failure, vomiting, weakness, myalgia, rhabdomyolysis, respiratory failure, ataxia, delirium, coma, central pontine myelinolysis, seizures, Wernicke encephalopathy (confusion, ataxia, ophthalmoplegia), liver failure, ATN, haemolysis, anaemia, thrombocytopaenia and reduced 2,3-DPG production.

Refeeding investigations should assess for: hypophosphataemia (<0.6mmol/L), hypokalaemia (<3.5mmol/L), hypomagnesaemia (<0.7mmol/L), hyperglycaemia, thiamine deficiency and trace element deficiencies. Management of refeeding syndrome involves controlled fluid, electrolyte, vitamin, and nutritional replacement with close monitoring. Electrolyte complications should be managed accordingly.

The American Society for Parenteral and Enteral Nutrition (ASPEN) has consensus criteria for identifying patients at risk of refeeding syndrome for adult patients:

- Moderate risk factors — two factors are required for a risk of refeeding: BMI 16–18.5kg/m², 5% weight loss in a month, none/negligible intake for 5–6 days (or reduced intake over certain time periods), minimally low levels of electrolytes (K^+, PO_4^{3-}, Mg^{2+}) or normal levels with recent replacement, evidence of mild/moderate loss of subcutaneous fat and muscle mass, higher-risk conditions, e.g. chronic alcohol use (moderate disease).
- Significant risk factors — one of the following is required for a risk of refeeding: BMI <16kg/m², weight loss (7.5% in 3 months of >10% in 6 months), none/negligible oral intake for >7 days (or reduced intake over certain time periods), moderate/significantly low levels of electrolytes, or minimally low with recent significant replacement, evidence of severe loss of subcutaneous fat and muscle mass, higher-risk conditions (severe disease).

References

1. Whereat J, Lobaz S, Hill S. Phosphate management in intensive care. ATOTW 507, 2023. Available at: https://resources.wfsahq.org/wp-content/uploads/ATOWatow-507-00_ED-1.pdf.
2. da Silva JSV, Seres DS, Sabino K, et al. ASPEN consensus recommendations for refeeding syndrome. *Nutr Clin Pract* 2020; 35(2): 178–95.

Answer 24: b

The Child-Pugh-Turcotte score is a specific score that provides mortality prediction in patients with liver cirrhosis. It was originally used to triage patients for liver transplantation but has been replaced by the MELD or UKELD (in the UK) score for this purpose as the elements of the Child-Pugh-Turcotte score were felt to be subjective and did not account for renal function.

The Child-Pugh-Turcotte score provides both a 1-year all-cause mortality as well as specific post-abdominal surgery mortality and provides three levels of severity (A to C).

SBA Paper 2: Answers

There are five elements that each can score up to 3 depending on the severity of the abnormality:

- Encephalopathy (West Haven grading system).
- Ascites.
- Bilirubin.
- Albumin.
- Prothrombin time prolongation or INR.

Once stratified the score can be used to predict mortality from liver disease as follows:

- Child-Pugh A (5–6 points): 0% 1-year all-cause mortality, 10% post-abdominal surgery mortality.
- Child-Pugh B (7–9 points): 20% 1-year all-cause mortality, 30% post-abdominal surgery mortality.
- Child-Pugh C (10–15 points): 55% 1-year all-cause mortality, 70–80% post-abdominal surgery mortality.

References
1. Tsoris A, Marlar CA. Use of the Child Pugh score in liver disease. StatPearls [Internet]; 2020. Available at: https://www.ncbi.nlm.nih.gov/books/NBK542308/.

Answer 25: c

	Actual outcome +ve	Actual outcome -ve
Test outcome +ve	A	B
Test outcome -ve	C	D

Figure 2.6. 2 x 2 table: actual outcome and test outcome.

There are several calculations related to data that allow us to describe how useful a given test is based on results from a trial.

The sensitivity of a test is the ability of a test to correctly identify a positive outcome (where it exists) and can be used to rule out a condition if the sensitivity of a test is high. If the sensitivity is high, you can be confident that if the test is negative the patient does not have the condition being tested for. It is calculated by the number of correctly identified positives (A) divided by the total number of actual positive outcomes (A+C). Therefore, sensitivity = A/(A+C) and is expressed as a percentage.

The specificity is the ability of the test to correctly identify a negative outcome (where it exists) and can be used to demonstrate the presence of a condition. If a test is highly specific, then a positive result confirms the presence of the disease in question with a high level of certainty. This is calculated as the number correctly identified as negative by the test (D) divided by the total number that are negative (B+D). Therefore, specificity = D/(B+D) and is expressed as a percentage.

The above can be recalled using the 'SPin and SNout' rule — SPecificity rules things IN, SeNsitivity rules things OUT.

The positive predictive value (PPV) is the certainty that a positive test result correctly predicts the presence of the disease as a percentage. It is calculated by A/(A+B).

The negative predictive value (NPV) is the certainty that a negative test result correctly predicts the absence of a disease as a percentage. It is calculated by D/(C+D).

The odds ratio (OR) is a ratio of the odds of a certain outcome in the treatment group compared to the odds of the same outcome in the control group.

References
1. Spoors C, Kiff K. Statistics for the anaesthetist. In: Spoors C, Kiff K, Eds. *Training in anaesthesia: the essential curriculum*. Oxford: Oxford University Press; 2010: chapter 24: pp. 561–72.

SBA Paper 2: Answers

 Answer 26: c

The gold standard for fluid resuscitation after burns is the Parkland formula. Fluid resuscitation is advised if over 15% total body surface area (TBSA) is affected (superficial burns not included). The use of technology to assist burns calculations is now common and the 'Mersey Burns' app is commonly used in the UK.

The Parkland formula is 2–4ml/kg/%TBSA burn of warm, isotonic balanced crystalloid over the 24 hours after the burn injury with half delivered in the first 8 hours and the remaining half over the next 16 hours. The fluid calculation is started from the time of the burn not the time of arrival in hospital.

Some centres advocate starting with Parkland and then using urine output to guide fluid therapy, aiming for a minimum of 0.5ml/kg/hr but ideally closer to 1ml/kg/hr, especially if there is a suspicion of significant muscle injury and risk of rhabdomyolysis (e.g. electrical burns).

A retrospective review performed in Germany found that a restrictive fluid regime was associated with higher survival compared to either the Parkland formula or a more liberal fluid regime than the Parkland. Pragmatically, the Parkland formula should be used to guide initial fluid resuscitation with regular patient review and adjustment of fluid therapy according to any changes in the clinical picture.

References
1. McGovern C, Puxty K, Paton L. Major burns: part 2. Anaesthesia, intensive care and pain management. *BJA Educ* 2022; 22(4): 138–45.
2. Daniels M, Fuchs PC, Lefering R, *et al*. Is the Parkland formula still the best method for determining the fluid resuscitation volume in adults for the first 24 hours after injury? — a retrospective analysis of burn patients in Germany. *Burns* 2021; 47(4): 914–21.

 Answer 27: b

Thromboelastography is a point-of-care test that provides measurement of the viscoelastic properties of whole blood from initial clot formation through to fibrinolysis. The most used systems in the UK are TEG® and ROTEM®, and these produce similar-shaped curves (albeit with different names for the measurements)(Figure 2.7).

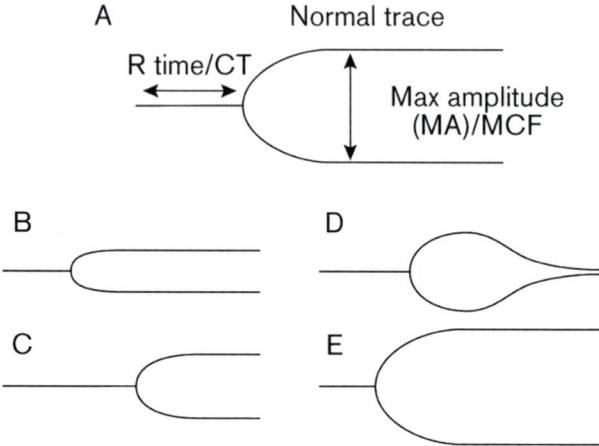

Figure 2.7. Normal and pathological thromboelastography curves.

Trace A represents a 'normal' curve. The thromboelastography is run with several different factors to allow assessment of different parts of the clotting cascade, e.g. tissue factor for EXTEM measurements (extrinsic pathway). The normal ranges for each element will be slightly different as they are measuring different components of the clotting cascade.

The initial straight line up until the curve starts is the time to the initiation of a clot, known as the R time (TEG®) or clotting time/CT (in ROTEM®). The normal range for this with whole blood is 4–8 minutes. This element represents the function of soluble clotting factors in the plasma.

The period of time taken for the amplitude of the clot to go from 2mm to 20mm is known as the K time or CFT (clot formation time). The normal range is 1 to 4 minutes. This represents the clot kinetics and prolongation of this element is usually due to fibrinogen deficiency.

The angle of the curve from the start of clot formation (2mm) up until the horizontal midline is called the alpha angle in TEG®. This represents the speed of fibrin build-up and is dependent on fibrinogen. The normal range is 47 to 74°.

The widest part of the trace is called the maximum amplitude (MA) or maximum clot firmness (MCF). The normal range is 55 to 73mm. This is a factor of the number and function of platelets as well as the fibrinogen concentration.

The CL30 or LY30 is the percentage decrease in clot size compared to MA/MCF at 30 minutes. A greater than 8% reduction implies there is an issue with excessive fibrinolysis. The normal range is 0–8%.

Abnormalities seen include the following:

- Trace B: is seen with thrombocytopaenia. There is a normal R time and alpha angle, some increase in K time and a reduced MA (so the clot is smaller). Both TEG® and ROTEM® are insensitive to aspirin and clopidogrel, so are not an appropriate way of analysing platelet function in the presence of antiplatelet drugs. There are point-of-care platelet assessment devices, but they are not commonplace. Management is with platelet transfusion if the patient is actively bleeding.
- Trace C: is seen with a deficiency or inactivity of soluble clotting factors. Causes include coagulopathy from blood loss, use of anticoagulants and haemophilia. There will be a prolongation of the R and K time, with a decreased MA; if combined with platelet deficiency then the MA will be smaller still. In the presence of fibrinogen deficiency there will be a reduction in the alpha angle. Management of this is with the use of FFP or prothrombin factor concentrate with cryoprecipitate if there is a reduced alpha angle.
- Trace D: occurs with excessive fibrinolysis. A normal R, K and MA are seen but a CL30 of >8% and a CL60 (lysis at 60 minutes) of >15% are seen. This can be caused by thrombolytic therapies. Tranexamic acid can help manage this if occurring in the context of bleeding (it is the intended effect of thrombolysis medication so does not need treating in this scenario).
- Trace E: is representative of hypercoagulability and has a shortened R time and increased MA.

Although the tracings of TEG® and ROTEM® are similar and recognition of the patterns can be done with either, they are not interchangeable, and treatment given should be based on the measurements taken.

References
1. Srivastava A, Kelleher A. Point-of-care coagulation testing. *Contin Educ Anaesth Crit Care Pain* 2013; 13(1): 12–6.
2. Nickson C, Lala H. Thromboelastogram (TEG). Life in the fast lane (LITFL); 2023. Available at: https://litfl.com/thromboelastogram-teg/.

● Answer 28: a

Environmental sustainability is a vital consideration in modern medicine with the triple bottom line (people, planet and profit) being discussed in many different areas of healthcare and procurement. Intensive care is one of the most carbon-intensive areas of the hospital and knowledge of the constituents of the carbon footprint and consideration of ways to reduce it are intrinsic to our work.

A life cycle analysis showed that the daily carbon footprint of an ICU bed in the UK is around 100kg CO_2e (CO_2 equivalent). The largest constituent of this is energy (60%), followed by consumables (12%), food (8%), with the remaining elements analysed (staff travel, equipment, gases and waste) contributing around 5% each. Interestingly, the carbon footprint of an ICU bed in the USA is significantly higher at around 160kg CO_2e per bed per day. The highest contributor in the USA is consumables, followed by energy use. The life cycle analysis for the UK was performed in 2015 and given the efforts to decarbonise the energy within the UK, the figure is hopefully now lower than this.

References
1. Prasad PA, Joshi D, Lighter J, *et al*. Environmental footprint of regular and intensive inpatient care in a large US hospital. *Int J Life Cycle Assess* 2021; 27(1): 38–49.

● Answer 29: b

The National Tracheostomy Safety Project has produced guidelines for the management of emergencies in patients with tracheostomies *in situ*, and also in patients who are post-laryngectomy and therefore obligate neck breathers (see Figures 2.8 and 2.9).

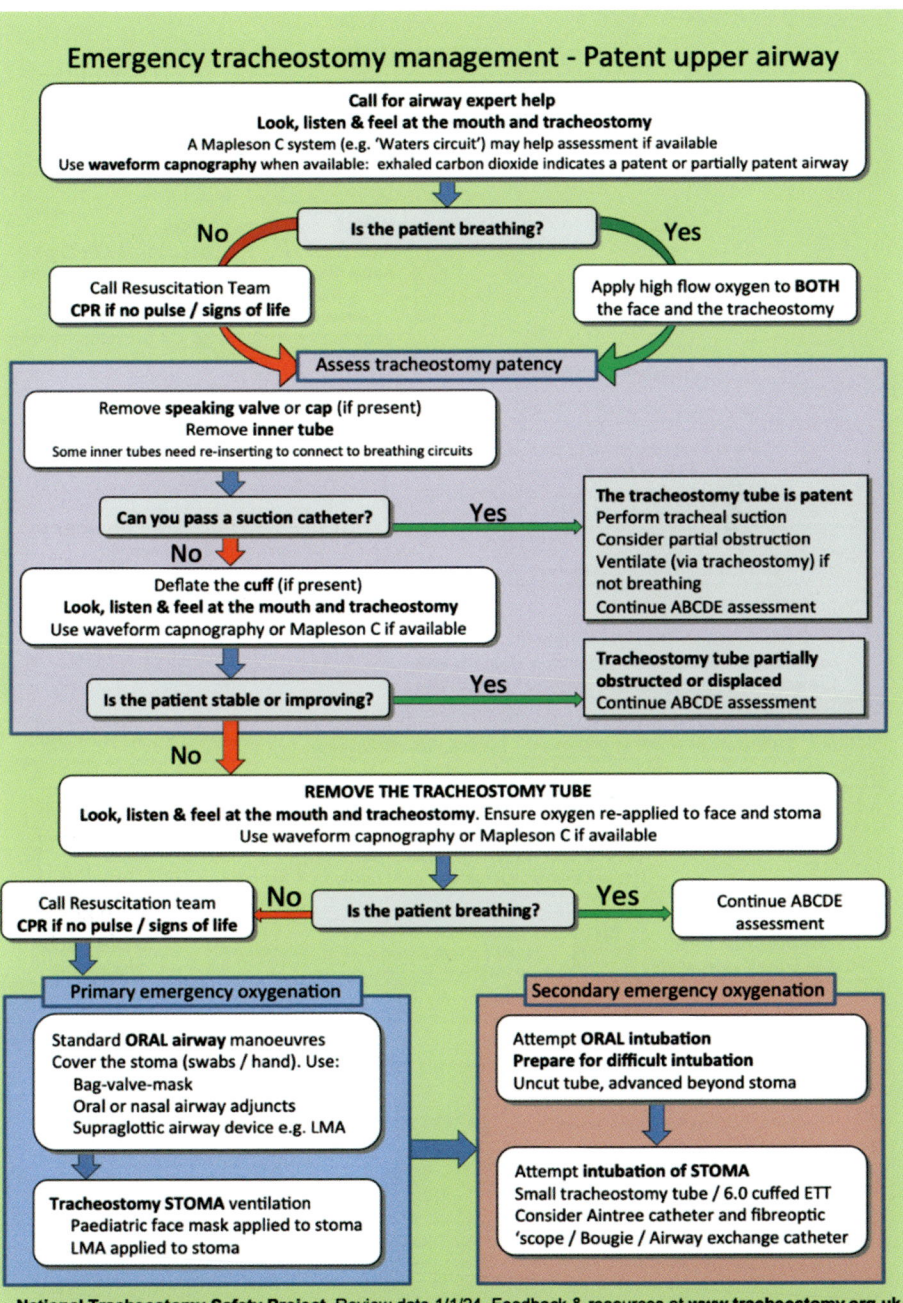

Figure 2.8. Emergency tracheostomy management. *Reproduced with permission from the National Tracheostomy Safety Project.*

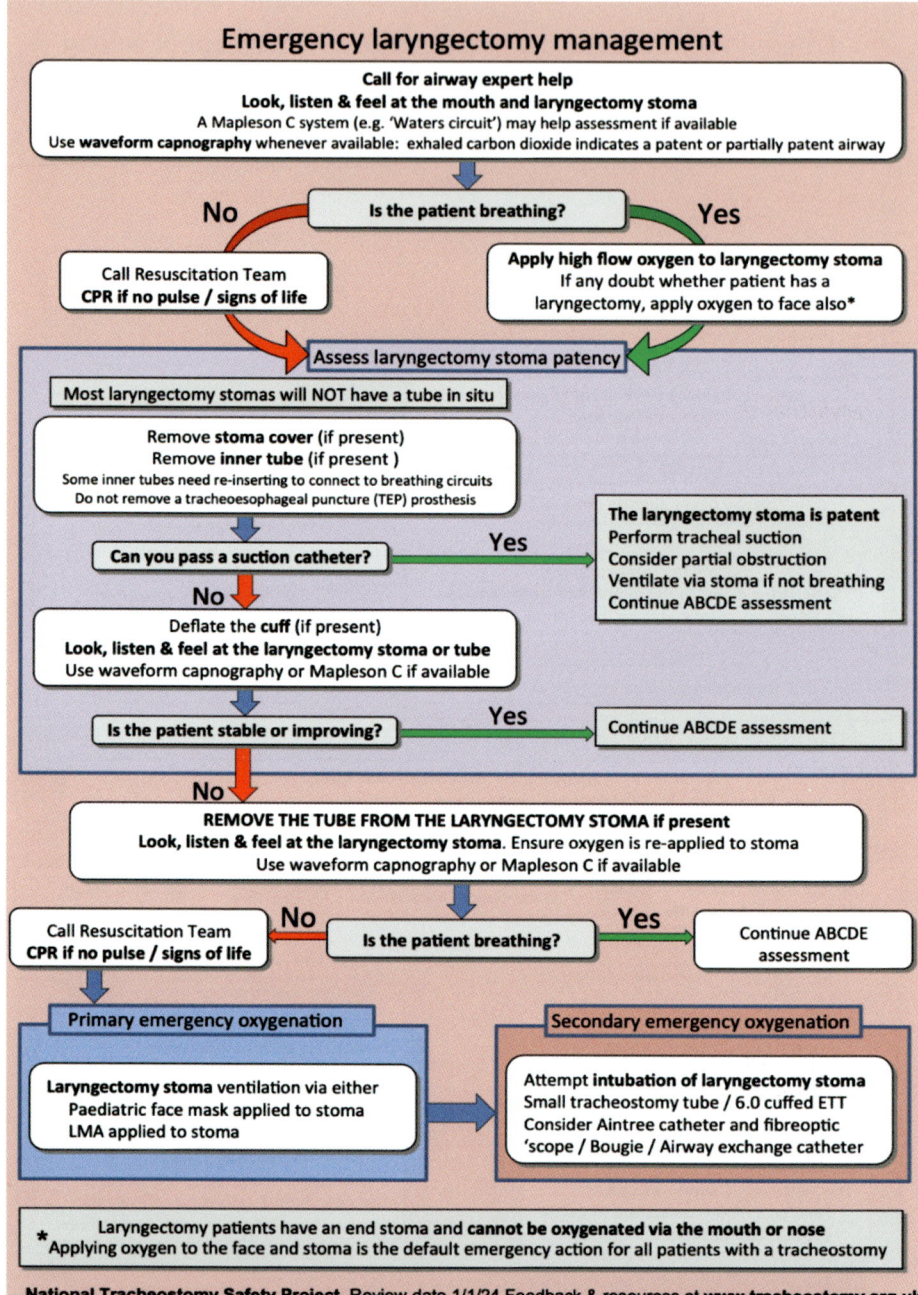

Figure 2.9. Emergency laryngectomy management. *Reproduced with permission from the National Tracheostomy Safety Project.*

SBA Paper 2: Answers

Following the algorithm, the next step in the management of this patient is to pass a suction catheter down the tracheostomy to assess patency.

References
1. National Tracheostomy Safety Project. Emergency tracheostomy management — patent upper airway. Available at: https://tracheostomy.org.uk/NTSP-Algorithms-and-Bedheads#.

Answer 30: e

Myasthenia gravis (MG) is an autoimmune disease in which autoantibodies to Ach receptors and other postsynaptic membrane molecules (such as muscle-specific kinase MuSK) result in reduced neuromuscular junction transmission. This manifests clinically as fatigable weakness of skeletal muscle. The condition can be well managed with acetylcholinesterase inhibitors and immunosuppression, but patients may present to the ICU prior to diagnosis, with a known diagnosis in a myasthenic crisis or as part of a perioperative admission.

Several commonly used drugs in critical care may result in worsening weakness of patients with MG. The most significant of these are neuromuscular blocking drugs (NMBDs). MG patients are relatively resistant to suxamethonium and are very sensitive to non-depolarising NMBDs. The autoantibodies attach to Ach receptors, making less available and thus higher doses of suxamethonium are required for a clinical effect. Conversely, much smaller doses of non-depolarising NMBDs are needed as these act via competitive antagonism of Ach at the neuromuscular junction.

In a patient already treated with acetylcholinesterase inhibitors this can complicate matters further, so if NMBDs cannot be avoided, the use of incremental small doses using a nerve stimulator to guide effect is advised. Rocuronium is the preferred NMBD as use of its reversal agent sugammadex avoids the need for additional acetylcholinesterase inhibitors.

There are a number of other drugs that are known to exacerbate patients with MG and these should be avoided, or used with caution if there is no alternative and include:

- Antibiotics such as aminoglycosides, fluoroquinolones, macrolides.
- Other drugs including beta-blockers, botulinum toxin, desferrioxamine, iodinated X-ray contrast, magnesium, procainamide and statins.

Sedative agents such as propofol and short-acting opioids like alfentanil are safe for use in patients with MG.

References
1. Daum P, Smelt J, Ibrahim IR. Perioperative management of myasthenia gravis. *BJA Educ* 2021; 21(11): 414–9.

Answer 31: c

There are several subgroups of antiviral agents, classified according to which stage in the viral life cycle they target.

Nucleoside analogues work after being taken up into a cell infected with a virus and only affect those cells infected with the virus. Examples include aciclovir, famciclovir (active against HSV/VZV), ganciclovir, cidofovir and valganciclovir (active against CMV).

Other antivirals with activity against herpes viruses include foscarnet, which is a pyrophosphate analogue that reversibly inhibits viral DNA polymerase. It is also active against CMV.

The neuraminidase inhibitors are active against the influenza viruses (A and B). They work by preventing release of new virus from infected cells. Examples include oseltamivir (oral preparation) and zanamivir (the IV equivalent). There is resistance seen to oseltamivir in H1N1 and H5N1 infections although this is not an issue seen with zanamivir. Treatment with these drugs reduces the time to functional recovery and can decrease the risk of hospitalisation from lower respiratory tract infections.

The human herpes viruses (HHVs) are large double-stranded DNA viruses. Infection tends to be lifelong with periods of latency occurring after the primary infection. They are classified based on which cell type is involved with the latent infections and are also numbered 1 to 8.

Alpha herpes viruses are rapidly growing and latent in neurones. They include herpes simplex 1 (HHV1) which affects orofacial areas, HHV2 which affects genital areas and varicella zoster (HHV3) which causes chickenpox and shingles. Beta HHVs are slow-growing and become latent in secretory glands and the kidneys. This group includes *Cytomegalovirus* (HHV5), exanthem subitem or 'sixth disease' (HHV6) and HHV7 which is carried widely but has no associated clinical syndrome. Gamma HHV are latent in lymphoid tissues and include the Epstein-Barr virus (HHV4) — which has an association with the development of lymphoma — and HHV8 which causes an infectious mononucleosis and Kaposi sarcoma in the immunocompromised.

References
1. Virgincar N, Ajayi A. Miscellaneous drugs: antiviral agents. In: Waldmann C, Rhodes A, Soni N, Handy J, Eds. *Oxford desk reference: critical care*, 2nd ed. Oxford: Oxford University Press; 2019: chapter 16: pp. 252–3.
2. Gillespie S, Bamford K. Herpes viruses. In: Gillespie S, Bamford K, Eds. *Medical microbiology and infection at a glance*, 2nd ed. Oxford: Blackwell Publishing; 2003; chapters 27 and 28: pp. 60–3.

● Answer 32: d

The ECG changes encountered with hypokalaemia have poor correlation with plasma levels; however, changes are more often seen when the K^+ is below 3mmol/L and include: T wave flattening or inversion, ST segment depression and the development of U waves. Conduction deficits are also common with a lengthening of the PR interval and the appearance of QT prolongation due to the presence of U waves. The true QRS width remains unchanged in hypokalaemia.

A shortened QT interval is seen in hypercalcaemia and the other abnormalities listed are associated with hyperkalaemia.

For the initial management of hypokalaemia and to help identify a cause, the following hypokalaemia algorithms may be useful (see Figures 2.10, 2.11, 2.12 and 2.13).

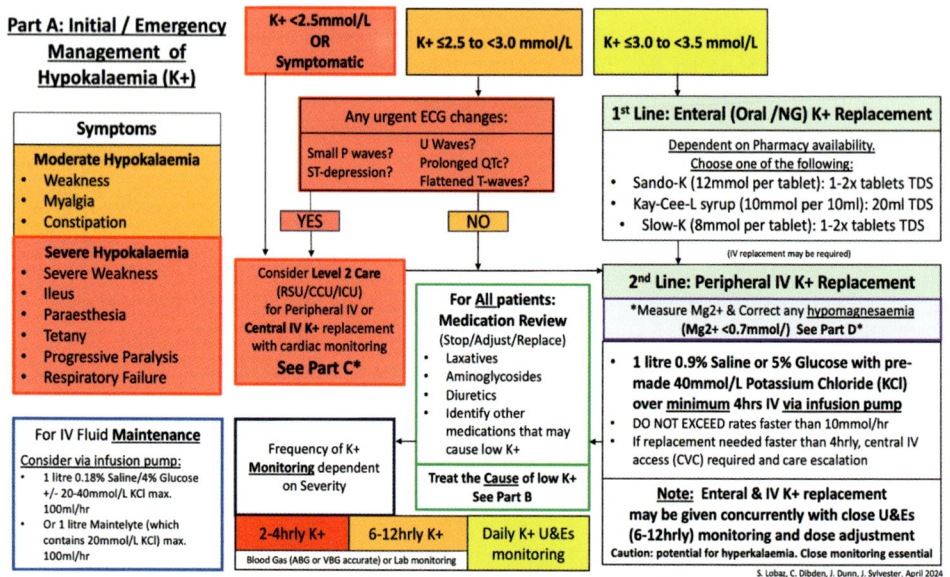

Figure 2.10. Management and investigation of hypokalaemia: emergency management. *Reproduced with permission from Lobaz S, Dibden C, Dunn J, et al.*

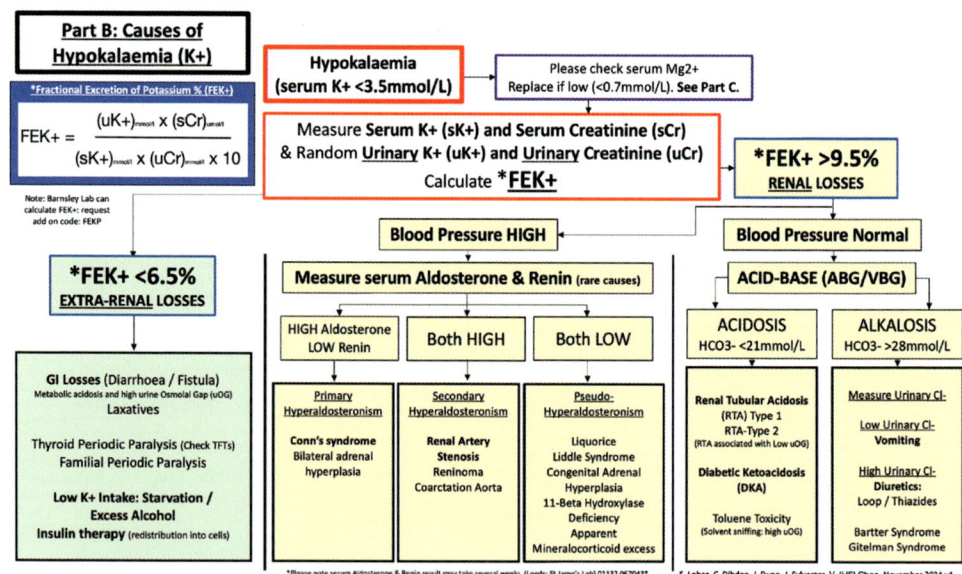

Figure 2.11. Management and investigation of hypokalaemia: causes of hypokalaemia. *Reproduced with permission from Lobaz S, Dibden C, Dunn J, et al.*

Part C: IV replacement of Hypomagnesaemia (Mg2+)

> *If hypokalaemia (K+), correct any
> hypomagnesaemia
> (Mg2+ <0.7mmol/l)

Mg2+ replacement:
- Compatible with 0.9% saline or 5% glucose fluid
- Do not combine Mg2+ and K+ replacement in the same IV fluid bag
- Ampoules: 1g (4mmol) in 2ml amps & 5g (20mmol) in 10ml amps

Peripheral IV Mg2+ Administration:
- Prescribe 8mmol in 100ml compatible fluid IV over 2 hours
- Rates exceeding 8mmol/hr require cardiac monitoring

Level 2 / Critical Care:
Central CVC Mg2+ Administration with cardiac monitoring:
- Dose & Rate dependent on Mg2+ deficit: <0.5mmol/l is severe
- Higher doses can be given if severe via central venous line (CVC)
- Prescribe 20 or 40 mmol in 100ml compatible fluid CVC over 2hours
- Do not exceed maximum rate 36mmol/hr

Figure 2.12. Management and investigation of hypokalaemia: IV replacement of hypomagnesaemia (Mg^{2+}). *Reproduced with permission from Lobaz S, Dibden C, Dunn J, et al.*

Part D: Critical Care Management of Hypokalaemia (K+)

Enteral Replacement:
- Sando-K (12mmol per tablet: 2 tabs Oral / NG TDS) or alternatives:
  - Slow-K (8mmol/each): 1-2 tablets Oral onlyTDS

Measure & Correct any Hypomagnesaemia (Mg2+ <0.7mmol/L). See Part C.

Peripheral IV Replacement:
- Use pre-made crystalloid fluid bags with 20 or 40mmol/L potassium chloride (KCl): 1000ml 0.9% saline or 5% glucose or 0.18% saline/4% Glucose depending on clinical circumstances
  - *Give IV no faster than **10mmol per hour** when given peripherally via infusion pump
  e.g. over 2hrs for 20mmol/L or 4hrs for 40mmol/L*

Central CVC Replacement ONLY
- Potassium Chloride (KCl) 100mmol in 50ml syringe
  0.9% saline (2mmol/ml), rate 0-10ml/hr (0-20mmol/hr)
- 2-4hrly K+ monitoring (via ABG) depending on situation
- Adjust K+ replacement rate accordingly
- Rates >20mmol/hr via CVC increases risk of arrhythmias and should only be exceeded with caution in rare circumstances. Cardiac monitoring required (Max 30mmol/hr or 15ml/hr)

Diuretics – hypokalaemia secondary to diuretics e.g. furosemide:
Consider changing to K+ sparing diuretics (e.g. Amiloride or Spironolactone)

Phosphate Replacement & Concurrent Hypokalaemia (e.g. refeeding syndrome):
Consider: Potassium Acid Phosphate: 13.6% vials
(contains 1mmol/mL K+ for every 1mmol of phosphate)

Moderate Hypophosphataemia (Phosphate = 0.4-0.6mmol/L):
- Peripheral IV: 20mmol in 500mL, or 40mmol in 1L
  of glucose 5% over 24hours (21 to 42mL/hour)
- CVC: 50mmol in 50mL syringe neat over 24 hours (2.1mL/hour)

Severe Hypophosphataemia (Phosphate <0.4mmol/L):
- Peripheral IV: same as above
- CVC: 50mmol in 50mL syringe neat over 12 hours (4.2mL/hour)

S. Lobaz, C. Dibden, J. Dunn, J. Sylvester, V. (HS) Chan. November 2024 v4

Figure 2.13. Management and investigation of hypokalaemia: critical care management. *Reproduced with permission from Lobaz S, Dibden C, Dunn J, et al.*

References

1. Spoors C, Kiff K. Body compartments and fluid balance. In: Spoors C, Kiff K, Eds. *Training in anaesthesia: the essential curriculum*. Oxford: Oxford University Press; 2010: chapter 11: pp. 289–316.
2. Assadi F. Diagnosis of hypokalemia. A problem-solving approach to clinical cases. *Iran J Kidney Dis* 2008; 2(3): 115–22.
3. www.uptodate.com. Clinical manifestations and treatment of hypokalemia in adults. UpToDate, 2024. Available at: https://www.uptodate.cn/contents/clinical-manifestations-and-treatment-of-hypokalemia-in-adults.
4. Lobaz S, Dibden C, Dunn J, *et al*. Management of hypokalaemia in adults guideline, 2025. Barnsley Hospital NHS Foundation Trust.

● Answer 33: b

Thiamine — also known as vitamin B1 — acts as a catalyst in energy generation from amino acids and ketoacids. It also has an important role in propagating nerve impulses and maintaining the myelin sheath. Deficiency of thiamine can be from poor intake or absorption (diets high in processed grains, gastric bypass surgery, malnutrition and chronic alcoholism), increased losses (diarrhoea, diuretic use, renal replacement therapy, vomiting) and increased thiamine requirements (pregnancy, lactation, hyperthyroidism and refeeding syndrome). It takes approximately 4 weeks to deplete thiamine stores.

There are several different clinical syndromes associated with thiamine deficiency as described below. Initially deficiency will present with anorexia, irritability and short-term memory problems.

Wernicke's encephalopathy (WE) is the triad of nystagmus, ophthalmoplegia and ataxia in addition to confusion. It is the most common form of thiamine deficiency in adult and older children. WE symptoms may resolve if detected and treated promptly with thiamine replacement.

Korsakoff syndrome is WE with the addition of memory loss and psychosis. Typically, confabulation is seen in these patients. Korsakoff syndrome shows little to no improvement once thiamine deficiency has been corrected.

Dry beriberi is characterised by symmetrical peripheral neuropathy with motor and sensory involvement and reduced reflexes, typically affecting the lower legs.

SBA Paper 2: Answers

Wet beriberi is heart failure related to impaired energy metabolism coupled with dysautonomia. It results in a high-output congestive heart failure with dilated cardiomyopathy, tachycardia and peripheral oedema. There is also a low-output cardiac failure with lactic acidosis and cyanosis variant called Shoshin beriberi.

Wet and dry beriberi may occur in isolation or patients may display a degree of both. With thiamine replacement, heart failure symptoms often will resolve within days; the peripheral neuropathy may improve or completely resolve.

References

1. Wiley KD, Gupta M. Vitamin B1 thiamine deficiency (beriberi). StatPearls [Internet]; 2019. Available at: https://www.ncbi.nlm.nih.gov/books/NBK537204/.
2. bestpractice.bmj.com. Vitamin B1 deficiency. BMJ Best Practice, 2025. Available at: https://bestpractice.bmj.com/topics/en-gb/633.

● Answer 34: e

The European Resuscitation Council in combination with the European Society of Intensive Care Medicine (ESICM) have produced guidelines for post-resuscitation care which were updated in 2021. This document contains guidance for neuro-prognostication after cardiac arrest which has been adopted into the UK resuscitation guidance for post-resuscitation care.

The guidelines recommend targeted temperature management (TTM) at 32–36°C for the first 24 hours, followed by rewarming with avoidance of hyperthermia (keep temperature under 37.7°C) for the first 72 hours post-ROSC. An assessment of the patient can then be made after 72 hours if this is still required. If the patient is unconscious (without another cause for this) with a motor score of ≤3, then the presence of at least two of the following indicates that a poor outcome is likely:

- No pupillary and corneal reflexes at ≥72 hours.
- Bilaterally absent N20 SSEP wave.
- Highly malignant EEG at >24 hours.
- Neuron-specific enolase (NSE) >60µg/L at 48 hours and or 72 hours (increasing levels with time further supports poor outcome).

- Status myoclonus ≤72 hours.
- Diffuse and extensive anoxic injury on brain CT/MRI.

If only one or none of the above list are present, then the advice is to continue to observe and re-evaluate daily.

References
1. Nolan JP, Sandroni C, Böttiger BW, *et al.* European Resuscitation Council and European Society of Intensive Care Medicine guidelines 2021: post-resuscitation care. *Resuscitation* 2021; 161(161): 220–69.

Answer 35: b

The rationale behind irradiation of blood products (in addition to leukodepletion) is to minimise the risk of transfusion-associated graft-versus-host disease (TA-GvHD). In the UK, blood products are routinely leucodepleted (all cellular components bar granulocytes are removed) to minimise this risk, but leucodepletion alone does not completely eliminate this risk. In patients at high risk for TA-GvHD, blood products need to be irradiated. The most common symptoms of TA-GvHD are rash, fever, elevated LFTs, pancytopenia and diarrhoea.

There is guidance from the British Society for Haematology on the use of irradiated blood products. In an emergency, blood product administration should not be delayed whilst waiting for irradiated units to become available and leucodepleted units should instead be used. Irradiation involves exposure of the products to either X-rays or gamma rays. Exposed red blood cells will have increased rates of potassium leakage and haemolysis, which only becomes relevant if large-volume red cell transfusions are given. There is no effect on irradiated platelets.

Conditions that require irradiated products include: intrauterine blood transfusions, allogeneic haematopoietic stem cell transplantation (from the point of conditioning chemotherapy up until the patient is off immunosuppression, patients free of active chronic GvHD, and over 6 months post-transplant), autologous stem cell transplant (during harvesting and transplant immunosuppression), Hodgkin lymphoma, purine analogue or alemtuzumab treatment and during CAR T-cell therapy and for 3 months afterwards.

SBA Paper 2: Answers

References
1. Foukaneli T, Kerr P, Bolton-Maggs PHB, *et al*. Guidelines on the use of irradiated blood components. *Br J Haematol* 2020; 191(5): 704–24.

● Answer 36: d

Carbon monoxide (CO) is a gas formed by hydrocarbon combustion. It is odourless and non-irritating, so undetected inhalation is common; the most frequent source of poisoning is smoke inhalation (with or without associated fire). Carbon monoxide binds to haemoglobin to form carboxyhaemoglobin (COHb) with around 240 times the affinity of oxygen and causes a conformational change in the haemoglobin that prevents oxygen offloading from the other three sites of the molecule. It also disrupts peripheral oxygen utilisation via binding to myoglobin, cytochromes and nicotinamide adenine dinucleotide phosphate (NADPH) reductase resulting in a hypoxia despite adequate PaO_2 and a lactic acidosis.

Minor symptoms include nausea and vomiting, dizziness and headache. The classic 'cherry red lips' are neither a sensitive nor specific sign and are not universally present. Major symptoms include altered conscious level, confusion, chest pain due to myocardial ischaemia (results in higher mortality), ventricular arrhythmias, pulmonary oedema and seizures. Up to 40% of patients with significant CO exposure can experience a delayed neuropsychiatric syndrome with cognitive deficits, personality changes, movement disorders and focal neurological deficits seen. This usually occurs in patients who lost consciousness during the acute exposure and can last for over a year post-poisoning.

Diagnosis cannot be made with standard pulse oximetry (as COHb has a similar absorption pattern to oxyhaemoglobin) so co-oximetry of a blood gas sample is undertaken. This provides a percentage of COHb present — smokers may have a baseline level of up to 10%; 3% or under is normal for non-smokers.

The mainstay of treatment of CO poisoning is oxygen therapy, typically via a non-rebreathe (NRB) face mask. The half-life of COHb is around 250 minutes breathing room air which is reduced to 90 minutes on a NRB oxygen mask. Oxygen therapy should be continued until symptoms attributable to CO poisoning have resolved.

In isolated CO poisoning, oxygen is the only therapy required. However, consideration should be given to other causes of these symptoms, with appropriate investigations and management. Hyperbaric oxygen therapy is a useful treatment for severe poisoning but requires access to a hyperbaric chamber. This often necessitates transfer to one of the few hyperbaric centres in the UK. Indications for hyperbaric oxygen therapy include:

- COHb >25%.
- >15% if the patient is pregnant.
- >10% with evidence of persistent neurological involvement, severe metabolic acidosis or end-organ ischaemia despite oxygen therapy (and may even be indicated even if CO level has normalised).

Hyperbaric treatment consists of FiO_2 1.0 at 2.5–3 atmospheres of pressure, which reduces the COHb half-life to around 30 minutes, and significantly increases the dissolved oxygen reducing tissue hypoxia.

References
1. www.uptodate.com. Carbon monoxide poisoning. UpToDate, 2024. Available at: https://www.uptodate.com/contents/carbon-monoxide-poisoning.

Answer 37: b

MBRRACE-UK (Mothers and Babies: Reducing Risk through Audits and Confidential Enquiries across the UK) has two surveillance reports: one for perinatal mortality and one for maternal mortality. It reports this data across overlapping 3-year periods (triennia). The latest data include updates up until the end of 2023. It divides deaths into direct, indirect, coincidental and late. Direct deaths are those directly resulting from the pregnancy that would not have occurred if the pregnancy did not occur. The most common cause of direct death is venous thromboembolism (VTE) and that has been the case since the reports began in 1985. In the latest report, suicide is second followed by sepsis. Historically, haemorrhage has been the second or third most common cause.

Indirect deaths are not directly due to the pregnancy, but the pregnancy has exacerbated the problem. The most common indirect death is cardiac disease and has been for the last 10 years. The report covering 2019–2021 showed an equal number of deaths from cardiac disease and COVID-19. During 2020 and 2021, maternal mortality attributable to COVID-19 was more than any other single cause.

Coincidental deaths (0.92%) are those that would have occurred regardless of pregnancy such as homicide and road traffic collisions.

Late deaths (13%) are not specifically defined in the report but are death from 6 weeks postpartum onwards.

The rates of maternal death have been decreasing over time but this is not a linear trend and a large increase from 8.79 to 10.9 deaths per 100,000 was seen in the latest triennia. The other worrying finding was the mortality difference between ethnic groups, with Asian women having twice the mortality of white women, and black women four times the mortality. In addition, patients from the most socioeconomically deprived areas have twice the mortality of those from the least deprived.

References
1. MBRRACE-UK. Lessons learned to inform maternity care from the UK and Ireland Confidential enquiries into maternal deaths and morbidity 2018–2020, 2022. Available at: https://www.npeu.ox.ac.uk/mbrrace-uk/reports.

Answer 38: a
Normal intra-abdominal pressure (IAP) in a critically ill patient is 5–7mmHg. There are many pathologies within critical care that can cause an increase in this pressure. Risk factors can be divided into:

- Reduced abdominal wall compliance (e.g. burns, trauma, prone positioning, surgery).
- Increased intraluminal contents (e.g. ileus, bowel obstruction).
- Increased intra-abdominal contents (e.g. pancreatitis, haemo/pneumoperitoneum, ascites, tumours), capillary leak (e.g. massive transfusion, sepsis with large-volume fluid resuscitation).

Patients with risk factors or in whom there is a suspicion of raised IAP should have their IAP measured and monitored. The standard approach for measurement is via the bladder with a specialist catheter tubing after instillation of up to 25ml of saline with the patient supine.

Intraabdominal hypertension (IAH) is graded by the World Society of Abdominal Compartment Syndrome (WSACS) as follows: grade I 12–15mmHg, grade II 16–20mmHg, grade III 21–25mmHg and grade IV >25mmHg. Abdominal compartment syndrome (ACS) is a sustained IAP of >20mmHg with associated new organ dysfunction (typically renal impairment).

The management of IAH and ACS can be categorised according to the aetiology:

- Improve abdominal wall compliance (increase sedation, analgesia, neuromuscular blockade, optimised patient positioning).
- Reduce intraluminal contents (NG tube on drainage, flatus tube, use of prokinetics).
- Reduce intra-abdominal contents (paracentesis, percutaneous drainage), management of fluid balance (diuretics, RRT, rationalise fluid input).
- Optimise end-organ support — aim for an abdominal perfusion pressure (APP) of 50–60mmHg (APP = MAP – IAP), optimise ventilation, recruitment manoeuvres.

If the patient has primary ACS (ACS related to injury or disease in the abdomen or pelvis requiring surgical or radiological intervention), or the IAP remains >20mmHg with progressive organ dysfunction despite all above management, then consideration of surgical decompression — leaving the patient with a total or partially open abdomen — may be warranted.

References

1. Kirkpatrick AW, Roberts DJ, De Waele J, *et al*. Intra-abdominal hypertension and the abdominal compartment syndrome: updated consensus definitions and clinical practice guidelines from the World Society of the Abdominal Compartment Syndrome. *Intensive Care Med* 2013; 39(7): 1190–206.

2. Popwicz P, Dayal N, Newman RK, Dominique E. Abdominal compartment syndrome. StatPearls [Internet]; 2024. Available at: https://www.ncbi.nlm.nih.gov/books/NBK430932/.

Answer 39: b

Fire is thankfully a rare event in hospital, but knowledge of the processes and risks is important. Guidelines for the Provision of Intensive Care Services (GPICS), UK, version 2.1, has a section on fire preparedness recommendations. To create fire, the presence of the 'fire triad' is required:

- Oxidizer (produces oxygen or combusts material more than air — typically oxygen and nitrous oxide).
- Ignition source (device capable of creating a spark or flame such as electrical sockets, defibrillator, etc.).
- Fuel (substance with potential energy that can be released as heat when in a combustion reaction with an oxidant).

All staff should undergo annual fire safety training that covers evacuation procedures with nominated staff trained on fire extinguisher use. Ventilation of ICUs where there is use of high-flow oxygen should be a minimum of 10 air changes per hour to prevent development of an oxygen-rich environment. There should be laminated fire and evacuation cards for each area of the ICU next to the fire call points.

There must be oxygen shut-off valves, ideally for different sections of the ICU, so that cessation of oxygen supply to a specific area can be achieved without shutting off supply to the entire clinical area. Oxygen cylinders must be stored in bed brackets (cylinder sparks from turning on oxygen have been responsible for fires in the past). The safe order of connecting oxygen to a patient is:

- Connect tubing and mask to the oxygen cylinder.
- Turn on the cylinder and select flow away from the patient's bed (blankets/clothing).
- Place the mask on the patient's face.

There should be evacuation equipment for every bed space that is easily accessible.

Further information is provided in section 6 of the GPICS document.

References

1. Miles LF, Scheinkestel CD, Downey GO. Environmental emergencies in theatre and critical care areas: power failure, fire, and explosion. *Contin Educ Anaesth Crit Care Pain* 2015; 15(2): 78–83.
2. The Faculty of Intensive Care Medicine (FICM) and the Intensive Care Society (ICS). Guideline for the Provision of Intensive Care Services. Version 2.1, 2022. Available at: https://ics.ac.uk/resource/gpics-v2-1.html.
3. Kelly FE, Hardy R, Hall EA, *et al.* Fire on an intensive care unit caused by an oxygen cylinder. *Anaesthesia* 2013; 68: 102–18.

Answer 40: e

The Royal College of Anaesthetists (RCOA) National Audit Project 4 (NAP4) revealed that intubation in the ICU had an increased rate of adverse outcomes due to a combination of the patient population and environmental factors. The Difficult Airway Society (DAS) produced guidelines in collaboration with intensivists and anaesthetists to provide recommendations for practice and an algorithm for use in ICU patients (Figure 2.14).

The scenario in the question falls into the plan B/C section of the DAS guidance, which focuses on 'rescue oxygenation' and preparation for failure. As such the first four answers are all reasonable, including oxygenation via a supraglottic airway. Nasal fibreoptic intubation, however, would not be appropriate.

References

1. Cook T, Woodhall N, Frerk C. NAP4. Major complications of airway management in the United Kingdom. The Royal College of Anaesthetists and the Difficult Airway Society, 2011. Available at: https://www.rcoa.ac.uk/sites/default/files/documents/2023-02/NAP4%20Full%20Report.pdf.
2. Higgs A, McGrath BA, Goddard C, *et al. Guidelines for the management of tracheal intubation in critically ill adults. Br J Anaesth* 2018; 120(2): 323–52.

SBA Paper 2: Answers

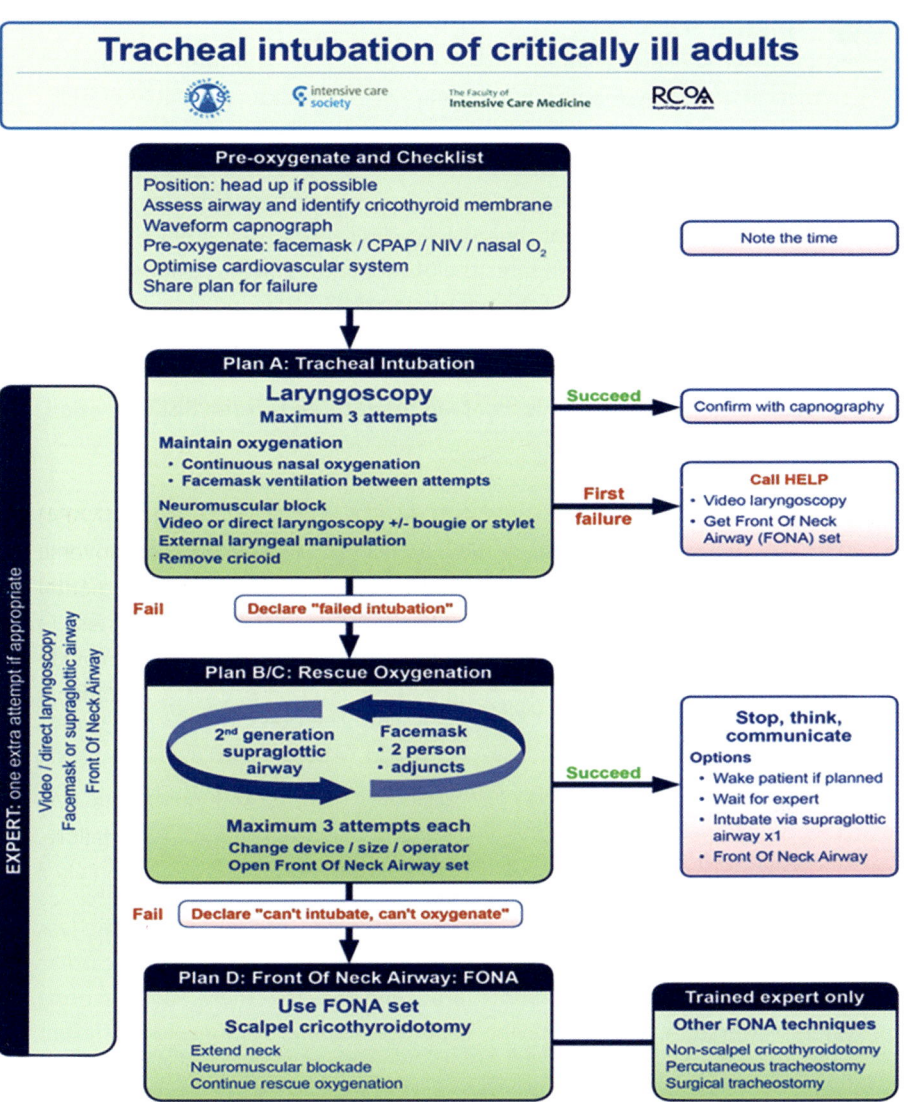

Figure 2.14. Tracheal intubation of critically ill patients. *Reproduced with permission from the Difficult Airway Society.*

● **Answer 41: c**

Physiological scoring systems are used to assess and monitor several healthcare-related outcomes but primarily are used to predict mortality. They are broadly divided into organ dysfunction/failure scoring systems (which use repeated measurements over time to track trends, e.g. SOFA) and severity of illness scoring systems (which are taken at a single point in time such as ICU admission or enrolment to a clinical trial, e.g. APACHE, SAPS). Severity of illness scoring compares the observed data with previous patients with the same score to predict the population rather than individual mortality so should not be used as the basis for clinical decision making.

The utility of scoring systems is assessed using three factors: discrimination, calibration and validity.

Discrimination is measured using the AUROC (area under the receiver operating characteristic curve). Models that perfectly predict mortality will have a score of 1 and those which are no better than guessing 0.5. Strong discrimination is a score of over 0.8 and excellent over 0.9. A score of 0.9 means that 90% of the time it will correctly predict if the patient will survive. The AUROC for commonly used scoring systems are as follows: APACHE II 0.85, APACHE III 0.9, ICNARC 0.86, SAPS II 0.86. The quick SOFA (qSOFA) uses three criteria and can predict the likelihood (AUROC of 0.81) of hospital mortality (not ICU mortality) in a patient with suspected infection.

Calibration of a scoring system is how close the predicted mortalities given are to actual figures within a given population — for example, ICNARC is designed for use with the UK population. A scoring system may become less well calibrated when heterogenous patient groups such as post-cardiac surgery and general ICU patients are cohorted together. Some scoring systems overcome this by having separate scoring systems for different patient populations.

Validity is how accurate a model is compared to reality and is a function of discrimination and calibration. A very narrow scope score such as qSOFA has good discrimination and calibration for patients with suspected infection outside of the ICU but cannot be used to predict the risk of death in ICU patients suspected of infection.

SBA Paper 2: Answers

References

1. Barlow CJ, Pilcher D. Severity scoring and outcome prediction. In: Bersten AD, Handy JM, Eds. *Oh's intensive care manual*, 8th ed. London: Elsevier; 2019: part 1, chapter 3: pp. 19–33.

● Answer 42: c

Management of a patient awaiting organ donation can generate uncertainty as to which interventions would be deemed acceptable from an ethical and moral standpoint. The Donation Actions Framework document produced by NHS Blood and Transplant (in collaboration with a wide number of stakeholder organisations) provides helpful guidance on management of the patient who may or is proceeding to donation after brainstem death (DBD) or after circulatory death (DCD). These guidelines are designed to help clinicians make decisions in the best interest of the patient and are only valid for use in the UK.

The Donation Actions Framework document provides several examples of what is felt (by the consensus group) to be 'very likely, likely, unlikely or very unlikely' to be in the patient's best interests at four different time points: before death and consent, before death after consent, after death before consent and after death and consent.

Actions which are a continuation of ICU treatment that aim to maintain cardiorespiratory stability (ventilation, vasopressor support including insertion of a central line, bedside testing including bloods) are all felt to be 'very likely or likely' to be in the patient's best interests. In addition, it is felt that information gathering and sharing with the organ donation team (including screening blood tests) is also 'likely' to be in the patient's best interests after consent or in a patient known to be willing to donate.

More invasive interventions prior to consent (e.g. biopsy, angiography) or treatments specifically for the management of organs for retrieval prior to consent (e.g. methylprednisolone) are felt to be 'unlikely' to be in the patient's best interests, along with anything that goes against the wishes of the patient and family.

There are a few actions which are felt to be against professional, ethical and legal guidance. These include taking blood and other samples for the purposes of transplantation when it is not known if the patient/family are likely to consent to organ donation, any action that is against the wishes of the patient, any actions that could restore cerebral perfusion and function (before death after consent in DCD donation), any interventions which carry risk of serious harm and starting CPR, ECMO or normothermic regional perfusion.

These guidelines are designed to help clinicians make decisions in the best interest of the patient and in line with what the patient's wishes would have been based on discussions with the family. This guidance is only valid for use in the UK and relates to UK donation practice.

References

1. Donation Actions Framework, 2022. Available at: https://nhsbtdbe.blob.core.windows.net/umbraco-assets-corp/27065/donation-actions-framework-v10-june-2022.pdf.

Answer 43: b

Antiplatelets are commonly encountered drugs in ICU practice used primarily for the prevention of coronary heart disease and stroke. There are several different mechanisms involved in platelet activation and aggregation and the antiplatelet agents available act via actions on these different receptors and mechanisms, including:

- Irreversible acetylation of the cyclooxygenase (COX) enzyme, which is responsible for converting arachidonic acid to prostaglandin H2 (a precursor to a variety of other prostaglandins). Aspirin selectively acts on COX-1 at low doses which provides antiplatelet action.
- Phosphodiesterase inhibition which prevents the breakdown of cyclic adenosine monophosphate (cAMP), which in turn leads to increased intracellular calcium and inhibition of platelet action. Dipyridamole acts via this mechanism.
- Glycoprotein IIb/IIIa (GPIIb/IIIa) receptor antagonism. GPIIb/IIIa receptors sit on the platelet surface and when activated undergo conformational change which results in binding of fibrinogen and von Willebrand Factor (vWF) leading to platelet aggregation. Drugs that bind to this receptor will prevent this and include abciximab (a monoclonal antibody — given as an IV bolus, then infusion, and acts

rapidly but the effects last 48 hours), eptifibatide and tirofiban (IV bolus, then infusion, inhibits platelets within 15 minutes, half-life of a few hours once stopped).
- P2Y12 ADP receptor blockers prevent platelet activation by blocking adenosine diphosphate (ADP) binding and subsequent activation of GPIIb/IIIa receptors. Clopidogrel and prasugrel are irreversible antagonists of the P2Y12 ADP receptor (so last the lifetime of the platelet, 7–10 days), whereas ticagrelor is a reversible antagonist with rapid onset after oral loading and a terminal half-life of 7–9 hours.
- Prostaglandins are naturally occurring compounds that inhibit platelet adhesion by stimulating adenylate cyclase which converts adenosine triphosphate (ATP) to cAMP. This increases intracellular calcium and inhibits the mechanism that leads to degranulation and GP IIb/IIIa expression. Epoprostenol (prostacyclin PGI2) is a prostaglandin that may be used as an anticoagulant in CRRT circuits.

References

1. Ramalingam G, Jones N, Besser M. Platelets for anaesthetists — part 2: pharmacology. *BJA Educ* 2016; 16(4): 140–5.
2. Peck T, Hill S, Williams M. Drugs affecting coagulation. In: Peck T, Hill S, Williams M, Eds. *Pharmacology for anaesthesia and intensive care*, 3rd ed. Cambridge: Cambridge University Press; 2008: chapter 23: pp. 335–46.

Answer 44: e

In patients with subarachnoid haemorrhage (SAH), vasospasm and delayed cerebral ischaemia (DCI) are significant causes of morbidity and mortality for those patients surviving the initial aneurysmal rupture. DCI is multifactorial and vasospasm is one of the causes. Other mechanisms proposed for DCI include failure of cerebral autoregulation, blood brain barrier disruption and micro-thrombosis.

The intervention with the best evidence to prevent cerebral vasospasm is the early use of enteral nimodipine, which has a class 1 recommendation based on a grade A level of evidence. Nimodipine should be continued even if it is causing hypotension (provided this can be managed with standard medical interventions) as temporarily stopping nimodipine significantly increases DCI risk. Interventions with a class 2 recommendation include: maintaining euvolaemia, elevation of BP targets in patients with symptomatic vasospasm, intra-arterial vasodilator therapy in patients with severe vasospasm, and cerebral angioplasty to reverse severe vasospasm. Treatments with no benefit (class 3) are routine use of statins and routine use of IV magnesium. Prophylactic hypervolaemia and hypertension is not recommended and has been shown to cause harm.

References
1. Hoh BL, Ko NU, Amin-Hanjani S, *et al.* 2023 guideline for the management of patients with aneurysmal subarachnoid hemorrhage: a guideline from the American Heart Association/American Stroke Association. *Stroke* 2023; 54(7): e314–70.

Answer 45: c

Clostridioides difficile (formally *Clostridium difficile*) is a Gram-positive anaerobic bacillus that is part of the gut flora in colonised patients or can be acquired through the faecal-oral route, most commonly in healthcare settings. It can cause a colitis that can lead to toxic megacolon and significant illness and death. Antibiotics are the main cause of symptomatic disease as they disrupt the natural gut flora and promote *C. difficile* overgrowth.

Antibiotics that are most frequently associated with *C. difficile* proliferation are fluroquinolones (e.g. ciprofloxacin), clindamycin, broad-spectrum penicillins, cephalosporins (2nd, 3rd and 4th generation as a treatment course although not as a one-off surgical prophylaxis) and carbapenems (e.g. meropenem). Longer courses of other broad-spectrum antibiotics can also cause *C. difficile*. It is recommended that any antibiotic course is targeted and duration limited.

Treatments for *C. difficile* include oral vancomycin (there has been an increase of metronidazole-resistant *C. difficile*, so this is no longer first-line treatment) and oral fidaxomicin. Metronidazole may be added in if initial treatment has not been effective. Probiotics are recommended alongside antibiotic treatment. A faecal transplant can be considered for patients with recurrent episodes of *C. difficile*.

References
1. National Institute for Health and Care Excellence (NICE), guideline NG199. *Clostridioides difficile* infection: antimicrobial prescribing, 2021. Available at: www.nice.org.uk/guidance/ng199.

2. www.uptodate.com. *Clostridioides difficile* infection: prevention and control. UpToDate, 2025. Available at: https://www.uptodate.com/contents/clostridioides-difficile-infection-prevention-and-control.

● Answer 46: d

Acquired long QT syndrome is most commonly caused by medications. Prolongation of the QT interval comes with a risk of the development of polymorphic VT or torsade de pointes (TdP). The proposed mechanism of this is the development of early afterdepolarisations due to the prolongation of repolarisation. The mechanism of QT prolongation is blockage of the IKr current (via potassium channels) which is the major current responsible for ventricular repolarisation. Most of the causative drugs affect repolarisation of different cell types at different rates (e.g. endocardial, myocardial and epicardial cells) and the resulting dyssynchrony of repolarisation is what increases the risk of TdP.

Many medications can cause prolongation of the QT interval but have a variable risk of leading to TdP development. Additional risk factors for TdP include being female, age over 65, history of heart disease and electrolyte abnormalities (low K^+, Mg^{2+} and Ca^{2+}). Drugs with the highest risk of TpD associated with a prolonged QTc (up to 10%) are the class Ia antiarrhythmics (quinidine, procainamide) and class III antiarrhythmics (sotalol, ibutilide). There are also case reports of TpD associated with methadone, tricyclic antidepressants and haloperidol.

Amiodarone and verapamil regularly prolong the QTc but as they uniformly inhibit IKr across the different ventricular myocardial cell types, they have a low incidence of TpD.

References
1. Li M, Ramos LG. Drug-induced QT prolongation and torsades de pointes. *Pharm Ther* 2017; 42(7): 473–7.

● Answer 47: b

The definitions for the diagnosis of pulmonary hypertension (PH) were updated in 2022 in guidelines produced by the European Society of Cardiology and European Respiratory Society.

PH is defined as a mean pulmonary artery pressure (mPAP) of >20mmHg at rest across all causes of PH. In patients with pre-capillary PH, the pulmonary arterial wedge pressure (PAWP) is ≤15mmHg; in those with elements of post-capillary PH (left heart disease) the PAWP is >15mmHg.

Patients will present with symptoms of the underlying cause. PH-specific symptoms include exertional dyspnoea, fatigue, bendopnoea (dyspnoea on bending forwards), palpitations, haemoptysis and peripheral oedema.

PH is classified into five groups based on aetiology:

- Group 1: pulmonary arterial hypertension (PAH). This is rare and mainly idiopathic but can be inherited or secondary to drugs. This would be classified as precapillary.
- Group 2: associated with left heart disease such as heart failure with preserved ejection fraction (HFpEF), heart failure with reduced ejection fraction (HFrEF) or valvular disease. This is the most common cause of PH and would be classified as postcapillary.
- Group 3: PH secondary to lung disease. Mild PH is common with advanced parenchymal and interstitial lung disease; patients with chronic hypoxia of other causes (e.g. living at altitude) would also be classified in this group. This is the second most common cause of PH and is classified as precapillary.
- Group 4: PH due to pulmonary artery obstruction, classically chronic pulmonary embolism (also known as chronic thromboembolic PH or CTEPH). This is a rare cause of PH and would be classified as precapillary.
- Group 5: PH with unclear or multifactorial causes, e.g. haematological disease, systemic and metabolic diseases (sarcoid), complex congenital cardiac disease. PH in this group can be mixed precapillary and postcapillary in addition to isolated precapillary.

References

1. Humbert M Kovacs G, Hoeper MM, *et al.* 2022 ESC/ERS guidelines for the diagnosis and treatment of pulmonary hypertension. *Eur Respir J* 2023; 61(1): 2200879.

SBA Paper 2: Answers

● **Answer 48: c**

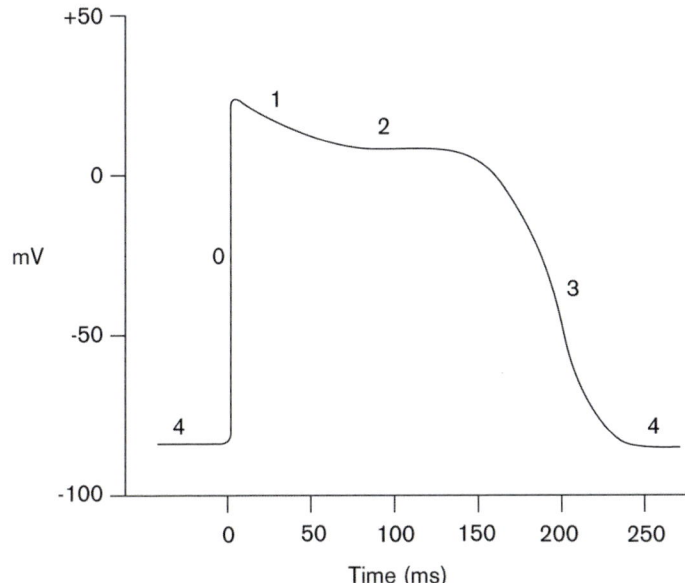

Figure 2.15. Cardiac muscle action potential curve.

The action potential (AP) in cardiac muscle tissue is different to that in the nerve cells. It is longer in duration and has a distinct plateau phase during which depolarisation is maintained resulting in an absolute refractory period of around 200ms. This means that cardiac muscle cannot experience tetany. The cardiac AP can be divided into five phases (Figure 2.15):

- Phase 0: this phase starts when fast sodium channels open and Na^+ rapidly moves into the cell increasing the membrane potential to just above 0 from its resting membrane potential of –95 to –85mv.
- Phase 1: repolarisation begins due to a rapid decrease in Na^+ permeability and opening of K^+ channels with K^+ efflux.
- Phase 2: L-type (slow) Ca^{2+} channels open causing Ca^{2+} to move into the cell, offsetting the K^+ efflux and causing a plateau phase.

- Phase 3: L-type Ca^{2+} channels close and K^+ efflux continues moving the membrane potential back towards baseline.
- Phase 4: Na^+/K^+ pump restores the resting gradient by moving three Na^+ ions out of the cell for every two K^+ ions moved in.

References
1. Power I, Kam P. Physiology of excitable cells. In: Power I, Kam P, Eds. *Principles of physiology for the anaesthetist*, 2nd ed. London: Hodder Arnold; 2008: chapter 1: pp. 1–38.

Answer 49: d

Bacterial toxins cause damage to host cells and are divided into two broad groups: endotoxins and exotoxins.

Endotoxins are lipopolysaccharides (LPSs) which are part of the cell wall of Gram-negative bacteria. LPS endotoxins are released when the cell lyses and cause symptoms associated with Gram-negative sepsis including hypotension, tachycardia, fever, tachypnoea and organ hypoperfusion. They do not stimulate an adaptive immune response and so repeated endotoxin syndromes may occur. They act by causing the release of tumour necrosis factor alpha (TNF-α) and interleukin 1.

Exotoxins are most commonly described as types 1 to 3 as below, but they may also be classified according to the tissue susceptible to the toxin (e.g. neurotoxins, enterotoxins and cytotoxins).

Type 1 exotoxins are polypeptide toxins typically released by Gram-positive cocci and are responsible for toxic shock syndrome (TSS seen with *Staphylococcus aureus* and *Streptococcus pyogenes*). They act as 'superantigens' bypassing the normal mechanism of T4 lymphocyte activation and attach directly to major histocompatibility complex II and T cell receptors. This leads to rapid activation of a large numbers of T4 lymphocytes and a highly exaggerated immune response with a clinical syndrome of severe hypotension, shock and multi-organ dysfunction.

Type 2 exotoxins are polypeptide toxins typically released by Gram-positive anaerobes (such as *Clostridium perfringens* and *C. difficile*). They act by destroying cell membranes and extracellular matrices which damages cells and propagates infection along tissue planes. This damage also stimulates the immune system to release inflammatory cytokines.

Type 3 exotoxins are polypeptide toxins typically released by Gram-positive anaerobes (such as *Clostridium tetani* and *Clostridium botulinum*). These are also known as A-B toxins as they have two parts: A is the active component that causes cell damage, and B is the binding component that dictates which cells are affected. Some bacteria have a secretion system that allows them to inject exotoxins directly into host cells. They produce recognisable specific clinical syndromes such as tetanus and botulism. These exotoxins can be used to make toxoids which do not affect the cells but do stimulate the immune response and are used as vaccines for these diseases.

Clindamycin and linezolid reduce toxin production in Gram-positive bacteria and so are used as adjuvant therapy in infections with exotoxin-producing bacteria.

References
1. Sheehan JR, Sadlier C, O'Brien B. Bacterial endotoxins and exotoxins in intensive care medicine. *BJA Educ* 2022; 22(6): 224–30.

Answer 50: e

A never event is defined as a 'serious incident (SI) that is wholly preventable because guidance or safety recommendations that provide strong systematic protective carriers are available at a national level and should have been implemented'.

The never events relevant to ICU practice are:

- Misplaced naso/orogastric tubes.
- Mis-selection of a strong potassium solution.
- Administration of a medication by the wrong route.
- Overdose of insulin due to abbreviations or incorrect device use.
- Mis-selection of high-strength midazolam during conscious sedation.
- Transfusion of ABO-incompatible blood components.
- Unintentional connection of a patient requiring oxygen to an air flowmeter.

Undetected oesophageal intubation was removed from this list following an update in 2021. The other complications listed in this question are serious incidents, and it may well be required to undertake a serious incident review into these events, but they are not classified as never events.

References

1. NHS Improvement. Never events list 2018 (updated February 2021). Available at: https://www.england.nhs.uk/publication/never-events/.
2. NHS Improvement. Never events policy and framework. Revised January 2018. Available at: https://www.england.nhs.uk/publication/never-events/.

SBA Paper 3: Questions

Question 1

You are asked to review a 57-year-old lady in the emergency department (ED) who has presented with severe chest and back pain. You are working in a hospital that does not have on-site cardiothoracic surgeons. A CT angiogram has shown an aortic dissection that originates at the aortic root and extends down to just beyond the coeliac artery.

On examination:

A: Maintaining own airway.
B: Sats 98% in room air, RR 20/min.
C: BP 145/90mmHg, HR 85/min, warm peripheries.
D: Alert and orientated, in pain which is partially controlled with IV morphine.
E: Urine present in catheter.

What is your management priority?

a   Referral and rapid transfer to a cardiothoracic centre for surgical intervention.
b   Further analgesia aiming for a pain score of <3.
c   BP management with labetalol aiming for an SBP of 100–120mmHg.
d   BP management with a GTN infusion aiming for an SBP of 100–120mmHg.
e   Referral to a cardiothoracic centre for consideration of endovascular intervention.

Question 2

You are undertaking a daily review of a patient on the cardiothoracic ICU. He had undergone coronary artery bypass grafting of three vessels 1 week ago. Overnight yesterday he had to go back to theatre for repair to one of the grafts; this included a second period on bypass. He is now extubated and on no cardiovascular or respiratory support. He is complaining of a sore leg. On examination you notice that his right foot (contralateral side to that used for vessel harvest) is very swollen, red and painful and clinically resembles a deep vein thrombosis (DVT). Pacing wires and two mediastinal drains remain *in situ*.

Blood test results are shown in Table 3.1.

Table 3.1. Blood test results.

	Today	Yesterday		Today	Yesterday
Hb	120g/L	125g/L	Na$^+$	135mmol/L	136mmol/L
WCC	12.3 x 10^9/L	14.2 x 10^9/L	K$^+$	4.5mmol/L	4.4mmol/L
Platelets	75 x 10^9/L	155 x 10^9/L	Urea	8.1mmol/L	9.2mmol/L
PT	10.5 seconds	10.8 seconds	Creatinine	110µmol/L	100µmol/L
APTT	35 seconds	38 seconds			
Fibrinogen	2.5g/L	3.0g/L			

An urgent Doppler of the right leg confirms a large proximal occlusive DVT.

What is the most appropriate next step in the investigation and management of this patient?

a   Therapeutic dalteparin.
b   IV heparin infusion.
c   Bloods for presence of PF4 antibodies.
d   Argatroban infusion.
e   Rivaroxaban.

Question 3

A 34-year-old, 80kg patient who has been on the ICU for 2 weeks, following a 30% total body surface area (TBSA) burn injury, has had multiple failed attempts to initiate gastric feeding. A decision has been made to commence total parenteral nutrition (TPN).

What statement regarding TPN for this patient is correct?

a   The EPaNIC study demonstrated that early TPN (day 3) resulted in better survival.
b   Given the TPN is likely to be short term, it can be given through a peripheral cannula.
c   It should consist of 1.3–1.5g/kg/day protein, with the remaining calories as 60% carbohydrate and 40% fats.
d   In relation to electrolytes, TPN only contains sodium, potassium and calcium.
e   This patient's energy requirements are likely to be lower than standard amounts.

Question 4

You are asked to review a patient already on the ICU, who had been admitted overnight for vasopressor support. The patient presented to the ED with a 48-hour history of widespread rash, which started initially as an erythematous rash on the neck and axillae, and then rapidly spread over 48 hours to the whole body. The patient is 24 years old and has Crohn's disease, for which he is on infliximab. He has no other past medical history. He had received treatment for bacterial conjunctivitis the week before admission (eye drops) and had been taking ibuprofen regularly for the past week, due to a flare-up of hip pain.

The nurses have asked you to review the patient, as when they last rolled him, they noticed his skin was coming away with gentle pressure. On examination there are no obvious blisters and generalised erythema is noted across his whole body which blanches with gentle pressure. There are some areas of superficial flaccid bullae, and where the skin has come away it looks shiny and moist. There is no evidence of oral or tongue blisters, but there is some residual crusting around the eyes.

What is the most likely diagnosis in this case?

a   Stevens-Johnson syndrome (SJS).
b   Toxic epidermal necrolysis (TEN).
c   Drug reaction with eosinophilia and systemic symptoms (DRESS).
d   Staphylococcal scalded skin syndrome (SSSS).
e   Toxic shock syndrome (TSS).

● Question 5

You are asked to review and assist with a patient currently in theatre undergoing a trauma laparotomy and splenectomy. The patient is a 24-year-old lady who had fallen whilst mountain biking and landed on the handlebars of her bike, sustaining rib fractures and a grade 4 splenic laceration. The other past medical history of note is of pernicious anaemia.

The anaesthetic team state that though induction was uneventful, she was a grade 3 view on direct laryngoscopy. They had also noted that the lady had had a goitre during their airway examination pre-operatively. She had a rapid sequence induction with propofol and rocuronium, sevoflurane and remifentanil were used for maintenance of anaesthesia. The splenectomy has been completed, and the surgeons are currently closing the abdomen.

During the course of the anaesthetic her temperature has risen, and it is now sitting at 39.5°C; this is despite cooled intravenous fluids and cold lavage by the surgeons into the abdominal cavity. She has also gone into fast atrial fibrillation (AF) with a rate of approximately 150–180 beats/min. There is no response to fluids or magnesium therapy, and there are now rising metaraminol (vasopressor) requirements. The lady is flushed and sweaty and has a bounding pulse on examination. A blood gas has been taken (FiO_2 of 50%) which is shown in Table 3.2.

Table 3.2. Arterial blood gas results.			
pH	7.30	HCO_3^-	21mmol/L
pCO_2	6.8kPa	Hb	98g/L
pO_2	18kPa	Glucose	11.5mmol/L
BE	−4mmol/L		

What is the next best step for the haemodynamic management of this patient?

a   IV propranolol.
b   Amiodarone loading.
c   Dantrolene 2mg/kg bolus.
d   100mg IV hydrocortisone.
e   Lugol's iodine.

 Question 6

A 78-year-old lady presents to the ED with new right-sided hemiparesis and slurred speech; visual fields are intact. The symptoms began 3½ hours ago. She presented to a hospital that has both thrombolysis and thrombectomy capabilities. A CT head scan shows no intracerebral bleeding, no ischaemic changes and possible clot within the left middle cerebral artery (MCA) (hyperdense MCA sign). Her blood pressure is 195/120mmHg and she has a heart rate of 80 beats per minute with the rhythm being atrial fibrillation.

Which of the following statements is correct?

a   She has had a total anterior circulatory stroke (TACS).
b   Her National Institutes of Health Stroke Scale (NIHSS) score is 15, which means she is not eligible for thrombolysis.
c   She should have immediate thrombolysis.
d   She should go for an urgent thrombectomy.
e   She should receive aspirin loading and be started immediately on a statin.

Question 7

You are called down to assist with a patient in the ED with chest pain. You are in a district general hospital, from which there is a 20-minute transfer time to the local percutaneous coronary intervention (PCI) centre. The patient started with chest pain 12 hours ago, which has got progressively worse and is ongoing. The ECG shows anterior Q waves in leads V2–4 with 4mm ST-elevation. Point-of-care echocardiography shows significant regional wall motion abnormalities (RWMAs) and an impaired left ventricular ejection fraction. You have been called to assess the patient for ICU admission for CPAP, given the increased oxygen requirement.

What is the best option for his management?

a   Thrombolysis and admission to the ICU for CPAP.
b   Transfer out for primary PCI at the nearest centre.
c   Transfer to the PCI centre, to enable PCI within the next 72 hours.
d   Dual-antiplatelet therapy (DAPT) and fondaparinux.
e   Await the troponin level, and if elevated proceed with thrombolysis.

● Question 8

You have been asked to review a patient on the ward with acute kidney injury (AKI), who weighs 80kg. The serum creatinine level on admission was 80μmol/L. Over the first 2 days of admission the creatinine has risen, being 160μmol/L and 200μmol/L on days 1 and 2, respectively. Urine output has been 25–30ml per hour for the last 12 hours.

Which one of the following statements is correct?

a   This patient falls into the risk category of the RIFLE classification system.
b   There is no need to review and adjust drug doses currently.
c   This patient falls into KDIGO stage 2 AKI.
d   This patient needs admitting for CRRT.
e   This patient falls into stage 1 of the AKIN criteria.

● Question 9

A 25-year-old lady is on the NICU with a severe traumatic brain injury (TBI). The CT head scan shows diffuse axonal injury (DAI). In addition, there is evidence of contusional bleeding and traumatic subarachnoid haemorrhage (SAH).

She is 3 days into her admission and has a multi-lumen intracranial pressure bolt *in situ* that has microdialysis and brain tissue oxygenation measurement capabilities, along with jugular bulb oximetry (SjO_2).

There have been multiple periods of instability during the first 3 days, with elevations in intracranial pressure (ICP) requiring treatment with paralysis agents and deep sedation.

The nursing staff have called you to say that they are concerned she is becoming unstable again as her ICP is starting to climb and her pupils are now unequal.

Which of the following results is unlikely given this situation?

a   A brain tissue oxygen level of 10mmHg.
b   Jugular bulb oximetry shows an SjO_2 of 85%.
c   P2 is larger than P1 on the ICP trace.
d   Lundberg A waves are seen on the ICP trace.
e   There is a lactate:pyruvate ratio of 45.

● Question 10

A 67-year-old man presents with increasing shortness of breath, frequent vomiting and a productive cough — a diagnosis of community-acquired pneumonia (CAP) is made. He has a history of chronic obstructive pulmonary disease (COPD) but good functional capacity and can walk his dog 2–3 miles a day. He says he hasn't managed to eat for a week. On admission he weighs 58kg and is 180cm tall.

He quickly deteriorates on admission to the ICU requiring an FiO_2 of 0.9 on 10cmH_2O CPAP; the P:F ratio is 11kPa so he is intubated. Bloods show raised inflammatory markers and a serum potassium of 3.2mmol/L but are otherwise normal. A nasogastric (NG) tube is placed at the time of intubation.

What is the best option with regards to nutrition?

a   No nutrition for the first 48 hours.
b   Place a PICC and start early total parenteral nutrition (TPN).
c   Standard NG feeding regimen.
d   Start NG feed at 50% of the standard regime.
e   Trophic feed only for the first 24 hours.

Question 11

A 23-year-old man with a severe learning disability presents to the hospital, having mistakenly eaten a dishwasher cleaning pod. He is in discomfort and clutching the centre of his chest. His airway shows some redness to the posterior oropharynx but no swelling; there are no added airway sounds and no change to his voice. Baseline observations show RR 32/min, oxygen saturations of 95% in room air, HR 120/min sinus rhythm and BP 100/60mmHg. He is cool peripherally. The man is cannulated and routine bloods are taken. A fluid challenge is given in addition to intravenous morphine.

What is the next priority in management?

a   Immediate intubation and ventilation.
b   A CT scan of the thorax to assess the degree of injury.
c   NG tube insertion to enable gastric lavage.
d   Broad-spectrum antibiotics.
e   Upper GI endoscopy.

Question 12

You are asked to review a 65-year-old, 60kg patient, who is day 9 following left lower lung lobectomy surgery. The patient is unable to have their chest drain removed due to a persistent air leak; a bronchopleural fistula (BPF) is suspected. The chest drain is on suction, and the lung remains inflated on radiography. Oxygenation had been improving but overnight the oxygen requirement has increased, and a repeat CXR shows partial reaccumulation of the pneumothorax. The patient is otherwise well, apyrexial, and there is no increased sputum load. On sedation hold they are alert, obey commands and have good peripheral and respiratory muscle strength. The current ventilator settings are as follows: hybrid mode — PRVC/PS, FiO_2 of 0.35, PEEP of 7.5cmH_2O, TV 480ml x 18/min rate, I:E 1:1.5, PS 5cmH_2O achieving TV 500ml, SV rate currently 20/min.

What can be done to optimise the patient's ventilation and reduce the leak from the BPF?

a   Extubate the patient onto high-flow nasal oxygen (HFNO).
b   Administer a muscle relaxant, set PEEP to 10cmH$_2$O, I:E to 1:1 and TV to 500 x 10/min rate.
c   Choose PS/CPAP mode, set PEEP to 5cmH$_2$O, and change PS to achieve a TV of 350ml.
d   Extubate the patient onto NIV.
e   Continue PRVC ventilation, decrease TV to 400ml, with a PEEP of 5cmH$_2$O, I:E 1:2 and set rate of 20/min.

● Question 13

You are asked to review a 21-year-old patient who has presented to the ED with significant hypoxia. He states that he has had a persistent sore throat for 3 weeks, and for the last week he has felt like his neck has become swollen.

Today he presented to the ED because he is coughing up blood. A CXR shows multiple well circumscribed areas with fluid levels, and bilateral pleural effusions. You admit the patient to the ICU for CPAP. On attempting to site a central venous catheter (CVC) you are unable to use the right internal jugular vein (IJV) due to clot visualised on ultrasound; a left-sided IJV CVC line is sited instead.

What is the most likely causative bacteria?

a   *Streptococcus pneumoniae*.
b   *Fusobacterium necrophorum*.
c   *Staphylococcus aureus*.
d   *Streptococcus pyogenes*.
e   *Klebsiella pneumoniae*.

● Question 14

You are called to the ED of a major trauma centre, as part of the 'code red' trauma team. The patient is already in the department having been dropped off by a friend in their car, after sustaining an isolated machete injury to the posterior aspect of the right leg. There was reported to be a large volume of blood in the footwell of the car. As you arrive there are attempts ongoing to site intravenous access, but these are unsuccessful, and the patient is very agitated. Primary survey is as follows:

C: Tourniquet on the right thigh, minimal ooze from the injury site, no other catastrophic bleeding.
A: Airway maintained with a non-rebreathe oxygen mask *in situ*.
B: Chest clear, equal air entry, O_2 saturations — unable to measure, RR 26/min.
C: Very cool peripherally, looks pale, no palpable radial pulse, weak central pulse, BP not recording, HR 140/min, sinus rhythm.
D: Agitated, with no evidence of head injury. Pupils are equal and reactive.
E: Temperature 35.5°C, no other wounds, no rashes.

Shortly after the primary survey you notice the heart rate starts to drop, and there is now no longer a palpable central pulse.

What is the next management priority?

a Cardiopulmonary resuscitation (CPR).
b Further efforts at peripheral IV access.
c Intraosseous access (IO) access followed by CVC insertion.
d Resuscitative endovascular balloon occlusion of the aorta (REBOA).
e Intubation.

● **Question 15**

A 54-year-old lady with primary pulmonary hypertension is admitted to the ICU after an emergency laparoscopic cholecystectomy. She had undergone the acute operation secondary to repeated episodes of cholecystitis, each requiring hospital management. She is on an infusion of iloprost (currently at 4µg/hr) started preoperatively, as advised by the pulmonary hypertension team. Intra-operatively she received 3L of fluid and the total fluid balance (including fluid received intraoperatively) is +500ml. You are asked to review her in the evening, 4 hours postoperatively, due to low blood pressure. She has a CVC line inserted and a calibrated LiDCO pulse power analysis device is in place. During your assessment, clinical examination is as follows:

A: Maintaining own airway.
B: Quiet lung bases, no added sounds, oxygen sats 94% on nasal high-flow O_2 50L/min, an FiO_2 of 0.4.
C: BP 85/50mmHg, HR 90/min, sinus rhythm, CVP 10cmH$_2$O, CI 2.8L/min/m², SVRI 1500 dynes/s/cm⁵/m², stroke volume variation (SVV) 5%, slightly cool peripheries, reduced radial pulse, strong central pulse, mild peripheral oedema. The iloprost infusion is running at 4µg/hr.
D: Alert and orientated, mild abdominal pain, receiving regular oral morphine.
E: Temperature 38.5°C, abdomen soft, mildly tender, port site dressings clean with no bleeding.

You start her on IV Tazocin® to cover infection. What is the best management of her hypotension?

a   Administer a fluid bolus.
b   Start noradrenaline.
c   Start milrinone.
d   Stop the iloprost infusion.
e   Administer diuretics.

● Question 16

You are called to review a patient who has just arrived in the ED. The patient had a witnessed collapse in the supermarket; there was bystander CPR and two shocks from an automated external defibrillator (AED). On arrival of the paramedics, the patient had return of spontaneous circulation (ROSC) and was spontaneously breathing; the GCS was 3. A laryngeal mask airway (LMA) was inserted, and the patient was transferred to hospital.

On examination:

A: LMA *in situ*, well seated.
B: Spontaneously breathing rate of 12/min, equal air entry, fine bibasal crepitations, O_2 sats 100% on 15L via a Waters circuit. Initial ABG: pH 7.15, PaCO$_2$ 7.4kPa, PaO$_2$ 32kPa, HCO$_3^-$ 21mmol/L, lactate 4.5mmol/L, glucose 5.5mmol/L.
C: BP 110/60mmHg, HR 80/min, ECG shows anterior ST-elevation of 4mm in leads V1–4, warm peripherally.

D: Pupils equal and reactive to light, flexion response to pain.
E: Temperature 36.8°C, no rashes or injuries.

What is the management priority here?

a   Intubation and ventilation.
b   Transfer to the cardiac catheter lab for primary PCI.
c   Bedside echo.
d   A fluid bolus of Hartmann's solution.
e   A 100ml 5% dextrose bolus.

Question 17

A 50-year-man who has suffered 40% TBSA burns in a house fire a week ago is currently intubated and ventilated on the ICU. On review in the morning:

A: Intubated.
B: An FiO$_2$ of 0.45, ventilated Vt 500 x 16/min rate, PEEP set at 8cmH$_2$O.
C: BP 120/60mmHg on 0.12µg/kg/min of noradrenaline, HR 105/min, sinus rhythm.
D: Sedated with propofol and alfentanil. On sedation holds he has been appropriate.
E: Abdomen is distended but soft, BNO for around 5 days, previously absorbing enteral feed well. He has a right femoral CVC line *in situ* for access.

The nurse asks you to review the patient that afternoon because he looks unwell. On examination:

A: As before.
B: Oxygen exchange is unchanged.
C: Noradrenaline requirement has increased slightly (0.16µg/kg/min), HR 115/min, CRT 3 seconds. Urine output has reduced to 20ml/hr.
D: As before.
E: Temperature 36.0°C, abdomen remains soft. There have been three aspirates over 500ml from his NG tube in the last 24 hours, hence the feed has been stopped. One area of burns looks slightly sloughy.

What is the best next step in management?

a   Start prokinetics.
b   Administer a fluid challenge.
c   Take a full set of cultures.
d   Measurement of intra-abdominal pressure.
e   Per rectum (PR) examination and subsequent enema if faecally loaded.

● Question 18

You receive a medical emergency team bleep to the labour ward. The history is of a gravida 1 (G1), para 0 (P1), patient, who has had an uneventful pregnancy. She was admitted this morning for induction of labour due to being term +7 days. Observations taken on admission show oxygen saturations of 98% in room air, RR 20/min, HR 85/min, BP 130/70mmHg, urine dipstick testing shows 1+ protein and nil else significant. The lady is in active labour contracting at the rate of 2 every 5 minutes. She had an epidural inserted 30 minutes previously and had a subsequent epidural top-up to facilitate artificial rupture of membranes. Following this she suddenly felt very unwell and became agitated; she subsequently had a large vomit.

On your arrival 5 minutes later, examination reveals:

A: Maintaining own airway.
B: Oxygen sats 96% on a NRB mask, RR 28/min, bilateral creps to midzones.
C: BP 80mmHg systolic (following a 500ml IV fluid bolus), HR 110/min, occasional atrial ectopics, cool peripherally.
D: Agitated, not orientated to time place or person repeatedly saying 'I don't feel well, I am going to die'.
E: Temperature 37.3°C, no rash but there is oozing from one of the IV cannula sites.

What is the most likely cause of this lady's collapse?

a   Local anaesthetic (LA) toxicity.
b   Pre-eclampsia with severe features.
c   Pulmonary embolus (PE).
d   Sepsis.
e   Amniotic fluid embolism (AFE).

Question 19

You are undertaking a daily ICU review on a 64-year-old man with pancreatitis. He is currently on day 13 of his admission. He was intubated on day 4 due to agitation, and had a tracheostomy sited on day 12 following two failed extubation attempts (failed due to a combination of agitation and desaturation). He underwent a CT abdomen yesterday that showed generalised peripancreatic fluid and no organised collections. Examination is as follows:

A: Tracheostomy.
B: PS/CPAP ventilation, PEEP of 8cmH$_2$O, PS 10cmH$_2$O above PEEP, an FiO$_2$ of 0.4, RR 22/min.
C: BP 90/60mmHg, MAP 70mmHg, HR 105/min, AF, warm peripherally, moderate peripheral oedema. No CVS support. Urine output 10ml/hr.
D: Alert, mouthing words, slightly confused.
E: Temperature 37.3°C, distended abdomen, tense but not painful. NG aspirates 300ml for the last two done, feed running at 40ml/hr. IAP 26mmHg.

His blood test results including an arterial blood gas are shown in Table 3.3.

Table 3.3. Blood test results.

	Yesterday	Today		Today
Na$^+$	134mmol/L	136mmol/L	pH	7.34
K$^+$	4.3mmol/L	5.1mmol/L	pCO$_2$	4.6kPa
Urea	5.8mmol/L	10.1mmol/L	pO$_2$	10.2kPa
Creatinine	120µmol/L	180µmol/L	HCO$_3^-$	17mmol/L
WCC	12.2 x 10^9/L	12.1 x 10^9/L	Lactate	3mmol/L
CRP	89mg/L	87mmol/L		

Which of the following is the best management of the complications of his abdominal compartment syndrome (ACS)?

a   Prokinetics.
b   Stop NG feeding.
c   Site a percutaneous drain.
d   Start noradrenaline.
e   Paralyse the patient.

Question 20

A 66-year-old lady presents to the ED having been found collapsed at home by her wife, surrounded by vomitus. There are concerns regarding a possible overdose as she was found with multiple empty medication packets, having only picked up her prescription the previous day. The patient's wife had been away overnight and had last spoken to her at 9pm the previous evening. The patient has a background of type 2 diabetes; on metformin and gliclazide. You have been called to urgently review the patient, as although she had initially improved following treatment of her hypoglycaemia (glucose 2.1mmol/L), she is now very agitated, and profoundly acidotic. On examination:

A: Maintaining own airway.
B: Oxygen sats 99% on a NRB mask, RR 26/min, chest clear.
C: BP 80/50mmHg, HR 110/min, ECG — sinus tachycardia, cool peripherally, thready peripheral pulse.
D: Pupils equal and reactive to light (PEARL), GCS 12: M-5, E-3, V-4.
E: Temperature 36.0°C, no rashes.

Arterial blood gas (ABG) results are shown in Table 3.4.

Table 3.4. Arterial blood gas results.

pH	6.9	Lactate	22mmol/L
pCO_2	2.2kPa	Na^+	140mmol/L
pO_2	40kPa	K^+	5.0mmol/L
HCO_3^-	14mmol/L	Cl^-	85mmol/L
BE	−20mmol/L	Glucose	4.1mmol/L

What is the most effective treatment for the management of this patient's acidosis based on the likely diagnosis?

a   Continuous veno-venous haemofiltration (CVVH).
b   Fluid resuscitation.
c   Haemodialysis (HD).
d   Sodium bicarbonate bolus.
e   High-dose insulin therapy.

● Question 21

In which of the following ICU patients, would a Liberty Protection Safeguards document need to be completed?

a   Day 1 out-of-hospital cardiac arrest (OOHCA) patient, currently sedated and ventilated.
b   Day 35 patient, tracheostomy wean (external CPAP) post-ARDS, critical illness weakness limiting mobilisation, otherwise alert and orientated.
c   Ward-fit patient, alert and orientated, staying on the ICU due to the lack of a ward discharge bed.
d   Ward-fit patient, confused and wandering the ward at night requiring quetiapine to keep him settled and in bed.
e   Day 34 patient with pancreatitis, tracheostomy wean (PS/CPAP) on clonidine for agitation, also on noradrenaline.

● Question 22

You are walking through the ED waiting room when you hear a cry for help. You run over to find a mother holding her 6-month-old baby which looks cyanosed and lifeless. The ward clerk is ringing the cardiac arrest team, and another staff member is bringing the resuscitation trolly. You take the baby, open the airway and there is no breathing effort. What is the next step in management?

a   Feel for a central pulse in the neck.
b   Feel for a central pulse in the brachial area.
c   Start CPR at a rate: 30 compressions to 2 breaths.
d   Five rescue breaths.
e   Start CPR at a rate: 15 compressions to 2 breaths.

SBA Paper 3: Questions

● Question 23
With regard to haemoglobin and abnormalities of haemoglobin, which of the following is correct?

a   HbA consists of two α chains and two β chains.
b   HbF has a right-shifted oxygen dissociation curve.
c   β thalassaemia is due to mutations in the α chain.
d   Sickle cell anaemia is due to substitution of valine for glutamic acid at position 6 of the α-chain.
e   A common cause of sickle cell crisis is hyperthermia.

● Question 24
Which of the following physiological processes do **not** involve phosphate?

a   Buffering within blood to maintain acid base homeostasis.
b   Bone mineralisation.
c   Oxygen binding to haemoglobin.
d   Conversion of ADP to ATP.
e   Plateau phase of the cardiac action potential.

● Question 25
Which of the following is **not** associated with an increased risk of ICU-acquired weakness?

a   An ICU length of stay of greater than 7 days.
b   Obesity.
c   Noradrenaline use.
d   Neuromuscular blockade infusion.
e   High lactate levels.

Question 26
Which of the following findings is most diagnostically significant in the diagnosis of infective endocarditis (IE)?

a   The patient is an active intravenous drug user.
b   Presence of Janeway lesions.
c   New valvular regurgitation on auscultation of heart sounds.
d   Fever of greater than 38°C.
e   Bacteria commonly associated with IE are isolated from two separate blood cultures.

Question 27
What is the correct personal protective equipment (PPE) for taking bloods from a patient with confirmed COVID-19?

a   Non-sterile gloves, disposable apron, surgical face mask, eye protection.
b   Sterile gloves, fluid-repellent gown, FFP-3 mask.
c   Non-sterile gloves, surgical mask, eye protection.
d   Non-sterile gloves, disposable apron, FFP-3 mask.
e   Sterile gloves, disposable apron, surgical face mask.

Question 28
Which of the following describes West Haven Grade 3 encephalopathy?

a   Unresponsive to painful stimuli.
b   Reduced attention span, disordered sleep.
c   Inappropriate behaviour, disorientated in time, lethargic.
d   Rousable to voice, marked confusion.
e   Abnormality on psychometric testing, alert and orientated.

Question 29
A 75-year-old patient who has been on the ICU for 3 weeks, following an emergency laparotomy for perforated diverticulum, went into AF on day 3.

Despite multiple attempts at electrical and chemical cardioversion, he has remained in rate-controlled AF. An echocardiogram has shown normal valves and good left ventricular function. There is a past medical history of hypertension. The patient is now approaching being ready for discharge home and you are considering his long-term anticoagulation needs, with regard to persistent AF. You calculate the CHA_2DS_2-VASc score as 3, and that he has a low bleeding risk (ORBIT score 1). What would be the best form of anticoagulation for this patient?

a   No anticoagulation.
b   DAPT (aspirin and clopidogrel).
c   Aspirin only.
d   Apixaban.
e   Warfarin.

● Question 30
Which of these features on an ECG with a broad complex tachycardia would lead you away from a diagnosis of ventricular tachycardia?

a   Capture beats.
b   Irregular rhythm.
c   Fusion beats.
d   An RSR pattern, with the first R wave taller than the second.
e   QRS complex >160ms.

● Question 31
In which of the following patient cohorts has the transfusion trigger stated been shown to improve outcome?

a   Acute GI bleed ≤70g/L.
b   Septic shock ≤70g/L.
c   Critical care ≤70g/L.
d   Post-myocardial infarction ≤80g/L.
e   Traumatic brain injury ≤70g/L.

Question 32

There is a 35-year-old woman on your unit with acute pancreatitis. Which of the following is most likely to be the causative factor?

a   Alcohol.
b   Hypertriglyceridemia.
c   Gallstones.
d   Related to an ERCP.
e   Trauma.

 Question 33

You are asked to urgently review a patient on the ICU who has developed a regular narrow complex tachycardia at a rate of 200/min. The patient is alert, but complaining of central chest pain and is dyspnoeic. BP is 90mmHg systolic, having been 130mmHg systolic unsupported prior to this. The patient now has supplemental oxygen and has a pink (20G) cannula in the dorsum of their hand. What is the next best step in management?

a   Larger IV access.
b   Vagal manoeuvres.
c   Adenosine 6mg as a rapid IV bolus followed by a flush.
d   Synchronised DC cardioversion with sedation.
e   Amiodarone 300mg IV over 30 minutes.

 Question 34

In which of the following clinical situations would it be appropriate to immediately proceed with brainstem death testing (BSDT)?

a   Loss of last brainstem reflex 4 hours ago in a patient with a devastating brain injury.
b   12 hours after the beginning of rewarming, following therapeutic hypothermia.
c   Loss of all brainstem reflexes 6 hours ago, in a patient 12 hours post-decompressive craniectomy.
d   Patient with ongoing myoclonus.
e   25 hours after loss of brainstem reflexes, in a patient with hypoxic brain injury.

SBA Paper 3: Questions

● **Question 35**
Which of the following would **not** be part of the routine assessment of a patient's capacity?

a   Does the decision the patient is making seem rational?
b   Does the person understand what decision they need to make and why?
c   Does the person understand the likely consequences of making or not making the decision?
d   Is the person able to understand, retain, use and weigh up the information relevant to the decision?
e   Can the person communicate their decision?

● **Question 36**
Regarding methods of data analysis, which of the following best describes the relative risk?

a   The difference between the risk occurring in the control group and the intervention group.
b   The ratio of the risk of something occurring in the intervention group compared to the control group.
c   The ratio of the odds of a certain outcome in the intervention group to the odds of that outcome in the control group.
d   The likelihood of the observed value being the result of change alone.
e   The number of patients that need the intervention to prevent one outcome event happening.

● **Question 37**
Which of the following findings on analysis of pleural fluid would favour a diagnosis of empyema?

a   pH 7.3.
b   High WCC with leukocyte predominance.
c   Glucose 2mmol/L.
d   Protein 25g/L (serum total protein 60g/L).
e   Pleural LDH 100 IU/L (serum LDH 200 IU/L).

Question 38

Which one of the following would represent an absolute contraindication to the use of an intra-aortic balloon pump?

a   Severe mitral regurgitation.
b   Aortic dissection.
c   Peripheral vascular disease treated with an arterial stent.
d   Sepsis.
e   Cardiomyopathy.

Question 39

A patient is on the critical care unit with group A streptococcal sepsis. They are intubated and ventilated, and requiring haemodynamic support with noradrenaline 0.45μg/kg/min and vasopressin at 2 units/hour. Over the last 6 hours the patient has been anuric and now has a serum potassium (K^+) level of 6.8mmol/L with associated ECG changes, consistent with hyperkalaemia. Which mode of renal replacement therapy is optimal for this patient?

a   Slow continuous ultrafiltration (SCUF).
b   Peritoneal dialysis (PD).
c   Continuous renal replacement therapy (CRRT) dose 40–45ml/kg/hr.
d   Intermittent haemodialysis (IHD).
e   CRRT dose 25–30ml/kg/hr.

Question 40

A patient on the ICU develops type 7 stools, opening their bowels eight times in the last 24 hours. Which of the following would be **least** likely to be the cause?

a   Omeprazole.
b   NG feed.
c   Lactulose.
d   IV magnesium replacement.
e   Ciprofloxacin.

SBA Paper 3: Questions

● Question 41
Which of the following infections is a notifiable disease?

a   *Clostridioides difficile*.
b   Group A streptococcal sepsis.
c   Norovirus.
d   *Pseudomonas aeruginosa*.
e   *Streptococcus pneumoniae* bronchitis.

● Question 42
Which of the following describes the mechanism of action of the quinolone antibiotics, such as ciprofloxacin?

a   Inhibit cell wall synthesis.
b   Inhibit protein synthesis targeting the 30s subunit of the bacterial ribosome.
c   Inhibit bacterial DNA gyrase.
d   Inhibit protein synthesis targeting the 50s subunit of bacterial ribosome.
e   Interfere with intracellular folate synthesis.

● Question 43
A patient on the ICU has been on CRRT for 5 hours via a vascular access catheter (vascath) placed in the right internal jugular vein (RIJV). They are anuric and have a potassium of 6.0mmol/L and a pH of 7.25; serum bicarbonate (HCO_3^-) is 14mmol/L. You have been told that the current vascath is alarming with high access pressures. When the nursing team have tried to switch lumens they are unable to aspirate or flush either one of the lumens. What is the best option with regards to ongoing management?

a   Site a left IJV vascath and continue CRRT.
b   Site a femoral vascath and continue CRRT.
c   Pause CRRT, remove the current vascath and re-site into the RIJV in 12 hours.
d   Trial a period off CRRT.
e   Site a right subclavian vascath and continue CRRT.

Question 44
Which of the following is correct with regard to thrombophilia?

a   Antiphospholipid syndrome (APS) antibodies include lupus anticoagulant and anticardiolipin antibody.
b   A cause of thrombophilia is a deficiency of Factor V Leiden.
c   Oestrogen excess can lead to acquired protein S resistance.
d   Around 98% of people with APS will develop thrombosis.
e   APS can cause an unexplained prolongation of the prothrombin time.

Question 45
You are looking after a postoperative patient on the ICU who has an epidural catheter *in situ*, that has been in for 4 days and is no longer required. The patient is on 75mg of aspirin every morning and prophylactic dalteparin at 6pm in the evening. You are planning to remove the epidural on day 5. Which of the following is the optimal approach to removal?

a   Hold aspirin in the morning, remove the epidural catheter 6 hours later, give prophylactic dalteparin 4 hours after removal.
b   Continue aspirin, remove the epidural catheter, give prophylactic dalteparin 4 hours after removal.
c   Hold aspirin in the morning, remove the epidural catheter 4 hours later, give prophylactic dalteparin 12 hours after removal.
d   Continue aspirin, remove the epidural catheter and give prophylactic dalteparin 6 hours after removal.
e   Continue aspirin, remove the epidural catheter and give prophylactic dalteparin 12 hours after removal.

Question 46
With regards to the insertion and management of tracheostomies, which one of the following is correct?

a   It is safe to have the cuff inflated with a speaking valve on.
b   The TracMan study showed improved outcomes with early tracheostomy insertion.
c   A single-lumen tracheostomy tube should be changed every 30 days.

d   The ideal position for tracheostomy insertion includes head and neck flexion.
e   The ideal location for insertion is between the 2nd and 3rd tracheal rings.

● Question 47

With regards to oesophageal Doppler cardiac output measurement, which one of the following is true?

a   You can safely use oesophageal Doppler with oesophageal varices.
b   You will get accurate readings in a patient with a thoracic epidural running.
c   A peak velocity (PV) of 60cm/s would be normal in a patient who is 75 years of age.
d   The corrected flow time (FTc) decreases in vasodilation.
e   Aortic cross-section is taken from a nomogram based on age and height only.

● Question 48

Regarding acute liver failure (ALF), which of the following is true?

a   An ammonia level of over 200µmol/L is associated with cerebral herniation.
b   Paracetamol overdose is the most common aetiology worldwide.
c   Hepatitis C is commonly associated with acute liver failure.
d   Mortality can be predicted using the CLIF-C ACLF score.
e   Can be classified as acute, subacute and delayed.

● Question 49

Regarding West Zones, in a lung unit that is functionally alveolar dead space, which of the following pressure relationships would apply? (A=alveolar, a=arterial v=venous).

a   Pa > PA > Pv.
b   Pa > Pv > PA.
c   Pv > Pa > PA.
d   PA > Pa > Pv.
e   PA > Pv > Pa.

Question 50

In a patient with no known drug allergies and normal renal function, which of the following antibiotic regimes would be the most appropriate first-line treatment for a patient with MRSA sepsis?

a   Tazocin®.
b   Aztreonam.
c   Vancomycin.
d   Co-trimoxazole.
e   Meropenem.

Answer overview: Paper 3

Question:		Question:	
1	a	26	e
2	d	27	a
3	c	28	d
4	d	29	d
5	a	30	b
6	d	31	a
7	b	32	c
8	c	33	d
9	b	34	e
10	d	35	a
11	b	36	b
12	a	37	c
13	b	38	b
14	c	39	e
15	b	40	d
16	a	41	b
17	c	42	c
18	e	43	b
19	d	44	a
20	c	45	b
21	d	46	e
22	d	47	c
23	a	48	a
24	e	49	d
25	b	50	c

3 SBA Paper 3: Answers

Answer 1: a

This lady has a type A dissection, as the dissection flap originates within the ascending aorta.

The management priority for patients with a type A aortic dissection is assessment and input from a cardiothoracic surgeon, as surgery is the definitive treatment. If the patient is in a hospital that does not have cardiothoracic services, urgent referral and transfer to a regional centre is a key part of management. Blood pressure control is another key aspect of management. Patients are often significantly hypertensive and blood pressure management should be undertaken in the same manner as for a type B dissection, e.g. aiming for a systolic BP (SBP) of 100–120mmHg and a HR of <60/min, first-line management being anti-impulse therapy with short-acting beta-blockers such as labetalol and esmolol. Blood pressure management should NOT delay referral and transfer to a cardiothoracic centre.

Surgery is predominantly open (endovascular repair has a very limited role in type A dissections). The patients will need to go onto bypass, and many will require deep hypothermia during the operation to aid in the preservation of cerebral function. The surgery involves excision of the intimal tear, eliminating the entry point of the false lumen and placing an aortic graft. In addition, there may be repair of the aortic valve if required.

Postoperatively, these patients will require ongoing antihypertensive therapy with a SBP target of <120mmHg.

For more information on the classification of aortic dissection and management of type B dissection please see page 44, Paper 1, Q12.

References

1. www.uptodate.com. Management of acute type A aortic dissection. UpToDate, 2024. Available at: https://www.uptodate.com/contents/management-of-acute-type-a-aortic-dissection.
2. www.uptodate.com. Surgical and endovascular management of acute type A aortic dissection. UpToDate, 2024. Available at: https://www.uptodate.com/contents/surgical-and-endovascular-management-of-acute-type-a-aortic-dissection.

Answer 2: d

This patient has a history of two periods of significant IV heparin exposure, with a subsequent precipitous drop in platelets associated with a new thrombosis. This constellation of findings is consistent with a diagnosis of heparin-induced thrombocytopaenia (HIT).

There are two types of HIT:

- Type 1 is non-immune-mediated and due to direct activation of platelets by heparin. It occurs within 2–3 days of exposure and resolves on stopping the heparin. It is not associated with an increased risk of thrombosis.
- Type 2 is immune-mediated. Platelet factor 4 (PF4) is a protein released from platelets which is involved in platelet aggregation but also binds to heparin and neutralises it. On activation of the heparin/PF4 complex, the body produces PF4 antibodies; when these antibodies bind to the complex, they cause platelet activation. Thrombosis occurs in 30–50% of cases. Risk factors include: high cumulative doses, unfractionated heparin and intravenous heparin use. The presence of PF4 antibodies in isolation does not mean the patient has HIT syndrome. Diagnosis requires the combination of antibodies and evidence of dysfunctional platelet activation.

The HIT score is used to stratify the risk of HIT (Table 3.5).

SBA Paper 3: Answers

Table 3.5. The HIT score.			
	0 points	**1 point**	**2 points**
Thrombocytopaenia	Platelet count drop <30% OR platelet nadir <10 x 10^9/L	Platelet count drop 30–50% OR nadir 10–19 x 10^9/L	Platelet count drop >50% AND nadir of >20 x 10^9/L
Timing of platelet fall from heparin commencement	Platelet count fall <4 days without recent exposure	Unclear but likely days 5–10 OR onset after day 10 OR onset ≤1 day with heparin in last 30–100 days	Clear onset between 5–10 days OR platelet fall ≤1 day with heparin exposure in the last 30 days
Thrombosis or other complications	None	Progressive/recurrent thrombosis, suspected thrombosis, non-necrotising skin lesions	New thrombosis OR skin necrosis OR acute systemic reaction post-IV heparin bolus
Alternative reasons for thrombocytopaenia	Definite	Possible	Nil apparent

Score 0–3 = Low probability
Score 4–5 = Intermediate probability
Score 6–8 = High probability — HIT is likely

This patient had a score of 8 points indicating a high probability of HIT. Bloods should be sent for PF4 antibodies and if present, proceed to functional assays (these can take several days and are not universally available). In the context of an intermediate or high HIT score, in a condition that needs anticoagulation, then HIT should be assumed and a non-heparinoid anticoagulant should be used for anticoagulation. These include commencing an argatroban infusion, danaparoid, bivalirudin, or a direct oral anticoagulant (DOAC). Once HIT is confirmed with antibodies and assays, then therapeutic anticoagulation needs commencing, regardless of the presence of thrombosis, as the patient has a high thrombotic risk.

In this patient, treatment is needed for the DVT. The only options that will provide safe anticoagulation in the context of a high probability of HIT are argatroban and rivaroxaban. This gentleman has invasive drains and lines *in situ* that will need removing; therefore, an argatroban infusion (which can be stopped to facilitate safe line removal) is the single best option.

References

1. Cartwright B, Mundell N. Anticoagulation for cardiopulmonary bypass, Part 2: alternatives and pathological states. *BJA Educ* 2023; 23(7): 256–63.
2. MDCalc. 4Ts score for heparin-induced thrombocytopenia. Available at: https://www.mdcalc.com/calc/1787/4ts-score-heparin-induced-thrombocytopenia.
3. www.uptodate.com. Clinical presentation and diagnosis of heparin-induced thrombocytopenia. UpToDate, 2025. Available at: https://www.uptodate.com/contents/clinical-presentation-and-diagnosis-of-heparin-induced-thrombocytopenia.

● Answer 3: c

In general, nutrition should be started on ICU patients within 24–48 hours of admission if possible. Aim for enteral nutrition (EN) initially (unless there is a specific surgical indication for parenteral nutrition [PN or TPN]).

The EPaNIC study (2011) compared early vs. late PN (3 days vs. 8 days); the late group had better survival and less requirement for CRRT, experienced fewer complications and had reduced health care costs.

European guidelines (European Society for Clinical Nutrition and Metabolism [ESPEN]) recommend considering PN at 24–48 hours if EN is inadequate. ASPEN (American Society for Parenteral and Enteral Nutrition) guidelines recommend PN at 7–10 days if EN is not providing >60% of the recommended nutritional requirement.

Although short-term PN can be given through a cannula, the formulation needs to have a lower osmolality (<900mOsmol/kg) to be tolerated, which means the formulation is slightly different. It is better to site a CVC or PICC early, when providing PN.

Feed should be made up of nitrogen (in the form of protein) 1.3–1.5g/kg/day; if a patient has an open abdomen, they may need up to 2g/kg/day. The remaining calories should be made up of 60% carbohydrates (dextrose) and 40% fats (lipids).

PN can contain a variety of different electrolytes, typically Na^+, Mg^{2+}, Ca^{2+}, K^+, PO_4^{3-}. It can also contain vitamins, minerals and trace elements. The exact constituents are decided in liaison with the pharmacist and nutritional team (the electrolytes above are unlikely to be in a standard off-the-shelf bag of PN).

There are some groups of patients who may have higher energy requirements as they become hypermetabolic — notably burns, major trauma, and sepsis patients. Dieticians have ways of calculating a patient's energy requirements such as the NUTRIC score, indirect calorimetry and nutritional index calculations (e.g. Harris Benedict and Schofield index).

References
1. www.uptodate.com. Nutrition support in critically ill adult patients: parenteral nutrition. UpToDate, 2025. Available at: https://www.uptodate.com/contents/nutrition-support-in-critically-ill-patients-parenteral-nutrition.

Answer 4: d

Dermatological emergencies are rare, but it is important to know about those that may require ICU treatment or occur as a result of ICU treatment.

Staphylococcal scalded skin syndrome (SSSS) occurs as the result of infection with an exotoxin-producing *Staphylococcus aureus* infection, for example, conjunctivitis, impetigo and cellulitis. It tends to occur in younger children without staphylococcal antibodies or in adults who are immunocompromised. It can also occur in immunocompetent patients where there is a very high staphylococcal burden. SSSS presents with a spreading erythematous rash, typically starting in the neck and axillae. The rash consists of generalised erythema, with areas of superficial bullae and a positive Nikolsky's sign (where the skin comes away with gentle pressure, often in large sheets). The staphylococci in question produce one or both exotoxins — epidermolytic A or B. This exotoxin cleaves desmoglein-1 which is responsible for binding the keratinocytes together in the second layer of the epidermis (the stratum granulosum), which explains why there is loss of the very top dermal layer only. There is no involvement of the mucosa in SSSS. Patients are likely to suffer fluid loss and will have difficulty in maintaining their core temperature; they often need managing in a burns unit or ICU, primarily for skin care and fluid balance management. Treatment is primarily with antimicrobial therapy in discussion with your local microbiology team.

Differential diagnoses include Stevens-Johnson syndrome (SJS) and toxic epidermal necrolysis (TEN). This is a spectrum of disease, with SJS having <10% TBSA involvement, SJS/TEN overlap 10–30% and above this it would be TEN. The most common aetiological cause for this is medications, with anticonvulsants, antibiotics and NSAIDs being amongst the most common causative agents. SJS and TEN can also occur secondary to infection or vaccination and having HIV or cancer increases your likelihood of developing it. It is immune-mediated and results in detachment of the epidermis from the papillary dermis at the epidermal-dermal junction, resulting in deeper skin lesions than with SSSS. There is also mucosal involvement which can involve any part of the GI tract. Management is removal of the causative agent and supportive management of the skin involvement.

Toxic shock syndrome (TSS) is another differential diagnosis. TSS is a systemic syndrome related to exotoxins from staphylococcal or streptococcal infection. These are usually secondary to an ongoing infection or retained foreign bodies (e.g. retained tampon). Patients have a widespread erythematous rash which blanches, a strawberry tongue, fever and hypotension. Of note there are no bullae and a negative Nikolsky's sign on examination.

References

1. bestpractice.bmj.com. Stevens-Johnson syndrome and toxic epidermal necrolysis — symptoms, diagnosis and treatment. BMJ Best Practice, 2022. Available at: https://bestpractice.bmj.com/topics/en-gb/237.
2. www.uptodate.com. Staphylococcal scalded skin syndrome. UpToDate, 2024. Available at: https://www.uptodate.com/contents/staphylococcal-scalded-skin-syndrome.

● Answer 5: a

There are several factors in the patient history that point towards this clinical situation being the result of a thyroid storm: female patient with an autoimmune disorder, goitre and an event known to precipitate a thyroid storm in patients with thyrotoxicosis.

The obvious differential diagnosis in this case would be malignant hyperpyrexia (MH); however, the case history fits more with thyroid disease than MH.

A thyroid storm is a medical emergency that is associated with high mortality if not promptly treated. Clinical features include those associated with underlying thyrotoxicosis (e.g. goitre, proptosis, weight loss, hyperpigmentation, thinning of the hair and increased sweating).

Symptoms and signs specific to a thyroid storm include: pyrexia (>38.5°C), tachycardia (HR exceeding 140/min, atrial fibrillation [AF] is common), agitation, anxiety or coma. Bloods show high T3/T4 levels with a low thyroid-stimulating hormone (TSH) level along with mild hyperglycaemia, mild hypercalcaemia, abnormal liver function tests (LFTs) and a leukocytosis or leukopaenia.

Treatment of a thyroid storm is focused on managing the precipitant (in this case it was trauma, so the splenectomy and haemostasis would be managing the precipitant), inhibition of thyroid synthesis and release and reduction of peripheral conversion of T4 to T3, along with supportive care which includes temperature management.

Inhibition of thyroid hormone synthesis is achieved by administering propylthiouracil (PTU) (this inhibits hormone synthesis and prevents conversion of T4–T3).

An hour after PTU is given, Lugol's iodine can be given, which inhibits the release of stored hormone. An alternative to PTU is carbimazole.

Propranolol is the beta-blocker of choice, as it will manage tachycardia and a reduction of the fast heart rate will improve cardiac output. In high doses, propranolol reduces conversion of T4 to T3 and is a good choice of agent for the management of AF in this patient group. Amiodarone can precipitate a thyroid storm and should not be used in this scenario. Glucocorticoids also reduce the conversion of T4 to T3 and should be given as part of the treatment for a thyroid storm.

Management of hyperpyrexia is supportive with the administration of cold IV fluids, external cooling devices and paracetamol. If the hyperpyrexia is refractory to these measures, CRRT and dantrolene can be considered.

References
1. Kerr D, Wenham T, Newell-Price J. Endocrine problems in the critically ill 2: endocrine emergencies. *BJA Educ* 2017; 17 (11): 377–82.
2. de Mul N, Damstra J, van Dijkum EJMN, et al. Risk of perioperative thyroid storm in hyperthyroid patients: a systematic review. *Br J Anaesth* 2021; 127(6): 879–89.
3. www.uptodate.com. Thyroid storm. UpToDate, 2025. Available at: https://www.uptodate.com/contents/thyroid-storm.
4. www.uptodate.com. Overview of the clinical manifestations of hyperthyroidism in adults. UpToDate, 2024. Available at: https://www.uptodate.com/contents/overview-of-the-clinical-manifestations-of-hyperthyroidism-in-adults.

Answer 6: d

Ischaemic stroke is less frequently managed on the ICU than haemorrhagic stroke.

The cause of 80–90% of strokes is ischaemia; the remainder are haemorrhagic.

The Oxford Bamford classification of ischaemic strokes is as follows:

- TACS/PACS (total or partial anterior circulation syndrome); affects the middle and anterior cerebral artery territories, all three of the following is TACS, two of three (or third one alone) is PACS:
    - unilateral weakness (+/-) sensory deficit;
    - homonymous hemianopia;
    - high cerebral dysfunction (dysphasia, visuospatial abnormalities).
- POCS — posterior circulation syndrome — one of the following:
    - loss of consciousness;
    - isolated homonymous hemianopia;
    - cerebellar or brainstem symptoms (reduced GCS, cardiorespiratory disturbance).

SBA Paper 3: Answers

- LACS — lacunar syndrome — subcortical stroke due to small-vessel disease. Classified as the absence of higher cerebral dysfunction (e.g. dysphasia) plus one of the following:
  - unilateral weakness;
  - pure sensory stroke;
  - ataxic hemiparesis.

Once confirmed on imaging it becomes an infarct and not a syndrome, e.g. PAC infarct not PACS.

Management is dependent on factors such as time from onset of symptoms to presentation to hospital, stroke severity and the vessels involved. Thrombolysis is indicated within 4½ hours of symptom onset (ideally under 3 hours) in the absence of haemorrhage in patients with an NIHSS score of 6–25. Absolute contraindications include: increased risk of bleeding (recent surgery, head injury) and/or reversible cause such as hypoglycaemia. Once after 3 hours, guidance is stricter as the risk benefit ratio changes, for example, a BP of >185/110mmHg becomes a contraindication.

Thrombectomy is indicated, in centres that offer this service, up to 6 hours after the onset of ischaemic stroke symptoms or at up to 24 hours if there is evidence of salvageable brain. Thrombectomy is indicated for proximal vessels only such as the internal carotid or middle cerebral artery. The NIHSS score must be over 5.

All ischaemic stroke patients should have aspirin 300mg on diagnosis and for the first 2 weeks, followed by 75mg daily. In addition, statins should be started after 48 hours, unless the patient is already established on them in which case they should be continued.

References

1. National Institute for Health and Care Excellence (NICE), guideline NG128. Stroke and transient ischaemic attack in over 16s: diagnosis and initial management, 2019. Available at: https://www.nice.org.uk/guidance/ng128/resources/stroke-and-transient-ischaemic-attack-in-over-16s-diagnosis-and-initial-management-pdf-66141665603269.
2. National Institute of Neurological Disorders and Stroke. NIH Stroke Scale. stroke.nih.gov. Available at: https://www.ninds.nih.gov/sites/default/files/2024-05/KnowStroke_NIHStrokeScale_May2024_508c.pdf.

3. Raithatha A, Pratt G, Rash A. Developments in the management of acute ischaemic stroke: implications for anaesthetic and critical care management. *Contin Educ Anaesth Crit Care Pain* 2013; 13(3): 80–6.

● Answer 7: b

There is NICE guidance in relation to this question.

In the case of a patient presenting with a STEMI (new LBBB does not feature as an ECG finding for STEMI within the NICE guidance), primary coronary intervention (PCI) should be offered to those presenting within 12 hours of symptom onset, if PCI can be delivered within 120 minutes. PCI should be considered if a patient presents more than 12 hours after onset of symptoms with continued myocardial ischaemia or cardiogenic shock (which are present in this clinical vignette).

Thrombolysis should be considered if presenting within 12 hours of symptom onset, and PCI is not possible within 120 minutes.

With regard to other drugs, all patients should be loaded with 300mg of aspirin. Glycoprotein IIb/IIIa inhibitors (e.g. tirofiban) or fibrinolytic drugs should not be given before PCI. If the patient is assessed to be not eligible for primary PCI or thrombolysis, then they should be given aspirin in combination with ticagrelor (or clopidogrel or aspirin alone, if there is a high bleeding risk). If treating a NSTEMI or unstable angina, fondaparinux should be given, unless going for angiography immediately. In this group of patients, undertake a GRACE score; if risk >3% (intermediate of high) then the recommendation is for angiography within 72 hours.

References

1. National Institute for Health and Care Excellence (NICE), guideline NG185. Acute coronary syndromes, 2020. Available at: https://www.nice.org.uk/guidance/ng185/resources/acute-coronary-syndromes-pdf-66142023361477.

● Answer 8: c

Historically, there are a number of classifications for acute kidney injury (AKI): RIFLE, AKIN, KDIGO 2012.

RIFLE:

- **R**: Risk. Creatinine (Cr) increased by 1.5x, urine output <0.5ml/kg/hr for 6 hours.
- **I**: Injury. Cr increased by 2x, urine output <0.5ml/kg/hr for 12 hours.
- **F**: Failure. Cr increased by 3x, urine output <0.3ml/kg/hr for 24 hours or anuric for 12 hours.
- **L**: Loss. Complete loss of renal function for >4 weeks.
- **E**: End-stage renal disease.

AKIN:

- 1: Cr increased by 1.5x, urine output <0.5ml/kg/hr for 6 hours.
- 2: Cr increased by 2x, urine output <0.5ml/kg/hr for 12 hours.
- 3: Cr increased by 3x, urine output <0.3ml/kg/hr for 24 hours or anuric for 12 hours.

If a patient needs CRRT, then it is classified as a stage 3.

KDIGO 2012 — this is the most up-to-date AKI classification system:

- Stage 1: Cr increase ≥26µmol/L within 48 hours or Cr rise ≥1.5–1.9x baseline and/or urine output <0.5ml/kg/hr for 6 consecutive hours. Avoid nephrotoxics, maintain normal haemodynamics, normoglycaemia and investigate the cause, e.g. renal tract ultrasound.
- Stage 2: Cr rise ≥2–2.9x baseline and/or urine output <0.5ml/kg/hr for 12 hours. Review medications and doses, consider CRRT.
- Stage 3: Cr rise ≥3x baseline or Cr increase ≥354µmol/L and/or initiated on CRRT (irrespective of stage at time of initiation) and/or urine output <0.3ml/kg/hr for 24 hours or anuria for 12 hours.

Effective initial management of AKI can be remembered with the acronym STOP-AKI:

- **S**epsis: a common cause of AKI. Follow local sepsis management protocols, e.g. the Sepsis-6 bundle (give oxygen, take blood cultures, give intravenous [IV] antibiotics, administer a fluid challenge, measure lactate, measure urine output).

- **T**oxins: review any medication and drug therapies. Stop/adjust/reduce dosage as appropriate. Common toxic medications include NSAIDs, gentamicin and iodine radiological contrast. Antihypertensive medications are not toxic per se, but often exacerbate AKI when already hypovolaemic, e.g. ACEis, ARBs. Other medications such as metformin can worsen AKI when a patient is dehydrated.
- **O**ptimise/obstruction: optimise blood pressure using IV fluids and vasopressors (if appropriate). Bladder scan (POCUS) the patient and exclude urinary retention, which is often a reversible cause of AKI. Consider further imaging including ultrasound and CT to exclude hydronephrosis and renal tract obstruction.
- **P**revention/post-**AKI** care: iodine radiological contrast should not be used unless the delays in emergency imaging outweigh the risk of contrast-induced nephropathy (see page 357, Paper 4, Q44 for more information). Plan post-AKI care to prevent recurrence and chronic kidney disease.

References

1. Kidney Disease: Improving Global Outcomes (KDIGO). KDIGO clinical practice guideline for acute kidney injury. Section 2: AKI definition. *Kidney Int* 2012; 2: 19–36.
2. Lopez J, Jorge S. The RIFLE and AKIN classifications for acute kidney injury: a critical and comprehensive review. *Clin Kidney J* 2013; 6(1): 8–14.

Answer 9: b

Knowledge of the intracranial pressure (ICP) trace and wave form interpretation is important (Figures 3.1 and 3.2). In health, P1 is the first and largest upstroke. It is caused by the percussion wave caused by arterial pressure. P2 is the tidal wave due to brain compliance — this is normally a small upstroke after a big downstroke from P1; if P2 exceeds P1, this is evidence of a reduction in brain compliance. P3 is the third small upstroke that represents the dicrotic wave from aortic valve closure.

Lundberg waves:

- A: plateau waves seen in patients with critical perfusion, reach 50–100mmHg and last 5–20 minutes — ALWAYS pathological.

- B: transient rises in ICP 20–30 above baseline in cycles of 0.5–2/min, can be seen in healthy individuals.
- C: not clinically relevant.

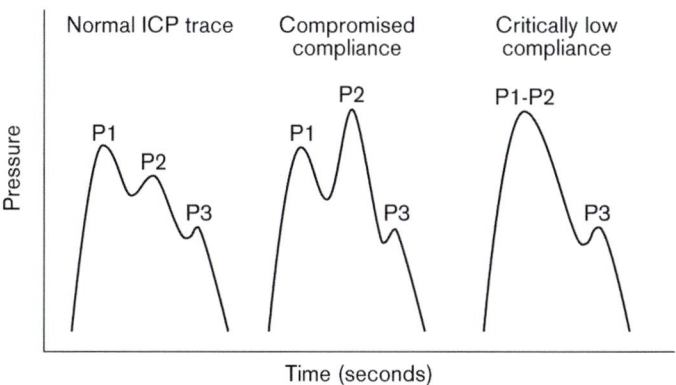

Figure 3.1. Normal and pathological intracranial pressure waveforms.

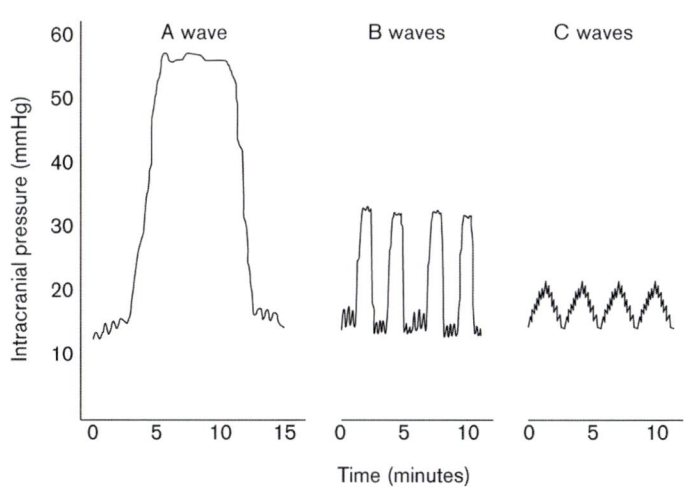

Figure 3.2. Lundberg intracranial pressure waves.

Normal brain tissue oxygenation (measured via a bolt) is 25–30mmHg, <20mmHg post-head injury, <5mmHg is associated with increased mortality; targeting >25mmHg may improve mortality.

Triple-lumen ICP bolts can have a microdialysis function to measure lactate, pyruvate and glucose. The LPR (lactate pyruvate ratio) can increase before ICP increases; normal is under 30 and above 30 is consistent with impaired cerebral oxidative metabolism and worse outcome.

Jugular bulb oximetry is the only advanced monitoring mentioned in the Brain Trauma Foundation (BTF) guidelines; a retrograde catheter (up the internal jugular vein [IJV]) is placed to sit in the dominant jugular bulb. The device measures global perfusion not localised perfusion (near-infrared spectroscopy or NIRS measures localised perfusion). BTF recommendations are to aim for an SjO_2 of over 50% to reduce mortality and improve outcomes.

References

1. Carney N, Totten AM, O'Reilly C, et al. Guidelines for the management of severe traumatic brain injury, 4th ed. Brain Trauma Foundation, 2016. Available at: https://static1.squarespace.com/static/63e696a90a26c23e4c021cee/t/640b5e97fa1ba a040e5c59af/1678466712870/Management_of_Severe_TBI_4th_Edition.pdf.
2. www.uptodate.com. Management of acute moderate and severe traumatic brain injury. UpToDate, 2024. Available at: https://www.uptodate.com/contents/management-of-acute-moderate-and-severe-traumatic-brain-injury.

Answer 10: d

This gentleman is at high risk of refeeding syndrome (three minor risk factors — see below).

With regard to refeeding syndrome, at risk patients have one major or two minor risk factors:

- Major: BMI <16, weight loss in the last 3–6 months >15%, 10 or more days without food, low Mg^{2+}, low K^+, low phosphate.
- Minor: BMI <18.5, weight loss in the last 3–6 months >10%, 5 or more days without food, alcohol abuse, diuretics, insulin, chemotherapy, proton pump inhibitors (PPIs).

There is no indication here to avoid nasogastric (NG) enteral feeding. The main reason to choose total parenteral nutrition (PN) initially would be a post-op surgical request. European guidelines (ESPEN) suggest PN should be started if EN is inadequate for 48 hours, whereas the American guidelines (ASPEN) recommend PN if EN is inadequate for 7–10 days. The definition of 'inadequate' is failure to provide over 60% of nutritional requirements. The EPaNIC study (2011) showed better survival with late PN in patients with malnutrition.

In almost all patients, aim to start nutrition within 24–48 hours of admission. Notable exceptions to starting to feed immediately would be in those having therapeutic hypothermia, and those patients on very high-dose vasopressors.

References
1. Casaer MP, Mesotten D, Hermans G, et al. Early versus late parenteral nutrition in critically il adults. *N Engl J Med* 2011; 365(6): 506–17.
2. Singer P, Blaser AR, Berger MM, et al. ESPEN practical and partially revised guideline: clinical nutrition in the intensive care unit. *Clin Nutr* 2023; 42(9): 1671–89.
3. Chowdry R, Lobez S. Nutrition in critical care. *BJA Educ* 2019; 19(3): 90–5.
4. Mehanna HM, Moledina J, Travis J, et al. Refeeding syndrome: what it is, and how to prevent and treat it. *BMJ* 2008; 336(7659): 1495–8.

● Answer 11: b

Caustic ingestion injury (strong acids and alkali) is normally accidental in paediatrics and intentional in adults.

Alkali ingestion may cause penetrating oesophageal injuries due to liquefaction necrosis, which can extend transmurally causing oesophageal perforation and mediastinitis. As alkalis are normally thick in consistency the injury tends to be limited to the oesophagus. If the alkaline substance does reach the stomach, it is partially neutralised by stomach acid. Damage typically occurs for 3–4 days following ingestion.

Acids typically cause pain on contact with the oropharynx, often stimulating both cough and a gag reflex, limiting the amount swallowed, but increasing risk of oropharynx and laryngeal injury. Acids are typically a thinner consistency hence once swallowed the acid passes directly into the stomach causing pylorospasm, often resulting in significant gastric injury. Generally, more superficial injury occurs than with alkalis.

Classification of caustic ingestion injury is as follows:

- 1st degree: superficial mucosal. Focal or diffuse erythema and oedema, lining sloughs off without scar formation.
- 2nd degree: into the submucosa. Ulceration followed by granulation resulting in scar formation and possible strictures.
- 3rd degree: transmural. Deep ulceration with perforation of the wall.

Complications of caustic injury include: bleeding in 3% (2–4 weeks post-ingestion), fistulisation, strictures of the oesophagus in up to a third of patients (steroids do not prevent strictures) and oesophageal squamous cell carcinoma (SCC) in 30%. Patients need long-term surveillance consisting of endoscopy every 2–3 years.

Management of caustic ingestion:

- Imaging with CT to assess for transmural damage and need for surgery.
- Endoscopy within 24 hours to guide management.
- Antimicrobials if there is presence of a perforation.
- No emetics or neutralising agents (can worsen injury and reaction also produces heat and thermal injury).
- Dilatation of stricture no earlier than 3 weeks post-injury.

References
1. www.uptodate.com. Caustic esophageal injury in adults. UpToDate, 2025. Available at: https://www.uptodate.com/contents/caustic-esophageal-injury-in-adults.

Answer 12: a
In patients with bronchopleural fistulas (BPFs) who are invasively ventilated, the volume of air leak is proportional to the mean airway pressure. Ventilation strategies should aim to reduce airway pressures to reduce leak fraction. Specific strategies include lower tidal volume (Vt) and PEEP (with permissive hypercapnia) or synchronized intermittent mandatory ventilation (SIMV) with a low set respiratory rate (RR).

SBA Paper 3: Answers

If the patient is able to, spontaneous ventilation with or without pressure support is often better than mandatory ventilation. The ideal is to liberate the patient from mechanical ventilation as soon as possible as this limits air leak even further.

The patient described seems appropriate for a trial of extubation. The slight increase in her FiO_2 requirement is likely due to an increase in the pneumothorax and air leak; this should improve once the patient is extubated. High-flow nasal oxygen (HFNO) once extubated will limit any positive pressure and therefore limit ongoing air leak.

References
1. www.uptodate.com. Management of persistent air leaks in patients on mechanical ventilation. UpToDate, 2024. Available at: https://www.uptodate.com/contents/management-of-persistent-air-leaks-in-patients-on-mechanical-ventilation.

Answer 13: b

This is a classic picture for Lemierre's syndrome — septic internal jugular vein (IJV) thrombophlebitis. It is a rare condition that tends to affect young adults with a slight male preponderance. Lemierre's syndrome typically starts with an oropharyngeal infection — most commonly tonsilitis, but it can also stem from other oral infections (dental) and sinusitis. Typically, around 1–3 weeks later, the infection spreads into the parapharyngeal space and you get thrombophlebitis of the IJV with or without associated clot. The carotid sheath can sometimes also be involved.

Pulmonary complications are common, such as necrotic cavitating lung lesions (due to septic emboli), pleural effusions, empyema, lung abscesses, pneumothorax and necrotising mediastinitis. Haematogenous spread to distant sites can also occur.

The causative bacteria are typically those from oral flora, most commonly the anaerobe *Fusobacterium necrophorum* (which can take over 5 days to grow in culture). Less common bacterial causes include *Enterobacteriaceae*, *Bacteroides*, *Streptococcus pyogenes* and Staphylococcal species.

References

1. Tiwari A. Lemierre's syndrome in the 21st century: a literature review. *Cureus* 2023; 15(8): e43685.

Answer 14: c

Traumatic cardiac arrest is considered a special cause of arrest within UK and European Advanced Life Support (ALS) guidance. If the cause of the cardiac arrest (despite it being a trauma patient) is likely to be non-traumatic in origin, then standard ALS algorithms should be followed with a focus on CPR and identifying the underlying cardiac rhythm.

In traumatic cardiac arrest, resuscitation should focus on the immediate simultaneous treatment of reversible cardiac arrest causes (4Hs and 4Ts) relevant to trauma. These are primarily hypoxia, hypovolaemia, tension pneumothorax and cardiac tamponade (with hypothermia, hypokalaemia/hyperkalaemia, thromboembolism and toxins less likely to be the cause). In the context of severe hypovolaemia, CPR can be done, but this should not impede management of the bleeding and administration of blood given the importance of an effective preload.

In this patient there is no evidence in the primary survey or history to suspect anything other than hypovolaemia. The patient is very shut down and so further attempts at peripheral intravenous (IV) access are unlikely to be successful. Intraosseous (IO) access will often be established quickly but rapid infusions can be difficult. The best option here is to insert an IO needle and begin to bolus blood, whilst simultaneously setting up and inserting a central venous (CVC) line to facilitate more rapid administration of blood. In a patient this shut down, insertion of a CVC line would be much more difficult with ongoing CPR and so stopping or not starting CPR until the CVC line is inserted would seem reasonable. Intubation and ventilation is also a priority but given the patient was breathing via a non-rebreathe mask prior to cardiac arrest, hypoxia is unlikely to be the primary cause of the arrest. In reality, interventions often occur simultaneously.

References

1. Lott C, Truhlář A, Alfonzo A, *et al*. European Resuscitation Council guidelines 2021: cardiac arrest in special circumstances. *Resuscitation* 2021; 161: 152–219.

Answer 15: b

Patients with pulmonary hypertension (PH) are very preload-sensitive and have the potential to deteriorate if they are underfilled or overloaded, with a very narrow fluid balance margin. Common causes of deterioration in PH patients are cardiac arrhythmias and sepsis. Patients with precapillary PH (for definitions of PH see page 175, Paper 2, Q47), are prone to developing atrial flutter which may have a slower rate than seen in conventional patients (i.e. a HR of 150/min) and is associated with a worse outcome. In this scenario, cardioversion should be prioritised over rate control. Suspected sepsis should be treated with early broad-spectrum antibiotics.

Management of patients with PH should begin with treatment of the precipitating factor (in this case sepsis, but it could be anaemia, venous thromboembolism [VTE], arrhythmia, etc.).

The subsequent aim should be to optimise right ventricular (RV) preload, with assessment of filling and fluid balance. Treatment may include either IV fluid boluses or diuretics. In this case, the patient seems optimally filled, with no evidence of fluid overload. Once preload has been optimised, the next step is to reduce RV afterload; this is primarily done using prostanoids (e.g. iloprost), endothelin receptor antagonists (e.g. bosentan) and drugs that act on the nitric oxide (NO) pathway (e.g. sildenafil). This patient is already on an iloprost infusion at a reasonable rate. Stopping this would improve their BP, but may risk decompensating the RV, so would not be advised as there are other options available for managing the hypotension.

Once RV afterload is optimised, and if the patient is still hypotensive, then you would aim to maintain perfusion pressures with vasopressors such as noradrenaline (known to be effective in patients with PH). Vasopressin can be added in addition, if the patient remains hypotensive despite noradrenaline. Although noradrenaline's action via α1-agonist effects may increase pulmonary vascular resistance, the β1-agonism appears to improve coupling between RV function and afterload. This patient has a low systemic vascular resistance index (SVRI), which would imply that the hypotension could be improved with vasopressors and would fit with the clinical diagnosis of sepsis.

If the patient is still hypotensive with poor perfusion despite all the above measures, the next step in management would be to improve RV contractility using dobutamine or milrinone.

In this patient, the lithium dilution cardiac output (LiDCO) readings show that cardiac output is reasonable, and so starting noradrenaline would be the best answer in this clinical scenario.

References
1. Condliffe R, Kiely D. Critical care management of pulmonary hypertension. *BJA Educ* 2017; 17(7): 228–34.

Answer 16: a

The management of an out-of-hospital cardiac arrest (OOHCA) patient after return of spontaneous circulation (ROSC) is laid out in guidelines, written by the Resuscitation Council UK and European Resuscitation Council. Following ROSC, the focus is on cardiorespiratory stability and identification of the cause of the arrest, so that specific treatments to prevent rearrest can be employed along with prevention of secondary brain injury.

Assessment and post-arrest management is undertaken in an A–E approach; the initial priority should be on securing an airway if the patient is not protecting their own airway. Ventilation should aim for oxygen saturations of 94–98% and a PaO_2 of 10–13kPa, and a $PaCO_2$ of 4.5–6kPa (ensuring a lung-protective ventilation strategy).

The management of circulation should include aiming for a MAP >65mmHg, using fluid IV challenges and vasopressors as required, insertion of an arterial line and establishing multiple IV access sites. Aim for a urine output of >0.5ml/kg/hr with a normal or decreasing lactate. Any seizures should be treated with IV levetiracetam (Keppra®) or sodium valproate. Temperature should be kept <37.7°C for the first 72 hours, and 32–36°C for at least the first 24 hours. In this case, the cause is a STEMI and so the patient should go urgently to the cardiac catheter lab for primary PCI.

In the scenario, all of the interventions listed are reasonable but there is no current indication for additional fluid therapy. The most urgent initial intervention is intubation and ventilation, as the patient is not currently awake enough to protect their own airway and they are not ventilating adequately for secondary neuroprotection.

References
1. Nolan JP, Deakin CD, Soar J, *et al.* Post-resuscitation care guidelines. Resus Council UK, updated July 2023. Available at: https://www.resus.org.uk/library/2021-resuscitation-guidelines/post-resuscitation-care-guidelines.
2. Perkins GD, Graesner J-T, Semeraro F, *et al.* European Resuscitation Council guidelines 2021: executive summary. *Resuscitation* 2021; 161: 1–60.

Answer 17: c

Identification of sepsis in a burns patient can be challenging. The most common organisms causing burn wound infections are *Staphylococcus* and *Pseudomonas*. There are likely to be local variations, so it is always important to manage these patients with input from hospital microbiology teams.

Burns patients are hypermetabolic; this means that their normal temperature runs between 37–38°C, and as such a temperature below 36.5°C or above 39°C would be concerning for sepsis.

Other signs of sepsis can include: tachycardia, tachypnoea, hypotension, oliguria, unexplained hyperglycaemia, thrombocytopaenia, and mental status change, as well as patients who were previously absorbing enteral feed no longer absorbing (e.g. with high residual volumes, abdominal distention, diarrhoea).

The clinical signs within the scenario suggest possible sepsis from wound infection; this should be investigated initially with a full set of cultures. If the patient was to deteriorate further then empirical antibiotics can be commenced, but as burns patients are at high risk of colonisation it is prudent (if safe) to identify the infecting organism first to allow for narrower-spectrum antibiotic treatment.

References
1. www.uptodate.com. Burn wound infection and sepsis. UpToDate, 2025.. Available at: https://www.uptodate.com/contents/burn-wound-infection-and-sepsis.

Answer 18: e

Amniotic fluid embolism (AFE) is a very serious, but thankfully rare, complication of pregnancy with significant morbidity and mortality. The mortality rate reported is variable but is likely to be between 20 and 50%. Between 2019 and 2021 in the UK, 8 women died of AFE which represents a rate of 0.39 for every 100,000 pregnancies.

No definite risk factors have been identified, but it is thought there is an association with C-section, instrumental vaginal delivery, augmentation of labour, pre-eclampsia and placental abnormalities such as placenta previa. In the main, AFE occurs during labour and delivery and up to 30 minutes postpartum, with the majority occurring during labour. It is thought that entry of amniotic fluid (containing foetal cells) into the maternal circulation leads to abnormal activation of the immune system, along with abnormal activation of clotting leading to disseminated intravascular coagulation (DIC).

AFE presents suddenly in the vast majority of patients with severe cardiorespiratory compromise (hypotension, hypoxia, tachypnoea) and/or cardiac arrest. There may be a short prodrome with the patient feeling anxious and having an impending 'sense of doom'. If the patient survives the initial cardiorespiratory event, they may go on to develop non-cardiogenic pulmonary oedema. The development of DIC is almost ubiquitous in patients who survive the initial phase and can result in major peripartum and postpartum haemorrhage. There will be foetal distress in all cases, meaning delivery of the foetus will need to be prioritised for both mother and baby.

There is no specific management for AFE, so focus is on resuscitation and management of any haemorrhage. Delivery should occur rapidly and ideally where the patient is (often not in theatre) to aid in maternal resuscitation. Tranexamic acid can be given in the context of haemorrhage and early activation of the major haemorrhage protocol is advised. In the context of a patient likely to need operative intervention (C-section or instrumental delivery) then management of coagulopathy by transfusion of products is advised. Give platelets if the level is <50 x 10^9/L, fresh frozen plasma (FFP) if the INR is deranged and cryoprecipitate or fibrinogen concentrates if the patient's fibrinogen is <2g/L.

References

1. www.uptodate.com. Amniotic fluid embolism. UpToDate, 2025. Available at: https://www.uptodate.com/contents/amniotic-fluid-embolism.

2. Metodiev Y, Ramasamy P, Tuffnell D. Amniotic fluid embolism. *BJA Educ* 2018; 18(8): 234–8.
3. MBRRACE-UK: mothers and babies: reducing risk through audits and confidential enquiries across the UK. Maternal, newborn and infant clinical outcome review programme. Saving lives, improving mothers' care. Lessons learned to inform maternity care from the UK and Ireland Confidential Enquiries into Maternal Deaths and Morbidity 2019–21. National Perinatal Epidemiology Unit, 2023. Available at: https://www.npeu.ox.ac.uk/assets/downloads/mbrrace-uk/reports/maternal-report-2023/MBRRACE-UK_Maternal_Compiled_Report_2023.pdf.

● Answer 19: d

The definition and management options for abdominal compartment syndrome (ACS) are available on page 165, Paper 2, Q38.

When deciding optimal management of ACS, there needs to be consideration of the following factors: what if there is any organ dysfunction as a result, the underlying disease process and any reversibility, the measured pressure and trends (sudden or gradual increase).

In this patient there is renal impairment, likely because of the raised intra-abdominal pressure; there is nothing in the history to suspect the patient is septic. Management therefore needs to result in better renal perfusion; although the other measures may reduce the IAP they are unlikely to significantly reduce it. Currently, the abdominal perfusion pressure (APP = MAP − IAP) is only 44mmHg, and guidance is that this should be 50–60mmHg; therefore, starting noradrenaline to aim for a MAP of around 80mmHg would be appropriate.

The patient's underlying pathology is that of pancreatitis. The CT showed fluid around the pancreas but not a focal collection that could be drained. It may be that with some more time this fluid becomes organised and then drainage would be possible, which would help reduce the IAP. Prokinetics may help, although the volumes on aspirates do not meet the threshold for prokinetic use as per the ESPEN guidelines. Stopping the NG feed may result in a marginal improvement in IAP, but this is not a longer-term solution, and nutrition is vital to recovery.

This patient is awake and self-ventilating, therefore measurement of the IAP may not be completely accurate, as any patient instigated increases in abdominal muscle tone will elevate the IAP. However, there is organ impairment likely as a result of high IAP, and measures should be undertaken to reduce this. As the patient is awake and weaning, the use of paralysis agents would not be the first choice as this would require sedation and impair ventilator weaning. Sedation and a muscle relaxant may be needed if all other measures to reduce the IAP fail, and the renal function is continuing to deteriorate.

References

1. De Laet IE, Malbrain MLNG, De Waele JJ. A clinician's guide to management of intra-abdominal hypertension and abdominal compartment syndrome in critically ill patients. *Crit Care* 2020; 24(1): 97.
2. Singer P, Blaser AR, Berger MM, *et al.* ESPEN guideline on clinical nutrition in the intensive care unit. *Clin Nutr* 2019; 38(1): 48–79.

Answer 20: c

Metformin toxicity is relatively unusual but is associated with high mortality and morbidity. Metformin is a commonly used drug for the treatment of type 2 diabetes and can be used for other indications. It is a biguanide which acts to decrease insulin resistance, hepatic glucose release and enhances peripheral glucose uptake. At toxic levels it induces cellular hypoxia and inhibits the mitochondrial transport chain, which means there is a bottleneck to the Krebs cycle outflow and the pathway from pyruvate downwards becomes saturated; therefore, there is preferential conversion of pyruvate to lactate with subsequent elevated lactate levels.

Lactic acidosis in a patient on metformin was classically referred to as metformin-associated lactic acidosis or MALA; however, more recently there have been further sub-categorisations which help to inform treatments:

- MILA: metformin-induced lactic acidosis is where high metformin levels are the primary cause of illness (and if levels were taken these would be very high). This could either be due to overdose of metformin, or accumulation of metformin due to renal failure (metformin is renally cleared). If there is an acute increase in metformin, these patients can become profoundly unwell, with lactates typically over 15mmol/L. If a slower build-up, then the patient may be relatively stable with some compensation.

SBA Paper 3: Answers

- MALA: metformin-associated lactic acidosis. This can be the umbrella term for all, but when subdivided it refers to patients who are on metformin long term, who develop an acute life-threatening illness such as sepsis, and metformin amplifies the degree of lactic acidosis, but is not the only cause of high lactate. If measured, the metformin levels would be elevated.
- MULA: metformin-unrelated lactic acidosis. Metformin levels are low. Differentiation from MALA is only by measurement of metformin levels, which are not widely available.

Management of patients with MILA (and some MALA) is with standard resuscitation initially with IV crystalloid fluids. If the lactate does not fall with fluids alone, then additional treatments may be required. The use of bicarbonate is controversial (due to an association with increased mortality) but is advised by Toxbase if acidosis persists, despite correction of hypoxia and fluid resuscitation. The treatment of choice for severe metformin toxicity is intermittent haemodialysis (IHD) (there is better clearance of metformin with IHD as compared to CRRT). The indications for IHD are a lactate >20mmol/L, pH ≤7.0 or a failure to improve with supportive care within 2–4 hours.

Rescue treatments include methylene blue and the standard insulin sliding scale (not high-dose therapy). These are not routinely recommended and are only used when all other treatments have failed and in consultation with toxicology experts.

References

1. Lalau J-D, Kajbaf F, Protti A, et al. Metformin-associated lactic acidosis (MALA): moving towards a new paradigm. *Diabetes Obes Metab* 2017; 19: 1502–2.
2. Rivera D, Onisko N, James Cao JD, et al. High risk and low prevalence diseases: metformin toxicities. *Am J Emerg Med* 2023; 72: 107–12.
3. www.uptodate.com. Metformin poisoning and toxicity. UpToDate, 2025. Available at: https://www.uptodate.com/contents/metformin-poisoning.
4. Toxbase.org. TOXBASE — the primary clinical toxicology database of the National Poisons Information Service. Poisons-index-A-Z/m-products/metformin. Available at: https://www.toxbase.org.
5. About EMCrit. Metformin toxicity — EMCrit Project. Internet book of critical care (IBCC), 2015. Available at: https://emcrit.org/ibcc/metformin/.
6. Goonoo MS, Morris R, Raithatha A, Creagh F. Metformin-associated lactic acidosis: reinforcing learning points. *BMJ Case Rep* 2020; 13(9): e235608. Corrected and republished in: *Drug Ther Bull* 2021; 59(8): 124–7.

● Answer 21: d

A patient is deprived of their liberty if they are not free to leave somewhere (in this case the hospital/ward) and are under constant supervision. They are not in a position to give consent for this situation either due to their condition or because of medications given.

If a patient is being kept in hospital against their will (for example, a patient with delirium who is wanting to leave, but does not have capacity and would be a risk to themselves if they left) and measures are being put in place to prevent them leaving, above and beyond talking them down, e.g. sedative medication, then a Mental Capacity Act Liberty Protection Safeguards form should be filled in (formally known as DOLS). This is also the case if a family member is wanting to remove their relative who lacks capacity, and this act would lead to patient harm.

The exception to a formal legal authority for this, is when a patient is on the ICU. The courts, up to and including the Supreme Court, have made it clear that necessary life-sustaining medical treatment means that although the patient cannot leave, this is not depriving them of their liberty as they are at immediate risk of dying anywhere other than the hospital, and the treatment they are receiving is the same as if the patient were able to consent.

References

1. Keene A, Troke B, on behalf of the Legal and Ethical Policy Unit. Midnight law: deprivation of liberty in intensive care. The Faculty of Intensive Care Medicine, 2021. Available at: https://ficm.ac.uk/midnightlaws.
2. Department of Health and Social Care. Guidance Liberty Protection Safeguards: what they are, 2021. Available at: https://www.gov.uk/government/publications/liberty-protection-safeguards-factsheets/liberty-protection-safeguards-what-they-are.

● Answer 22: d

The initial part of the ALS algorithm is slightly different for children as compared to adults, to reflect the fact that hypoxia is by far the leading course of cardiac arrest in children.

The European Paediatric Advanced Life Support (EPALS) has an algorithm for the management of a collapsed child. When alerted to a collapsed child, approach (ensuring your own personal safety), attempt to stimulate the child (with verbal and tactile stimulus — never shaking the child); if there is no response then shout for help and if in hospital, this would also involve putting out a cardiac arrest call.

Proceed to A — airway — assess if the patient is breathing by opening the airway and listening and looking for spontaneous breaths. In an infant (up to 1-year-old) this is with the neutral head position and in a child (over 1 year) with the 'sniffing the morning air' position. If there is no respiratory effort deliver 5 rescue breaths. These breaths must be 5 effective rescue breaths that result in good chest rise. After you have delivered the rescue breaths, if there are still no signs of life then start CPR at a rate of 15 compressions to 2 breaths. Once you have a cardiac rhythm monitor on (typically using pads and a defibrillator), you would then assess the rhythm and follow the EPALS algorithm. Feeling of a pulse is not specifically mentioned, but this can be done during the assessment of breathing.

References
1. Resus Council UK. European Paediatric Advanced Life Support, 5th ed. Resuscitation Council UK, 2021.

Answer 23: a

Haemoglobin in adults is predominantly formed of two alpha and two beta chains surrounding a haem group which has a porphyrin ring and a ferrous atom. This is known as HbA and makes up around 97% of adult haemoglobin. Once the first oxygen binds there is a conformational change in the haemoglobin, which allows the binding of three further oxygen atoms. HbF is the predominate haemoglobin in the foetal blood and consists of two alpha and two gamma chains. This has a higher affinity for oxygen than HbA so has a left-shifted oxygen dissociation curve.

There are many different haemoglobinopathies. Thalassaemia is due to mutations in either the alpha or the beta chain and can be classified based on this; alpha thalassaemia with impaired production of alpha chains due to gene deletions, and beta thalassaemia with mutations in the beta chains. Beta thalassaemia can then be subclassified based on whether the patient is 'transfusion-dependent' or not. There are four genes responsible for the alpha chain, and the severity is dependent on the number of genes affected; when all four genes are affected this results in hydrops fetalis which is not compatible with life.

Sickle cell haemoglobin (HbS) results from a single base mutation in the gene for beta chain production, resulting in a substitution of valine for glutamic acid. If the patient only has one abnormal gene, they have sickle cell trait (HbAS); if both are abnormal they have sickle cell anaemia (HbSS). As foetal haemoglobin has no beta chains, patients are often asymptomatic until around 6 months of age when the HbF levels drop to adult levels. HbS molecules result in a decrease in red blood flexibility and on exposure to certain precipitants (e.g. cold, infection, dehydration, acidosis, hypoxia) they will become rigid, and sickle-shaped, resulting in a painful sickle cell crisis. Longer term with repeated sickling, the cells are unable to return to a normal shape, resulting in anaemia from chronic haemolysis and long-term problems from repeated vaso-occlusive crises.

References
1. Murphy M, Pasi J, Roy N. Haematology. In: Kumar P, Clark M, Eds. *Kumar and Clark's clinical medicine*, 10th ed. London: Elsevier; 2020: chapter 16: pp. 320–78.

● Answer 24: e

Phosphate is vital to many processes within the body, and it makes up around 1% of total body weight. Phosphate homeostasis is tied in with calcium and is controlled by a number of factors including vitamin D, parathyroid hormone and calcitonin. Around 90% of the phosphate in the body is found in the bone. It is a vital constituent of ATP, cAMP, 2,3-diphosphoglycerate (DPG) and phospholipids among others and is involved in a vast array of physiological functions.

It is intrinsic to bone mineralisation and tooth structure.

ATP is the immediate source of cellular energy; by losing one phosphate group to form ADP (adenosine diphosphate), energy is released. ATP is then replenished via the Krebs cycle (into the electron transport chain and oxidative phosphorylation) and the anaerobic pathway (pyruvate to lactate).

In the form of 2,3-DPG it binds to the beta chains of haemoglobin, altering the conformation to reduce oxygen affinity and help to offload oxygen. Therefore,

SBA Paper 3: Answers

increasing 2,3-DPG levels causes a right shift in the oxygen dissociation curve (increased production in anaemia and high-altitude exposure).

One of the mechanisms of acid-base homeostasis is through buffering, and phosphate in the form of phosphoric acid (which has three base forms) and biphosphate acts as one of the buffers in blood, with the base monohydrogen phosphate acting as an important buffer within the urine.

References

1. Qadeer HA, Bashir K. Physiology, phosphate. StatPearls [Internet]; 2023. Available at: https://www.ncbi.nlm.nih.gov/books/NBK560925/.
2. Power I, Kam P. Respiratory physiology. In: Power I, Kam P, Eds. *Principles of physiology for the anaesthetist,* 2nd ed. London: Hodder Arnold; 2008: chapter 3: pp. 75–116.
3. Power I, Kam P. Acid-base physiology. In: Power I, Kam P, Eds. *Principles of physiology for the anaesthetist,* 2nd ed. London: Hodder Arnold; 2008: chapter 8: pp. 251–68.
4. Webster NR, Strachan D. Metabolic disorders: electrolyte disorders. In: Waldmann C, Rhodes A, Soni N, Handy J, Eds. *Oxford desk reference: critical care*, 2nd ed. Oxford: Oxford University Press; 2019: chapter 25: pp. 452–6.

● Answer 25: b

ICU-acquired weakness can be categorised as critical illness myopathy (CIM), critical illness polyneuropathy (CIP) or a combination of both. It is weakness that is a result of the intensive care illness and treatment, with no other neurological diagnosis to explain it.

With regard to risk factors, those that have been found in studies include: multi-organ failure, high Apache II score, lactate >2, use of noradrenaline, longer length of ICU stay (>7 days), longer periods of ventilation, use of neuromuscular blockade (aside from initial induction), status asthmaticus and liver transplantation. It was previously postulated that there was a link between glucocorticoid use and CIM; more recently, however, this is now not felt to be as big a risk factor as previously thought.

Studies have shown that if a patient is obese prior to ICU admission, this confers an ICU mortality benefit with less muscle mass loss and weakness.

References

1. Yang T, Li Z, Jiang L, Xi X. Hyperlactacidemia as a risk factor for intensive care unit-acquired weakness in critically ill adult patients. *Muscle Nerve* 2021; 64(1): 77–82.

2. Goossens C, Marques MB, Derde S, et al. Premorbid obesity, but not nutrition, prevents critical illness-induced muscle wasting and weakness. *J Cachexia Sarcopenia Muscle* 2017; 8(1): 89–101.
3. www.uptodate.com. Neuromuscular weakness related to critical illness. UpToDate, 2023. Available at: https://www.uptodate.com/contents/neuromuscular-weakness-related-to-critical-illness.

Answer 26: e

In 2023, the Infectious Diseases Society of America released an updated version of the Modified Duke Criteria for the diagnosis of infective endocarditis (IE), to reflect clinical changes in the recognition, causes and management of IE. Of note, intracardiac implantable electronic devices (CIED) now represent around 10% of cases of IE, and there has been a rise in the insertion of transcutaneous catheter-inserted valves. Several new bacteria have been added to the list of typical microorganisms.

The Duke criteria are divided into definite, possible and rejected IE.

Within definite there are pathological criteria which are based on either postmortem examination findings of the heart or examination of tissue/devices removed during an operation (typically valves — native or prosthetic, implantable devices, arterial thrombus, cardiac tissue).

The clinical criteria for definite and possible remain as major and minor criteria, with:

- Definite IE diagnosis when there is the presence of: 2 major, 1 major and 3 minor or 5 minor.
- Possible IE is the presence of: 1 major and 1 minor or 3 minor.
- Rejected IE is the presence of: a firm alternative diagnosis, lack of recurrence despite less than 4 days of antibiotics, no pathological evidence at surgery or autopsy (with <4 days antibiotics), and does not meet the criteria for possible IE.

Major criteria are as follows:

- Microbiological: positive blood cultures (microorganisms that commonly cause IE from two or more cultures, microorganisms that

occasionally/rarely cause IE from three or more cultures); positive PCR or equivalent for certain bacteria, *Coxiella burnetii* IgG isolated from one blood culture, IgM and IgG detected for *Bartonella*.
- Imaging: ECHO and/or CT showing vegetation, valve/leaflet perforation, abscess, pseudoaneurysm of intracardiac fistula; significant new valvular regurgitation on ECHO (compared to a previous ECHO); partial dehiscence of prosthetic valve compared to previous imaging; PET imaging showing abnormal metabolic activity on valve, aortic graft or implanted cardiac device.
- Surgical: evidence of IE on direct inspection of valve during heart surgery if imaging or further microbiological samples are not available.

Minor criteria are as follows:

- Predisposition: prior history of IE, prosthetic valve, previous valve repair, congenital heart disease, presence of moderate/severe regurgitation/stenosis, CIED, hypertrophic obstructive cardiomyopathy (HOCM), IV drug use.
- Fever: documented temperature >38°C.
- Vascular phenomena: clinical/radiological evidence of arterial emboli, pulmonary infarcts, brain/splenic abscess, mycotic aneurysm, intracranial haemorrhage, Janeway lesions, purulent purpura.
- Immune: +ve rheumatoid factor, Osler nodes, Roth spots, immune complex-mediated glomerulonephritis.
- Microbiological: positive blood culture but falling short of major criterion. Organism consistent with IE from sterile body site (not cardiac), single finding of skin bacteria by PCR on valve/wire with additional positive microbiology.
- Imaging: abnormal metabolic activity on PET scan within 3 months of implantation of prosthesis.
- Physical examination: new regurgitation on auscultation if ECHO not available.

References

1. Fowler VG, Durack DT, Selton-Suty C, *et al*. The 2023 Duke-International Society for Cardiovascular Infectious Diseases criteria for infective endocarditis: updating the Modified Duke Criteria. *Clin Infect Dis* 2023; 77(4): 518–26.

● Answer 27: a

The UK government has clear guidance on personal protective equipment (PPE) requirements when caring for someone with suspected or confirmed acute respiratory infection:

- Disposable gloves should be worn if there is likely to be contact with blood or bodily fluids; single use and type (sterile/non-sterile) appropriate to the task. They must be worn for aerosol-generating procedures (AGPs).
- A disposable apron should be worn if there is likely to be contact with blood or bodily fluids and must be worn if undertaking AGPs.
- A disposable fluid-repellent gown is only worn if there is likely to be extensive exposure to blood or bodily fluid. They should not be used as a default.
- Surgical face mask; wear for all interactions aside from AGPs.
- FFP3 mask; wear a fit-tested FFP3 mask when undertaking AGPs.
- Eye/face protection should be worn for all patient interactions; either as single or sessional use.

For PPE requirements for specific infections, refer to local trust and hospital guidance.

References

1. GOV.UK. PPE requirements when caring for a person with suspected or confirmed acute respiratory infection (ARI): text equivalent of poster. Available at: https://www.gov.uk/government/publications/infection-prevention-and-control-in-adult-social-care-acute-respiratory-infection/ppe-requirements-when-caring-for-a-person-with-suspected-or-confirmed-acute-respiratory-infection-ari-text-equivalent-of-poster.

● Answer 28: d

The West Haven grading for hepatic encephalopathy (HE) is widely used, and is the system used in a number of other scoring systems such as CLIF-SOFA and Child-Pugh.

The grading system is minimal followed by grades 1–4:

- Minimal: psychomotor testing reveals impaired processing speed and executive functioning. No conscious level impairment.
- Grade 1: shortened attention span, anxiety, mild confusion, disturbed sleep.
- Grade 2: lethargy, moderate confusion, inappropriate behaviour, lethargy/apathy.
- Grade 3: marked confusion, responsive to voice, very disorientated, strange behaviour.
- Grade 4: comatose and unresponsive to pain.

It is thought that this grading system may be difficult to assess clinically and there is an alternative classification of unimpaired, covert and overt hepatic encephalopathy proposed by ISHEN (International Society for Hepatic Encephalopathy and Nitrogen Metabolism). Unimpaired represents a patient with no HE, covert would be minimal and grade 1, and overt would be grades 2–4.

References
1. Weissenborn K. Hepatic encephalopathy: definition, clinical grading and diagnostic principles. *Drugs* 2019; 79(S1): 5–9.

Answer 29: d

Atrial fibrillation (AF) is the most commonly occurring arrhythmia in critical care. The incidence is around 13–14% for patients without a history of persistent or permanent AF. For some patients the AF is limited to their critical illness, but others will go on to develop permanent or persistent AF. An understanding of how to anticoagulate these patients once they are no longer critically ill is important.

NICE provides guidance on the management of anticoagulation in AF. Assessment of stroke and bleeding risks should be made in all patients with paroxysmal, persistent or permanent AF.

The CHA_2DS_2-VASc score should be calculated to assess stroke risk and the ORBIT bleeding risk score to assess bleeding risk. An ECHO should be undertaken to assess valvular function and help guide rate and rhythm control decisions.

Anticoagulation with a direct oral anticoagulant (DOAC) should be prescribed for those with a CHA_2DS_2-VASc score of over 2, or over 1 for men, considering their bleeding risk. If a DOAC is not tolerated or suitable then warfarin is advised. No treatment should be offered to people under the age of 65 with no risk factors, other than their sex (score of 0 for men and 1 for women). Aspirin as a monotherapy is not recommended for the prevention of stroke in patients with AF.

With regards to rate vs. rhythm control in AF, the guidance is to offer rate control as a first-line strategy for AF except in the following groups: AF has a reversible cause, heart failure primarily due to AF, new-onset AF, atrial flutter whose condition is considered suitable for ablation, and when rhythm control is more suitable based on clinical judgement. Rhythm control is often targeted for patients with new-onset AF in the ICU, who normally have a reversible cause such as sepsis. Rhythm control treatments include fluid boluses, IV magnesium, potassium replacement, digoxin, amiodarone and electrical cardioversion. New-onset AF lasting over 30 minutes is associated with an increased hospital mortality.

References

1. National Institute for Heath and Care Excellence (NICE), guideline NG196. Atrial fibrillation: diagnosis and management NICE guideline, 2021. Available at: https://www.nice.org.uk/guidance/ng196/resources/atrial-fibrillation-diagnosis-and-management-pdf-66142085507269.
2. Wetterslev M, Møller MH, Granholm A, *et al.* Atrial fibrillation (AFIB) in the ICU: incidence, risk factors, and outcomes: the International AFIB-ICU cohort study. *Crit Care Med* 2023; 51(9): 1124–37.
3. Bedford JP, Gerry S, Hatch RA, *et al.* Hospital outcomes associated with new-onset atrial fibrillation during ICU admission: a multicentre competing risks analysis. *J Crit Care* 2020; 60: 72–8.

● Answer 30: b

Broad complex tachycardias (QRS width is over 120ms) can be due to ventricular tachycardia (VT), SVT with bundle branch block, Wolff-Parkinson-White (WPW) syndrome or AF with either a bundle branch block or WPW.

There are a number of features that are suggestive of VT as the cause:

SBA Paper 3: Answers

- Very broad complex (QRS >160ms).
- Presence of p waves at a slower rate than the QRS complexes (AV dissociation).
- Regular rhythm (if irregular this points towards AF with aberrant conduction).
- Capture beats (normal QRS width beat as atrial beat has managed to go down the normal pathway).
- Fusion beats (sinus and VT beat coincide to produce an intermediate morphology complex).
- RSR complexes with taller left R wave (if right R wave taller this is likely to show SVT with RBBB).
- Concordance throughout the chest leads (all QRS are positive or negative).

There is also the Brugada algorithm which can be used to distinguish between VT and SVT in more difficult cases.

Whilst it is important to be able to work out the likely underlying rhythm, if a patient is unstable, this should not delay treatment. In this case, there is the presence of adverse features, and the patient is unstable warranting immediate cardioversion.

References

1. Burns E, Buttner R. Ventricular tachycardia — monomorphic VT. Life in the fast lane (LITFL); 2024. Available at: https://litfl.com/ventricular-tachycardia-monomorphic-ecg-library/.
2. Hampton J, Adlam D. The ECG in patients with palpitations and syncope. In: Hampton J, Adlam D, Eds. *The ECG in practice*, 5th ed. London: Elsevier; 2008: chapter 2: pp. 54–160.

Answer 31: a

A transfusion trigger of 70g/L is now standard for most conditions in the ICU. The landmark study on lower triggers was TRICC published in 1999. This study looked at using a trigger of <100g/L (aiming for 100–120g/L) vs. <70g/L (aiming for 70–90g/L) in ICU patients (excluding chronic anaemia, active blood loss and post-cardiac surgery). Overall, it showed non-inferiority with the restrictive group with a trend towards improved mortality for those <55 years old with APACHE II <30, and similar mortality in the groups with known cardiac disease.

Villanueva investigated transfusion triggers in patients with an acute upper GI bleed, comparing a threshold of 70g/L (aiming for 70–90g/L) to 90g/L (aiming for 90–110g/L). This showed that mortality was significantly reduced in the restrictive group. This was a single-centre study, in which all patients had an upper GI endoscopy within 6 hours, which is not standard practice in all centres.

The TRISS study (2014) looked at red cell transfusion thresholds in patients with septic shock, comparing 70g/L to 90g/L. The definition of septic shock was based on 1991 criteria (infection with SIRS, hypotension resistant to fluid resuscitation and organ dysfunction). This trial showed no significant difference in mortality or secondary outcomes between the groups; on subgroup analysis there was no significant difference in outcome in patients with cardiovascular disease.

The REALITY study (2021) investigated transfusion thresholds of 80g/L (target 80–100g/L) vs. 100g/L (target >110g/L post-transfusion) in patients with acute MI. The trial group had initially planned for 70g/L vs. 100g/L but changed it prior to recruitment of the first patient to maximise investigator adherence to the protocol. The results showed non-inferiority with a restrictive threshold with a trend towards better outcomes.

The HEMOTION study (2024) investigated thresholds of 70g/L vs. 100g/L in patients with moderate or severe traumatic brain injury (TBI). There was no statistically significant difference in outcomes between the groups so non-inferiority of the lower threshold. The study was powered to detect a difference of 10% in unfavourable outcomes; there was a 5.4% difference which may be significant, but it was not powered to detect this.

References

1. Hébert PC, Wells G, Blajchman MA, et al. A multicenter, randomized, controlled clinical trial of transfusion requirements in critical care. Transfusion Requirements in Critical Care Investigators, Canadian Critical Care Trials Group. N Engl J Med 1999; 340(6): 409–17.
2. Villanueva C, Colomo A, Bosch A, et al. Transfusion strategies for acute upper gastrointestinal bleeding. N Engl J Med 2013; 368(1): 11–21.
3. Holst LB, Haase N, Wetterslev J, et al. Lower versus higher hemoglobin threshold for transfusion in septic shock. N Engl J Med 2014; 371(15): 1381–91.
4. Ducrocq G, Gonzalez-Juanatey JR, Puymirat E, et al. Effect of a restrictive vs. liberal blood transfusion strategy on major cardiovascular events among patients with acute myocardial infarction and anemia. JAMA 2021; 325(6): 552–60.
5. Turgeon AF, Fergusson DA, Clayton L, et al. Liberal or restrictive transfusion strategy in patients with traumatic brain injury. N Engl J Med 2024; 391(8): 722–35.

SBA Paper 3: Answers

Answer 32: c

Severe pancreatitis accounts for around 2.4% of the ICU bed occupancy in England and Wales and has an in-hospital mortality of around 40%.

Pancreatitis has a variety of aetiologies; the most common cause is gallstones, which accounts for 40–70% of cases. Gallstones are a very common condition and more prevalent in women; therefore, there is a higher prevalence of this as a cause of pancreatitis. However, the risk of developing pancreatitis in men with gallstones is higher than in women. The lifetime risk of acute pancreatitis in a patient with gallstones is around 2%.

Alcohol is the cause of pancreatitis in around 25–35% of cases. Less than 10% of patients with chronic alcohol use develop acute pancreatitis. Hypertriglyceridaemia, with serum levels above 11mmol/L, can cause acute pancreatitis and accounts for between 1–14% of cases. Pancreatitis is the most common complication of undergoing an endoscopic retrograde cholangiopancreatography (ERCP). If the ERCP is complex, and is therapeutic as opposed to diagnostic, this increases the risk. Trauma is an uncommon cause of pancreatitis due to the pancreas being a retroperitoneal organ and so is partially protected from blunt force abdominal trauma. Other rare causes of pancreatitis include medications in under 5%, hypercalcaemia, infections, cancer, vasculitis, hypothermia, and autoimmune causes amongst others.

References

1. MacGoey P, Dickson EJ, Puxty K. Management of the patient with acute pancreatitis. *BJA Educ* 2019; 19(8): 240–5.
2. www.uptodate.com. Etiology of acute pancreatitis. UpToDate, 2025. Available at: https://www.uptodate.com/contents/etiology-of-acute-pancreatitis.

Answer 33: d

Within the ALS guidelines produced by the Resuscitation Council UK, there is a tachycardia algorithm (Figure 3.3). In the scenario the patient is experiencing cardiac chest pain and has a low BP so they would be classed as 'unstable' and so first-line management is synchronised DC cardioversion with sedation.

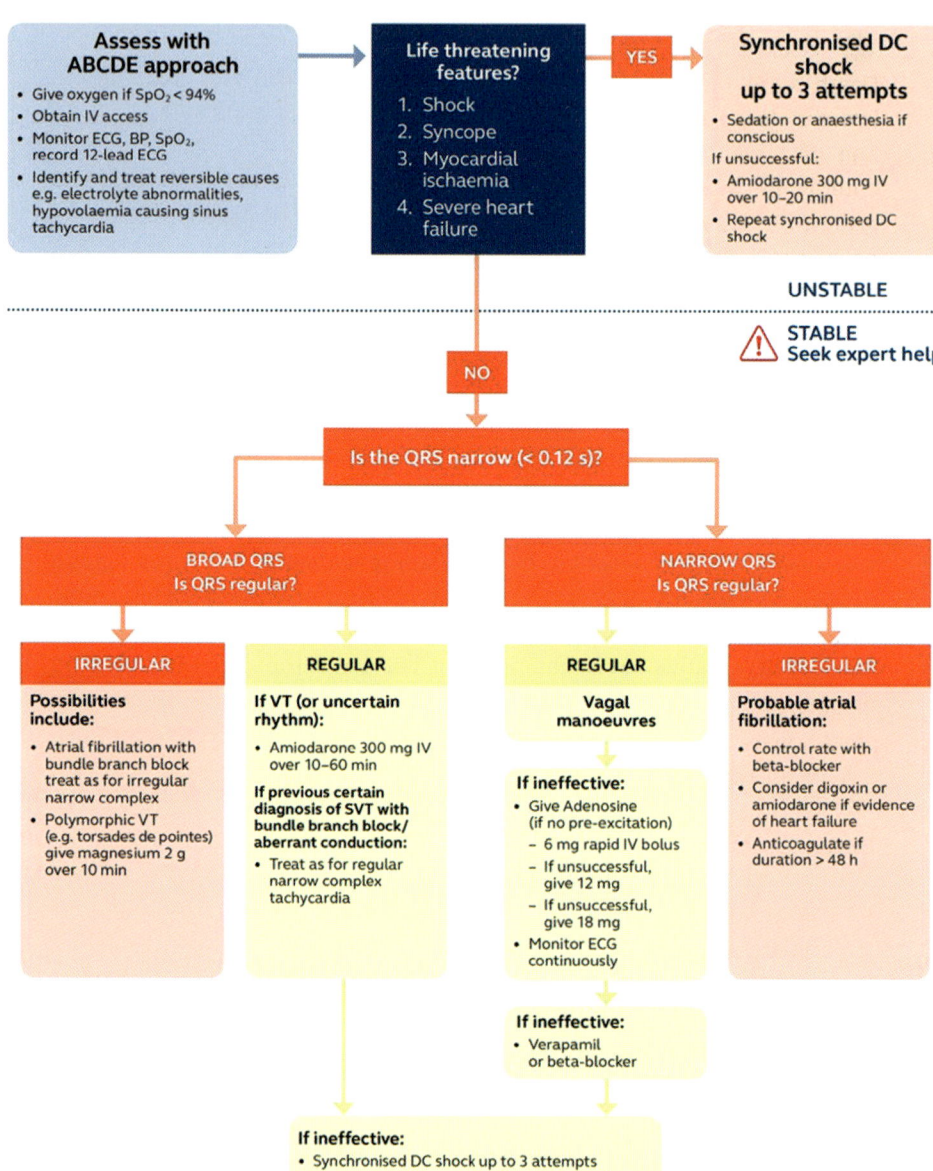

Figure 3.3. ALS tachycardia algorithm (with pulse). *Reproduced with permission from the Resuscitation Council UK.*

Answer 34: e

Death is the irreversible loss of the capacity to breathe, combined with the irreversible loss of the capacity for consciousness. Death can be diagnosed by one of three criteria: somatic, cardiovascular and neurological. Somatic criteria are used when the patient is ascertained to be dead by visual inspection alone (e.g. decomposing or decapitated) and can be used by the police and paramedics. Cardiovascular criteria are the most commonly used and is how death is diagnosed when the heart has stopped beating.

Neurological criteria involve brainstem death testing (BSDT) and forms part of the clinical management of patients on a ventilator in whom a diagnosis of neurological death is suspected. This is done to guide onward clinical management which includes, but is not exclusively for, the purpose of facilitating organ donation.

The Academy of Medical Royal Colleges (AoMRC) in the UK has produced recommendations for the diagnosis of death by neurological criteria, which have been endorsed by the Faculty of Intensive Care Medicine (FICM) and the Intensive Care Society (ICS). This guidance has been most recently updated in January 2025. The testing should be undertaken by at least two medical practitioners, one of whom must be a consultant, and all must have at least 5 years full registration with the GMC.

To consider undertaking BSDT, four sets of preconditions must be satisfied:

- Precondition 1: the patient must have an irreversible devastating brain injury of known aetiology, have a GCS of 3, with no observed brainstem reflexes and is on a ventilator. The nature of the brain injury must be one that can result in permanent cessation of brainstem function and has been diagnosed with neuroimaging.
- Precondition 2: there must have been a long enough period to exclude the potential for recovery. BSDT should not be undertaken less than 6 hours after the loss of the last brainstem reflex. In patients who have a hypoxic brain injury or are post-cardiac arrest, testing should not be undertaken until at least 24 hours after the loss of the last reflex. If the patient has been hypothermic (including therapeutic) then there should be at least a 24-hour observation period following rewarming

(core temperature should be greater than or equal to 36°C) prior to testing. If there is any uncertainty about the possibility for recovery, then the observation time should be extended.

- Precondition 3: you must exclude any potentially reversible causes of coma or apnoea. These include measurement of Na^+, K^+, PO_4^{3-}, Mg^{2+}, glucose, temperature, ammonia (if relevant to clinical picture) and hormonal assays if an endocrine cause is suspected. Residual neuromuscular blockade should be excluded with a train-of-four monitor or quantitative neuromuscular monitoring. You should be satisfied that there is no residual effect of depressant/sedating medications; drug levels can be sent if needed. In patients with preexisting neuromuscular disorders, consideration must be given to the impact of the drugs given prior as these may have longer lasting effects. If there is a known or suspected high spinal cord injury that is causing apnoea, then further investigation would be needed prior to proceeding with BSDT, and ancillary testing may be required alongside BSDT.
- Precondition 4: additional caution is required in the following uncommon circumstances: those who have received steroids to reduce brain oedema (e.g. tumour, abscess, meningitis or trauma), aetiology primarily isolated to the posterior fossa or brainstem and therapeutic decompressive craniectomy patients and other conditions where intracranial compliance may be significantly increased.

Ancillary testing is not routinely required and is undertaken if it has not been possible to either satisfy all the preconditions or undertake all the clinical tests within the BSDT framework (for example, if both ears or both eyes cannot be examined). The primary ancillary test would be CT angiography looking for the absence of cerebral blood flow.

If the patient is having any seizure activity that results in peripheral movement, then this demonstrates intact neural connections, and therefore the patient is not dead and BSDT should not be considered at that time.

With regard to BSDT there are several updates in the new 2025 guidance: with the apnoea test the starting $PaCO_2$ must be at least 5.3kPa (and may need to be higher still in those with a higher baseline value); the target $PaCO_2$ for the end of the test should be ≥2.7kPa higher than the starting value and at least 8kPa. The apnoea test runs for a minimum of 5 minutes and ends once the target PaCO$_2$ has been reached (and the pH is <7.3). The temperature for testing must now be 36°C or over (previously over 34°C), the lower Na$^+$ limit has been increased from 115 to 125mmol/L, there must be some formal assessment of neuromuscular blockade and both eyes and ears must be examinable. The official time of death is now at the completion of the second set of tests.

References

1. The Academy of Medical Royal Colleges (AoMRC) and the Faculty of Intensive Care Medicine (FICM). Form for the diagnosis of death using neurological criteria, 2025. Available at: https://ficm.ac.uk/sites/ficm/files/documents/2024-12/Form%20for%20the%20Diagnosis%20of%20DNC%20-%20adults%20and%20children%20over%202%20years%20-%20January%202025.pdf.

Answer 35: a

Capacity is regarded as the ability to make a particular decision at the time it needs to be made; assessment of capacity or lack off is made on an individual decision basis. For example, a patient with dementia may have the capacity to decide if and what they want for a meal, but not the capacity to decide about major surgery.

The starting assumption should be that a patient has the capacity to make all decisions unless it is established that they lack capacity. The decision a patient makes should not necessarily influence your assessment of their capacity; people are allowed to make unwise decisions.

The assessment of a patient's capacity starts with the two-stage test: firstly, does the patient have an impairment in the way their mind is working either acute or chronic (e.g. delirium or dementia) and does this impairment mean that the patient is unable to make the decision in question at the time it needs to be made.

Assessing their ability to make a decision is done using the following questions:

- Does the person have an understanding of the decision they are required to make and why?

- Does the person have an understanding of the likely consequences of making or not making the decision?
- Is the person able to understand, retain, use and weigh up the information relevant to this decision?
- Can the person communicate their decision (with any communication aids that are needed, e.g. interpreter, speech and language therapist)?

If it is deemed that a person lacks the capacity for a certain decision it should not be assumed this will be the case for all subsequent decisions, and assessment of capacity should be done on a decision-by-decision basis.

References

1. Department for Constitutional Affairs, 2007. Code of Practice, Mental Capacity Act 2005. Available at: https://assets.publishing.service.gov.uk/media/5f6cc6138fa8f541f6763295/Mental-capacity-act-code-of-practice.pdf.

Answer 36: b

There are several different ways to analyse data; the following compare an intervention group to a control group:

- The difference between the risk occurring in the control group and the intervention group — absolute risk reduction.
- The ratio of the risk of something occurring in the intervention group compared to the control group — relative risk.
- Ratio of the odds of a certain outcome in the intervention group to the odds of that outcome in the control group — odds ratio.
- The likelihood of the observed value being the result of change alone — p value.
- The number of patients that need the intervention to prevent one outcome event happening — number needed to treat.

With regard to the p value, a value of <0.05 is generally regarded as statistically significant. This means that the difference observed could occur by chance in 5% of occasions — so a 5% risk of a false positive result.

References

1. Cross M, Plunkett E. Statistical principles. In: Cross M, Plunkett E. *Physics, pharmacology and physiology for anaesthetists*, 2nd ed. Cambridge: Cambridge University Press; 2014: section 12: pp. 347–76.

Answer 37: c

Pleural fluid sampling can be undertaken for a number of reasons. In the context of intensive care, pleural aspiration is often done to investigate the presence of infection within the pleural fluid.

Parapneumonic effusions can be classed as 'uncomplicated' and will be an exudate (high protein and LDH levels) with an elevated WCC with neutrophil predominance, but with a normal pH and glucose levels with no evidence of infection within the fluid.

A 'complex' parapneumonic effusion will be an exudate characterised by a high WCC with neutrophil predominance, acidic pH of <7.2, glucose <2.2mmol/L, and LDH >1000 IU/L. If there is frank pus, then this is termed an empyema.

To distinguish between a pleural effusion transudate and exudate there are a number of different calculations and methods that can be used which include:

- Light's criteria states that the fluid is an exudate if one or more of the following criteria are present: pleural fluid protein level is more than 50% of the serum level, pleural fluid LDH is more than 60% of the serum LDH and pleural fluid LDH is over two-thirds the upper limits of the normal lab value.
- PFO3 test (pleural fluid only 3); this test has the advantage of only needing pleural fluid and has a similar accuracy to Light's criteria. If one or more of the following are present then the fluid is an exudate: protein greater than >30g/L, cholesterol >1.42mmol/L and LDH >0.67 times the upper limit of the normal lab value.

The common causes of transudates include: congestive cardiac failure, liver cirrhosis, hypoalbuminemia and nephrotic syndrome.

The common causes of exudates include: malignancy, pleural infection, pulmonary embolism, and autoimmune pleuritis.

References

1. Roberts ME, Rahman NM, Maskell NA, *et al*. British Thoracic Society guideline for pleural disease. *Thorax* 2023; 78(Suppl 3): s1–42.

2. www.uptodate.com. Pleural fluid analysis in adults with a pleural effusion. UpToDate, 2025. Available at: https://www.uptodate.com/contents/pleural-fluid-analysis-in-adults-with-a-pleural-effusion.

Answer 38: b

Intra-aortic balloon pumps (IABPs) are the most commonly used circulatory mechanical assist devices, and provide temporary support (typically no more than 14 days). The indications for insertion are patients with inadequate cardiac output despite medical management in the following conditions: acute MI, cardiogenic shock, acute mitral regurgitation (MR) and ventricular septal defect (VSD), unstable angina, cardiomyopathy, peri-procedure and surgical support (angioplasty, surgery, weaning off bypass), sepsis.

Contraindications to IABP insertion can be divided into absolute and relative:

- Absolute contraindications include: significant aortic regurgitation, aortic dissection, aortic stents, and end-stage heart disease with no definitive treatment options.
- Relative contraindications include: uncontrolled sepsis, abdominal aortic aneurysm, tachyarrhythmias (difficultly in timing and effectiveness of inflation), severe peripheral vascular disease (ideally treat vascular disease first) and uncontrolled bleeding disorders.

References

1. Krishna M, Zacharowski K. Principles of intra-aortic balloon pump counterpulsation. *Contin Educ Anaesth Crit Care Pain* 2009; 9(1): 24–8.
2. www.uptodate.com. Intraaortic balloon pump counterpulsation. UpToDate, 2025. Available at: https://www.uptodate.com/contents/intraaortic-balloon-pump-counterpulsation.

Answer 39: e

Intermittent haemodialysis (IHD) is generally avoided in patients who are haemodynamically unstable, due to the rapid fluid removal and risk of significant hypotension in this patient group.

Slow continuous ultrafiltration (SCUF) uses low filtration rates and is very effective at removing volume but provides minimal solute clearance. It is used mainly for more stable patients who only require fluid balance management.

Peritoneal dialysis (PD) is not typically used in the ICU due to the risk of inadequate clearance, high risk of peritonitis, protein loss, interference with ventilation (through impaired diaphragm functioning) and hyperglycaemia.

Continuous renal replacement therapy (CRRT) is the modality of choice recommended in the KDIGO guidelines for unstable ICU patients with AKI. CRRT encompasses CVVH (continuous veno-venous haemofiltration), CVVHD (continuous veno-venous haemodialysis) and CVVHDF (continuous veno-venous haemodiafiltration). These all have similar dosing and blood flow rates but differ in the method of clearance and need for replacement fluid. CVVH uses convection only and so has no dialysate fluid and requires replacement fluid for a zero balance. CVVHD uses diffusion only, has dialysate fluid running and needs no replacement fluid. CVVHDF is a combination of the two.

The dosing of the CRRT is what the effluent flow rate aims to be and is presented in ml/kg/hr. The optimum dosage has been the subject of several trials and there is no mortality benefit to a higher flow rate (40ml/kg/hr compared to 25ml/kg/hr). Given that a higher rate is difficult to achieve, as it requires good vascular access to allow for the necessary flow rates, and an absolute minimum downtime from CVVH, common practice is to use dosing of around 25–30ml/kg/hr. KDIGO recommends delivering an effluent volume rate of 20–25ml/kg/hr (which will require a slightly higher prescription dose to allow for downtime and blood flow issues meaning the delivered dose is within range).

References
1. Kidney Disease: Improving Global Outcomes (KDIGO). KDIGO clinical practice guideline for acute kidney injury, 2012. Available at: https://kdigo.org/wp-content/uploads/2016/10/KDIGO-2012-AKI-Guideline-English.pdf.
2. RENAL Replacement Therapy Study Investigators; Bellomo R, Cass A, Cole L, et al. Intensity of continuous renal-replacement therapy in critically ill patients. *N Engl J Med* 2009; 361(17): 1627–8.
3. Bellomo R. Renal replacement therapy. In: Bersten AD, Handy JM, Eds. *Oh's intensive care manual,* 8th ed. London: Elsevier; 2018: chapter 48: pp. 617–23.

Answer 40: d

Diarrhoea is a common symptom experienced by ICU patients, with a prevalence of around 13%. It is defined as three or more loose stools per day, with a volume estimated to be >250ml per day. Diarrhoea has been shown to increase ICU mortality and ICU length of stay. There are multiple possible causes in ICU patients, with medications and NG feed contributing to a significant proportion (either as the sole cause or compounding the problem). In a study looking at diarrhoea in ICU patients, a fifth of patients with diarrhoea had recently received laxatives. In this study only 9% of patients had positive stool samples for either *C. difficile* or other bacteria, indicating that infective diarrhoea is likely to make up the minority of causes. Antibiotics can cause diarrhoea as a side effect and increase the risk of *C. difficile* infection due to the loss of gut flora. NG feed is a well-recognised cause of ICU diarrhoea, likely due to the high sodium content and osmolality. Other medications that cause diarrhoea include: proton pump inhibitors, H_2 receptor antagonists and magnesium-containing oral medications.

References

1. Tirlapur N, Puthucheary ZA, Cooper JA, et al. Diarrhoea in the critically ill is common, associated with poor outcome and rarely due to *Clostridium difficile*. *Sci Rep* 2016; 6: 24691.
2. Waldmann C, Rhodes A, Soni N, Handy J. *Oxford desk reference: critical care*, 2nd ed. Oxford: Oxford University Press; 2019.

 Answer 41: b

In the UK, there is a list of communicable diseases which need to be reported to the UK Health Security Agency, to detect possible disease outbreaks and epidemics as rapidly as possible. Diseases do not need to be confirmed with testing prior to notification; suspicion is all that is required to notify. Similar systems exist in most countries.

There is a list of notifiable diseases, and a list of notifiable organisms. Some examples of notifiable disease include: acute meningitis and encephalitis (*Neisseria meningitidis*, *Streptococcus pneumoniae*), acute infective hepatitis, botulism, cholera, Covid-19, food poisoning (*Bacillus cereus*, *Clostridium perfringens*), haemolytic uraemic syndrome, invasive group A *Streptococcus*

SBA Paper 3: Answers

(streptococci grown from an area that is usually sterile, e.g. blood), malaria, measles, tetanus and tuberculosis amongst others. *Streptococcus pneumoniae* and *Streptococcus pyogenes* are notifiable if they are invasive (bronchitis is not counted as an invasive disease).

References
1. Public Health England. Notifiable diseases and causative organisms: how to report. UK Health Security Agency, 2024. Available at: https://www.gov.uk/guidance/notifiable-diseases-and-causative-organisms-how-to-report#list-of-notifiable-diseases.

Answer 42: c

Antibiotics have a number of different mechanisms of action, meaning that not all antibiotics are effective against all bacteria. Gram-positive bacteria have a thick cell wall. Gram-negative bacteria in comparison have a thin cell wall but have an outer membrane, which protects it from substances entering the bacteria. There are channels within this membrane that can allow for the passage of drugs.

Cell walls are made up of peptidoglycans, which undergo cross-linking in the presence of penicillin-binding proteins, to create strength within the cell wall. Mechanisms of antibiotic action can be divided into broad groups:

- Drugs that act via inhibition of cell wall synthesis: beta-lactam antibiotics (penicillin, cephalosporins, monobactams [aztreonam] and carbapenems [meropenem]). These bind to the penicillin-binding proteins meaning new peptidoglycan cannot be synthesised and linked, and this leads to lysis of the bacteria. Some bacteria can produce beta-lactamase which means they are resistant to beta-lactams, so some antibiotics are combined with a beta-lactamase inhibitor, e.g. the tazobactam in Tazocin® or the clavulanic acid in Augmentin® (co-amoxiclav). Glycopeptides (vancomycin and teicoplanin) bind to a precursor of the peptidoglycan preventing cell wall synthesis.
- Drugs that act via inhibition of protein synthesis within the bacteria: protein synthesis within cells is undertaken by ribosomes and cytoplasmic factors. The ribosome is composed of two subunits — 50S and 30S — and antibiotics in this group target one of these. The 50S

unit is targeted by: macrolides (erythromycin, clarithromycin), clindamycin, linezolid and chloramphenicol. The 30S unit is targeted by: tetracyclines (doxycycline, tigecycline) and aminoglycosides (gentamycin and tobramycin).
- Drugs that interfere with nucleic acid synthesis: quinolones (ciprofloxacin, levofloxacin) inhibit the enzyme bacterial DNA gyrase; this means the bacteria are unable to synthesize new DNA. Sulfamethoxazole and trimethoprim inhibit different steps of folic acid metabolism within the bacterial cell; these can be combined (e.g. co-trimoxazole) to reduce resistance rates and improve efficacy. Rifampicin inhibits RNA synthesis.

References
1. Kapoor G, Saigal S, Elongavan A. Action and resistance mechanisms of antibiotics: a guide for clinicians. *J Anaesthesiol Clin Pharmacol* 2017; 33(3): 300–5.

Answer 43: b

In this scenario, the patient is still unstable from a renal perspective, and therefore either of the options to stop CRRT would not be appropriate. With regard to re-siting the line, KDIGO suggests a preferred order for central access points. The first choice would be the right internal jugular vein (RIJV) (straight course, least risk of stenosis and thrombosis), the next preference would be femoral vein (there is mixed evidence regarding infection risk of femoral catheterisation; the study quoted in KDIGO shows no significant difference), the third choice would be the left IJV and the last choice would be the subclavian vein with preference for the dominant side (leaving the non-dominant side free for long-term access if needed).

The reasons for this order are primarily due to functionality; RIJV catheters malfunction least often. Other considerations include infection (where the evidence is mixed) and reducing the risk of thrombosis/stenosis which is thought to be more likely to occur in lines that have more angulations (e.g. left internal jugular and subclavian lines).

References
1. Kidney Disease: Improving Global Outcomes (KDIGO). KDIGO clinical practice guideline for acute kidney injury, 2012. Available at: https://kdigo.org/wp-content/uploads/2016/10/KDIGO-2012-AKI-Guideline-English.pdf.

Answer 44: a

Thrombophilia describes a range of clinical conditions which result in an increased thrombosis risk (arterial and venous) and recurrent pregnancy loss and failure (with a morphologically normal foetus). They can either be inherited or acquired disorders. Inherited thrombophilias are present in 5% of the population.

The main acquired thrombophilia is antiphospholipid syndrome (APS). Most patients with APS will not develop thrombosis. It is due to a family of antibodies that are reactive with epitopes on proteins complexed to phospholipids; the most common of these are: lupus anticoagulant (also present in around half of patients with SLE), anticardiolipin antibody and anti-beta-2 glycoprotein I antibody. APS is diagnosed if there is a persistent positive antiphospholipid antibody or other associated antibodies when tested on two separate occasions, at least 12 weeks apart, in addition to the presence of at least one clinical manifestation: arterial, venous or small vessel thrombosis, more than one miscarriage (foetal loss), associated with a morphologically normal foetus.

Other thrombophilias include deficiency of antithrombin, protein C and protein S, and the presence of factor V Leiden.

Factor V Leiden is a mutation in factor V rendering it insensitive to actions of activated protein C. Prevalence is around 4–5%.

Protein C is a major physiological anticoagulant. Activated by thrombin, in combination with protein S and phospholipid, it degrades factors Va and VIIIa, thus reducing clot formation. Protein C deficiency can be inherited, but more commonly it is acquired due to conditions such as DIC, liver disease and infection. Protein C deficiency can also be a cause of warfarin-induced skin necrosis. Protein S deficiency is caused by pregnancy, oral contraceptive use, DIC, acute thrombosis and HIV, amongst other things.

References

1. Rahman A, Giles I. Rheumatology. In: Kumar P, Clark M, Eds. *Kumar and Clark's clinical medicine*, 10th ed. London, Elsevier; 2020: chapter 18: pp. 437–69.
2. www.uptodate.com. Evaluating adult patients with established venous thromboembolism for acquired and inherited risk factors. UpToDate, 2023. Available at:

https://www.uptodate.com/contents/evaluating-adult-patients-with-established-venous-thromboembolism-for-acquired-and-inherited-risk-factors.

 Answer 45: b

Neuraxial analgesia in the form of epidural catheters, and regional analgesia in the form of nerve block catheters are common in patients on intensive care, especially in the postoperative surgical group. Management of different anticoagulants and antiplatelet medications in patients with such catheters, is core knowledge for an intensivist. Incorrect management of anticoagulants may lead to an epidural haematoma, which if not managed urgently, could lead to permanent neurological injury and paralysis.

Medications that will need consideration of timing and potential omission include: dalteparin (therapeutic and prophylactic), unfractionated heparin, antiplatelet drugs (e.g. aspirin, clopidogrel, prasugrel), DOACs and warfarin (the last two are very unlikely to be relevant to elective postoperative patients, but may be relevant to emergency patients or non-surgical patients, such as rib fracture patients).

There are three separate time periods to consider:

- Time between medication administered and insertion of the catheter.
- Management of medications whilst the catheter is *in situ*.
- Time after removal of catheter until resumption of medications.

In addition, there needs to be consideration to the risk associated with bleeding. Deep nerve blocks and epidurals have a high risk of significant injury should bleeding occur. Deep nerve blocks are those in whom vascular compression would be difficult and bleeding may require invasive control, e.g. paravertebral, lumbar plexus and infraclavicular brachial plexus nerve blocks. In this group, consideration should always be made to the timing of anticoagulants.

Other blocks have a low risk of injury should bleeding occur and include superficial nerve blocks and those in whom compression is possible to control bleeding (e.g. parasternal intercostal, erector spinae plane [ESP], rectus sheath, fascia iliaca, etc.). In this group, in most situations, anticoagulants can be continued assuming they are within their target range. The management of timings as recommended by the European Society of Regional Anaesthesia (ESRA), American Society of Regional Anesthesia and Pain Medicine (ASRA), and the Association of Anaesthetists (AoA) is shown in Table 3.6.

Table 3.6. Administration of anticoagulants and antiplatelets for patients with an indwelling neuraxial or nerve catheter.

Medication	Time from last dose to needle insertion	Management whilst catheter indwelling	Time from catheter removal to dose
Aspirin 75mg	0 hours	Continue as normal	Next scheduled dose
Prophylactic LMWH	12 hours (24 hours if CrCl <30ml/min)	Wait 24 hours from insertion for first dose then give at normal intervals	4 hours
Therapeutic LMWH	24 hours, consider anti-Xa measurement (48 hours if CrCl <30ml/min)	Not to be given	24 hours (ASRA and ESRA), 4 hours (AoA) but increase to 24 if traumatic block
Unfractionated heparin (at IV infusion doses <100 IU/kg/day)	4–6 hours with normal coagulation testing	Caution advised, typically only for vascular and cardiac patients — follow local protocols	1 hour (ASRA and ESRA), 4 hours (AoA)
P2Y12 inhibitors (e.g. clopidogrel)	5 days ticagrelor 5–7 days clopidogrel	Not recommended	0–24 hours ticagrelor (ASRA 0, AoA 6, ESRA 24 hours) 75mg clopidogrel immediately (AoA 6 hours), 24–48 hours 300mg clopidogrel

References

1. Ashken T, West S. Regional anaesthesia in patients at risk of bleeding. *BJA Educ* 2021; 21(3): 84–94.
2. Kietaibl S, Ferrandis R, Godier A, *et al*. Regional anaesthesia in patients on antithrombotic drugs. *Eur J Anaesthesiol* 2022; 39(2): 100–32.

● Answer 46: e

A tracheostomy is a relatively common procedure within the ICU. They can be inserted percutaneously on the ICU by intensivists or surgically by ENT surgeons in theatre. The patient should be adequately anaesthetised and paralysed with the head and neck in extension. The skin incision is made at the midpoint between the cricoid and the sternum and the trachea entered ideally between the 2nd and 3rd tracheal rings at the 12 o'clock position.

There has been no evidence suggesting improved outcome with early tracheostomy insertion. The TracMan study compared insertion at day 1–4 vs. at >10 days and showed no difference in mortality or any of the secondary outcomes. A further study looking at ≥5 days vs. >10 days in stroke patients requiring ventilation also showed no difference in outcomes.

Tracheostomy tubes are shorter than endotracheal tubes (ETTs), with no bevel at the end and the cuff bonded closer to the tip.

There are a number of different tracheostomy tube types:

- Single lumen: previously used for short-term patients on the ICU; these are being phased out as they need to be changed every 7 days and are more likely to get blocked.
- Double lumen: most common type, with an outer and inner tube. The inner tube can be changed regularly and cleaned to stop secretion build-up. The outer tube is changed every 30 days.
- Fenestrated: a hole or multiple holes above the cuff to allow air to pass out through the cords on expiration and allow vocalisation. If an unfenestrated inner is put in, these patients can be ventilated.
- Variable flange: for patients with a large distance from the skin to the trachea. This could be due to obesity, postoperative swelling, or swelling from other causes such as burns. The length can be altered as

SBA Paper 3: Answers

- the swelling goes down without having to exchange for a different tracheostomy.
- Cuffed tracheostomy tube: those used in the ICU are normally cuffed to allow positive pressure ventilation and to protect the airway from aspiration.
- Uncuffed tracheostomy tube: used in patients who require a long-term tracheostomy with intact bulbar function.
- Supraglottic suction: now present in many ICU ETTs and tracheostomy tubes, with the aim to reduce ventilator-associated pneumonia (VAP) from micro-aspiration of biofilm.

Speaking valves are a one-way valve that fits over the end of the tracheostomy, or within the circuit (in line, e.g. Passy-Muir), which prevents airflow out from the tracheostomy lumen and instead directs airflow out through the trachea and the vocal cords, allowing vocalisation. As there is no airflow out of the tracheostomy lumen during expiration, the cuff MUST be down when these are in place.

References

1. Dawson S, Gratix A. Respiratory therapy techniques: tracheostomy. In: Waldmann C, Rhodes A, Soni N, Handy J, Eds. *Oxford desk reference: critical care*, 2nd ed. Oxford: Oxford University Press; 2019: chapter 1: pp. 39–40.
2. Young D, Harrison DA, Cuthbertson BH, Rowan K; TracMan Collaborators. Effect of early vs late tracheostomy placement on survival in patients receiving mechanical ventilation: the TracMan randomized trial. *JAMA* 2013; 309(20): 2121–9.
3. Bösel J, Niesen W-D, Salih F, *et al*. Effect of early vs standard approach to tracheostomy on functional outcome at 6 months among patients with severe stroke receiving mechanical ventilation: the SETPOINT2 randomized clinical trial. *JAMA* 2022; 327(19): 1899–909.

● Answer 47: c

Oesophageal Doppler is a method of semi-invasive cardiac output (CO) monitoring. It works using Doppler to measure the velocity of the blood travelling down the descending aorta, and an estimate of the aortic cross-sectional area (from a nomogram based on the patient's age, height and weight or using M mode to determine diameter) to calculate the cardiac output. This calculation is dependent on the following assumptions: 70% of the CO is going into the descending aorta, an equal velocity profile across the aorta, estimated cross-sectional area is close to the mean systolic diameter, there is negligible diastolic blood flow and accurate measurement of the velocity of the blood flow.

The probe sits 35–40cm from the mouth where the descending aorta is posterior to the oesophagus. They can be left in safely for up to 14 days. Contraindications to insertion include oesophageal varices, recent oesophageal surgery and severe agitation. They may be inaccurate in patients with coarctation of the aorta, a thoracic aortic aneurysm, a functioning thoracic epidural and in the presence of an intra-aortic balloon pump.

The oesophageal Doppler monitoring produces a velocity-time wave, from which certain haemodynamic variables can be inferred.

The peak velocity is the highest point of the wave and gives an estimate of contractility and decreases with age. At age 20, it is 90–120cm/s, at age 50, 70–100cm/s, and at age 70, 58–80cm/s.

The flow time (corrected to heart rate) or FTc is the duration of forward blood flow within the aorta; the normal value is 330–360ms. It is increased in vasodilation (up to 400ms is normal during a general anaesthetic). It is decreased in hypovolaemia, mitral stenosis, PE and with the use of vasopressors.

CO — the area under the wave is the stroke distance (SD), which when multiplied by the aortic diameter gives an estimated stroke volume (SV); this multiplied by the heart rate gives a CO measurement.

As with most haemodynamic monitoring, the oesophageal Doppler has limited usefulness as a single measurement but should be used to look at trends over time, and in response to interventions such as fluid challenges.

References

1. Hamilton M, Price J. Cardiovascular monitoring: oesophageal Doppler. In: Waldmann C, Rhodes A, Soni N, Handy J, Eds. *Oxford desk reference: critical care*, 2nd ed. Oxford: Oxford University Press; 2019: chapter 7: pp. 126–7.

2. Sturgess D, Watts R. Haemodynamic monitoring. In: Bersten AD, Handy JM, Eds. *Oh's intensive care manual*, 8th ed. London: Elsevier; 2018: chapter 16: pp.134-49.

Answer 48: a

Acute liver failure (ALF) is due to massive parenchymal liver injury in a patient who has no pre-existing liver disease. It causes significant morbidity and mortality with only 40% having spontaneous recovery, with liver transplantation the only option for recovery for the majority of the remaining 60%. There are several classification systems which divide liver failure into hyperacute, acute or subacute (O'Grady and King's), or fulminant and subfulminant (Bernuau). These categories are based on the time between the onset of jaundice and the onset of encephalopathy. Hyperacute is less than 7 days, acute between 8–28 days and subacute 29 days up to 8 weeks.

The aetiology of ALF various throughout the world, with paracetamol toxicity being the primary cause in the UK and USA, and viral hepatitis (B and E) being the primary cause in India, France and Japan, accounting for up to 70% of ALF worldwide. Hepatitis C is a significant cause of chronic liver disease (CLD) but not of ALF. A definite cause can be found in around 80% of cases; the remaining are considered to be 'seronegative' hepatitis and are either caused by infections that have not been identified or autoimmune causes.

ALF patients' presentations differ slightly, dependent on the underlying cause.

Hyperacute liver failure (paracetamol, hepatitis A+B) progresses rapidly, and encephalopathy may present prior to jaundice. In addition, patients have severe coagulopathy, organ dysfunction with significant vasodilatation and are at high risk of intracranial hypertension and cerebral oedema. Regarding cerebral oedema, patients with high-grade encephalopathy are at the highest risk and high ammonia levels increase the risk; an ammonia level of over 200µmol/L is associated with cerebral herniation. Due to this risk, patients with ALF need to have neuroprotective care such as their head placed in a neutral position, the bed positioned at 30°, neuroprotective ventilation, etc.

Acute liver failure (hepatitis A, B, E, drug reactions) has a slower onset with jaundice occurring prior to encephalopathy, with high levels of transaminases and coagulopathy.

Subacute liver failure (seronegative, drug reaction) is associated with smaller rises in transaminases and often patients present with established ascites. These patients can have a worse outcome than the other two groups.

A more common cause of acute deterioration in liver function is acute-on-chronic liver failure (ACLF). This is an acute decompensation in a patient with known CLD (present for over 6 months), precipitated most commonly by a GI bleed or infection. Patients have symptoms of worsening liver disease (ascites, encephalopathy, variceal bleeds) and associated organ failure. ACLF carries a high, short-term mortality and this can be calculated using the CLIF-C ACLF scoring, which is a shortened version of the SOFA score specifically for this patient group.

References
1. Willars C, Ashraf HH, Damodaran A, Wendon J. Liver failure. In: Bersten AD, Handy JM, Eds. *Oh's intensive care manual*, 8th ed. London: Elsevier, 2018; chapter 44: pp. 573–93.
2. Rovegno M, Vera M, Ruiz A, Benítez C. Current concepts in acute liver failure. *Ann Hepatol* 2019; 18(4): 543–52.

● Answer 49: d

Blood flow varies throughout the lung and is affected by body position. In the upright position, blood flow decreases in a linear fashion from the bottom to the top, with very low blood flows in the apex. Dependent areas of the lung receive better blood flows, so when you are upright the flow is better in the bases; if you are supine, it is better in the posterior portions of the lungs and if you are prone it is better in the anterior portions of the lungs. The relationship between the alveolar pressure (PA), the arterial pressure (Pa) and the venous pressure (Pv) is described using West zones of the lung (Figure 3.4).

In zone 1, pulmonary arterial pressure is below alveolar pressure which results in no blood flow through the lungs. This is referred to as alveolar dead space as it is ventilated but NOT perfused. This does not happen in health but may occur if arterial blood pressure is very low (severe haemorrhage, sepsis) or the alveolar pressure is very high (positive pressure ventilation).

In zone 2, pulmonary arterial pressure is higher than alveolar pressure, and venous pressure is lower than them both; this means blood flow is dependent

SBA Paper 3: Answers

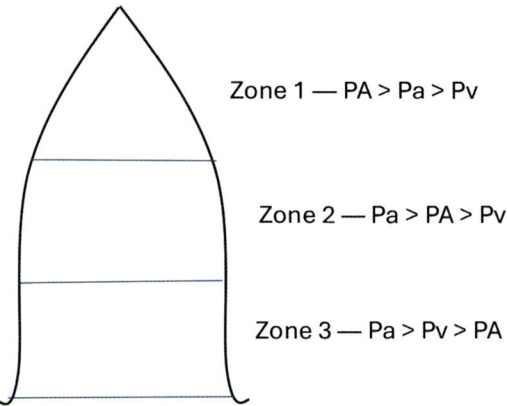

Figure 3.4. West's lung zones.

Zone 1 — PA > Pa > Pv

Zone 2 — Pa > PA > Pv

Zone 3 — Pa > Pv > PA

on the arterial alveolar difference. Ventilation and perfusion are well matched in this zone.

In zone 3, pulmonary arterial pressure is the highest, then venous pressure and then alveolar pressure. Blood flow is determined by arterial venous gradient. Increase in blood flow is mainly due to distension of the capillaries. The extreme end of this would be when you had no ventilation into a lung unit, but good blood flow, and this situation is called shunt.

Shunt is when blood returns back to the left side of the heart without having travelled through a ventilated area of the lung. Small volume shunt exists in health due to blood flow to the bronchi that drains back via the pulmonary veins, and coronary venous drainage. If a lung unit stops being ventilated effectively, the oxygen content decreases (for example, with lobar collapse or consolidation). This does not cause significant shunt due to hypoxic pulmonary vasoconstriction which causes arteriolar vasoconstriction in the hypoxic region, therefore redirecting blood to a better ventilated area.

References

1. West J. *Respiratory physiology: the essentials*, 8th ed. London: Wolters Kluwer/Lippincott Williams and Wilkins; 2008.

Answer 50: c

Methicillin-resistant *Staphylococcus aureus* (MRSA) incidence has been falling in the UK but remains a cause of infection amongst patients on the ICU. It is associated with high morbidity when causing deep-seated infections like

Table 3.7. Antibiotic management of MRSA infections.

Infection	First line	Alternative first line	Second line	Additional comments
Severe skin and soft tissue	Vancomycin or teicoplanin	Linezolid and daptomycin	Tigecycline (if sensitive)	
Complicated UTI	Vancomycin or teicoplanin	Daptomycin		Avoid linezolid as not renally excreted
Bone and joint	Vancomycin or teicoplanin		Daptomycin or linezolid	
Bacteraemia	Vancomycin	Linezolid	Daptomycin or teicoplanin	Co-trimoxazole (Septrin™) not first line but can be used as step-down treatment
Pneumonia (non-necrotising)	Linezolid	Vancomycin		Avoid daptomycin (inactivated by surfactant)
Necrotising pneumonia (PVL *Staph.*)	Linezolid or vancomycin			Clindamycin/rifampicin can be added for antitoxin effect
Meningitis	Vancomycin (plus rifampicin for severe infection)			If IV fails may need intraventricular vancomycin

SBA Paper 3: Answers

osteomyelitis. Unlike other resistant bacteria (like extended-spectrum beta-lactamases [ESBL]) there are a reasonable number of options when it comes to antibiotics.

The advice varies slightly depending on the site of the infection as shown in Table 3.7 (based on UK guidance).

Other antibiotics that will be effective against MRSA are clindamycin, doxycycline and ceftaroline (fifth-generation cephalosporin).

References

1. Brown N, Goodman A, Horner C, *et al*. Treatment of methicillin-resistant *Staphylococcus aureus* (MRSA): updated guidelines from the UK. *JAC Antimicrob Resist* 2021; 3(1): dlaa114.

4 SBA Paper 4: Questions

Question 1

You are called to review an ICU patient due to concerns regarding their arterial blood gas (ABG). The patient is a 34-year-old, 60kg man who was hit by a car and sustained a severe traumatic brain injury (TBI). He has been on the ICU for 4 days with repeated episodes of raised ICP. He has required multiple boluses of sedation, and two boluses of hypertonic saline. Review of the patient is as follows:

A: Endotracheal tube (ETT).
B: PRVC 400ml x 20, PEEP of 8cmH$_2$O, SpO$_2$ 98% on an FiO$_2$ of 0.4.
C: BP 110/70mmHg on noradrenaline 0.6µg/kg min, HR 120/min, AF (new onset), urine output 15ml/hr.
D: PEARL size 3mm, RASS −3, propofol 1% 35ml/hr, alfentanil 0.4µg/kg/min, midazolam 4mg/hr.
E: Temperature 38.2°C, abdomen soft, absorbing feed.

Blood test results are shown in Table 4.1.

Table 4.1. Blood test results.

	Yesterday	Today		Yesterday	Today
Hb	110g/L	111g/L	AST	60 U/L	250 U/L
WCC	8.5 x 10^9/L	10 x 10^9/L	ALT	70 IU/L	300 IU/L
Platelets	120 x 10^9/L	110 x 10^9/L	Bilirubin	15µmol/L	22µmol/L
Na$^+$	135mmol/L	136mmol/L	CK	200 U/L	5000 U/L
K$^+$	4.8mmol/L	5.6mmol/L	Triglycerides	4mmol/L	8mmol/L
Creatinine	80µmol/L	170µmol/L	Amylase	60 U/L	400 U/L
Urea	5.4mmol/L	8.9mmol/L			

The most recent arterial blood gas results are shown in Table 4.2.

Table 4.2. Arterial blood gas results.			
pH	7.25	HCO_3^-	16mmol/L
pCO_2	4.7kPa	Lactate	6mmol/L
pO_2	12kPa		

What is the most important management for the likely underlying condition?

a   CRRT.
b   Change sedation regime to midazolam and alfentanil only.
c   Glucose infusion.
d   Fluid challenge.
e   Add vasopressin.

● Question 2

You are working in a regional hospital which has a burns unit. A steel worker is bought into the ED following an industrial accident in which there was a fire within a contained space. The paramedics reported thick smoke at the scene and there is a strong suspicion of an inhalational injury. The patient is a 45-year-old male and normally fit and well. You are called to assess the airway. He has facial erythema with some blistering, soot in his nostrils and his tongue and mouth look red. There are limited burns elsewhere and the total body surface area (TBSA) affected is estimated at 8%. You intubate and ventilate him with an uncut ETT and transfer him sedated to the ICU.

What is the next most important step regarding management of his airway burns?

a   Bronchoscopy with BAL.
b   Triple nebuliser therapy (salbutamol, heparin and NAC).
c   Transfer to a burns centre.
d   Ventilation at 8–10ml/kg IBW.
e   Fluid resuscitation using the Parkland formula.

Question 3

A 46-year-old female patient has presented with a devastating brain injury secondary to spontaneous intracerebral haemorrhage. Forty-eight hours following admission she has stopped triggering the ventilator and has bilateral fixed and dilated pupils. After 6 hours the decision is made to undertake brainstem death testing (BSDT).

On examination:

A: Intubated.
B: FiO_2 of 0.4, PaO_2 10.5kPa, $PaCO_2$ 5.8kPa, TV 6ml/kg.
C: BP 110/70mmHg, HR 110/min, sinus rhythm, urine output 400ml/hr.
D: Pupils fixed and dilated, size 7mm, no sedative agents.
E: Temperature 36.1°C.

Blood test results are shown in Table 4.3.

Table 4.3. Blood test results.

Hb	78g/L	Na^+	157mmol/L
WCC	18 x 10⁹/L	K^+	3.4mmol/L
Platelets	130 x 10⁹/L	Mg^{2+}	0.7mmol/L
Glucose	3.5mmol/L	PO_4^{3-}	0.35mmol/L

Which of the above parameters need to be optimised prior to brainstem death testing?

a PaO_2.
b $PaCO_2$.
c Na^+.
d PO_4^{3-}.
e Glucose.

Question 4

A patient has been intubated on the ICU for 8 days with a community-acquired pneumonia (CAP). Sputum culture is positive for *Streptococcus pneumoniae*. Ventilatory weaning had been progressing well, but the patient is now pyrexial with an increase in oxygen requirements for 2 days. Antimicrobials were escalated to piperacillin-tazobactam from co-amoxiclav 48 hours previously when she became more unwell.

A chest radiograph suggests a large left pleural effusion with significant loss of lung volume. A lung US estimates the volume of the effusion at 1.5L. A diagnostic aspiration from this effusion is as follows: appearance — purulent, pH 7.15, glucose 1.5mmol/L, protein 45g/L.

What is the most appropriate next action?

a   Escalate antibiotics to meropenem, aztreonam and metronidazole.
b   Insert a Seldinger fine-bore chest drain.
c   Insert a wide-bore chest drain.
d   Perform a VATS procedure.
e   Continue current antimicrobial therapy and repeat imaging in 24 hours.

Question 5

You are asked to review a patient in the ED who has presented with acute shortness of breath. The patient has a history of rheumatoid arthritis for which they receive infliximab, and a weaning course of prednisolone (currently 5mg/day) following a recent flare-up. The patient reports increasing shortness of breath over the last few days, with reduced exercise tolerance, fevers and an unproductive cough.

The following are found on examination:

A: Maintaining own airway.
B: Bilateral inspiratory crackles in mid and lower zones, SpO_2 95% on 15L/min oxygen, ABG: PaO_2 11kPa and $PaCO_2$ 4.2kPa, CXR — bilateral patchy infiltrates.
C: BP 110/60mmHg, HR 100/min, sinus rhythm, warm peripheries.

D: Alert and orientated.
E: Temperature 38.5°C, no rash, abdomen soft and non-tender.

What would be the most appropriate antimicrobial management for this patient?

a   Augmentin®, clarithromycin, 10mg prednisolone.
b   Augmentin®, co-trimoxazole 30mg/kg QDS, 40mg prednisolone.
c   Co-trimoxazole 30mg/kg QDS, 40mg prednisolone.
d   Augmentin®, clarithromycin, co-trimoxazole 30mg/kg QDS, 40mg prednisolone.
e   Augmentin®, co-trimoxazole 980mg OD, prednisolone 10mg.

● Question 6

A 35-year-old female is admitted to the neurology ward with acute weakness. The patient provides a history of a chest infection (for which they received erythromycin due to a penicillin allergy), and then progressive weakness of her arms and legs which began 24 hours later. The patient is normally fit and well but had noticed some double vision in the evenings over the weeks preceding admission to hospital.

You have been asked to review her as she is now really struggling to breathe. A forced vital capacity (FVC) has been performed which is 15ml/kg, and she seems to be pooling secretions with a reduced swallow.

Examination is as follows:

A: Maintaining own airway.
B: SpO_2 98% on an FiO_2 of 0.3, RR 30/min, shallow breaths, PaO_2 14kPa, $PaCO_2$ 7kPa.
C: BP 120/60mmHg, HR 85/min, sinus rhythm, warm peripheries.
D: Alert, distressed, ptosis and poor swallow noted. Power 2/5 upper limb and 3/5 lower limb, sensation and reflexes intact.
E: Temperature 37.2°C, abdomen soft.

What is the most likely unifying diagnosis?

a   Guillain-Barré syndrome.
b   Miller Fisher syndrome.
c   Lambert-Eaton syndrome.
d   Multiple sclerosis.
e   Myasthenia gravis.

● Question 7

A patient has been on the ICU for 2 weeks with ARDS secondary to pneumonia. The patient has a tracheostomy *in situ* and is starting a respiratory wean, is now off all sedation and antibiotics and is receiving furosemide 40mg TDS to treat significant peripheral oedema (overall fluid balance 9L positive). The patient had been absorbing enteral nutrition well until 24 hours previously but now has high NG aspirates with 2L drained in the last 24 hours. An ileus is suspected, and a CT abdomen demonstrates a grossly distended stomach with a possible narrowing at D2.

Examination is as follows:

A: Tracheostomy (size 8 cuffed).
B: PS/CPAP 10/8cmH$_2$O, RR 15/min, SpO$_2$ 95% on an FiO$_2$ of 0.35, chest clear on auscultation.
C: BP 140/80mmHg, HR 88/min, sinus rhythm, warm peripheries, moderate oedema throughout, urine output 40ml/hr, total fluid balance 9L positive, 24-hour balance negative 2500ml.
D: Alert and orientated.
E: Temperature 36.5°C, abdomen distended and non-tender.

Blood test results including an arterial blood gas are shown in Table 4.4.

Table 4.4. Blood test results.

Na$^+$	142mmol/L	pH	7.50
K$^+$	3.4mmol/L	pO$_2$	10.2kPa
Urea	10mmol/L	pCO$_2$	5.8kPa
Creatinine	120µmol/L	HCO$_3^-$	33mmol/L
Albumin	25g/L	BE	+9mmol/L
		Cl$^-$	80mmol/L

What is the likely underlying cause of this patient's alkalosis?

a   Frusemide.
b   Hypochloraemia.
c   Compensation for respiratory acidosis.
d   Hypoalbuminaemia.
e   Conn's syndrome.

● Question 8

A 32-year-old man is having a laparoscopic appendicectomy for a ruptured appendix. He has a past medical history of anxiety and depression for which he takes sertraline. The patient was hypotensive on the ward prior to theatre with a high temperature and raised inflammatory markers, and a central line was inserted prior to induction with alfentanil, ketamine and rocuronium. Anaesthesia has been maintained with sevoflurane and remifentanil, and the patient has also received dexamethasone, ondansetron and 5mg of morphine.

The theatre team contact critical care as they are finding the patient increasingly difficult to ventilate and note that he has rapidly escalating vasopressor requirements. His heart rate has continued to rise despite an adequate depth of anaesthesia and his temperature has increased to 40.5°C having been 38.4°C pre-operatively. The end-tidal CO_2 is also rising and is 10kPa on an ABG despite incremental increases in the minute ventilation. The patient is profusely sweating. The surgeons have asked for a further dose of muscle relaxant as they are struggling to visualise the appendix due to increased abdominal wall tone, and this is a technically complex operation due to the degree of inflammation around the appendix.

What would be the best next step in the management of this patient?

a   Ask the surgeons to stop and give an additional dose of antibiotics.
b   Switch to total intravenous anaesthesia (TIVA) and give dantrolene.
c   Cyproheptadine.
d   Bromocriptine.
e   Midazolam infusion.

Question 9

A 65-year-old lady presents to the ED with hypoxia and a reduced GCS. The patient's daughter states she has complained of being increasingly lethargic and feeling cold with around 5kg of weight gain over the last month. She has a history of pernicious anaemia and diet-controlled diabetes. She lives with her husband, is a non-smoker and drinks two gin and tonics each night. Earlier in the day she complained of some chest discomfort after a walk outside (external temperature 2°C) and has become increasingly drowsy since then.

On examination:

A: Maintaining own airway.
B: Quiet bases, SpO$_2$ 96% on an FiO$_2$ of 0.5, pH 7.3, PaCO$_2$ 6.0kPa, PaO$_2$ 9.2kPa, RR 16/min.
C: BP 110/90mmHg, HR 40/min, sinus rhythm, ECG showing 2mm ST elevation in V2–V4 and a QTc of 510ms, cool peripheries with dry skin and pedal oedema.
D: GCS 10/15 (E-3, V-3, M-4), blood sugar 3.5mmol/L.
E: Temperature 34.5°C.

Blood test results are shown in Table 4.5.

Table 4.5. Blood test results.

Hb	112g/L	Na$^+$	128mmol/L
WCC	4.2 x 10^9/L	K$^+$	4.5mmol/L
Platelets	150 x 10^9/L	Urea	6mmol/L
		Creatinine	100µmol/L

What is the most likely unifying diagnosis?

a   STEMI.
b   Exposure-related hypothermia.
c   Hypothyroidism.
d   Addison's disease.
e   Chronic alcohol use.

SBA Paper 4: Questions

 Question 10
You are called to see a 25-year-old lady who is having a seizure on the medical admissions unit. As you arrive the patient stops seizing, but her blood pressure is low, and she has been recorded as having a labile blood pressure and heart rate since admission. Her girlfriend provides a collateral history of feeling unwell for a week, during which time she had experienced visual and aural hallucinations, and increasingly bizarre behaviour leading to concerns that she may have had her drink 'spiked' during a recent night out. She has no previous psychiatric history or history of any recreational drug use and is awaiting an abdominal USS for non-specific abdominal pain and bloating.

On examination:

A: Nasal airway *in situ*.
B: RR 14/min, occasional short apnoeas, SpO$_2$ 100% on 15L/min oxygen via a NRB mask.
C: BP 80/50mmHg (160/90mmHg prior to seizure), HR 120/min, sinus rhythm, warm peripheries, no oedema.
D: GCS 9/15 (E-2, V-2, M-5), PEARL and 4mm, blood sugar 6.3mmol/L.
E: Temperature 37.2°C, fullness in lower abdomen.

What test would be most likely to lead you to the underlying diagnosis?

a   CT head.
b   MRI head.
c   Toxicology screen.
d   Lumbar puncture for culture and autoantibody screening.
e   EEG.

 Question 11
You are asked to urgently review a 65-year-old man on the ICU who has started vomiting fresh blood and is hypotensive. The patient is day 3 after admission for urosepsis and is requiring invasive ventilation, cardiovascular support with noradrenaline and CRRT for an AKI. The patient has a background of alcoholic liver disease with cirrhosis (Child-Pugh stage B), type 2 diabetes and hypertension. The patient has an urgent upper GI endoscopy

which shows gastric stress ulceration; this is controlled with an adrenaline injection and the patient stabilises.

Blood test results are shown in Table 4.6.

Table 4.6. Blood test results.

Hb	75g/L	Na$^+$	128mmol/L
WCC	18 x 10^9/L	K$^+$	4.8mmol/L
Platelets	85 x 10^9/L	Urea	18mmol/L
PT	45 seconds	Creatinine	150µmol/L
APTT	40 seconds	Albumin	30g/L
Fibrinogen	1.8g/L		

Which of the following is the **least** important risk factor for the GI bleeding?

a   Mechanical ventilation over 48 hours.
b   Coagulopathy.
c   Child-Pugh B cirrhosis.
d   Acute kidney injury.
e   Shock.

● Question 12

You are on a day shift on the cardiac ICU when you are called to review a patient, who was bought round from theatre 4 hours previously having had a right intrapericardial pneumonectomy for lung cancer. The patient has suddenly deteriorated and is now hypotensive and hypoxic. Nursing colleagues report an extended non-productive coughing episode.

On examination:

A: Own airway, extremely distressed, moaning and clutching their chest.
B: SpO$_2$ 75% on an FiO$_2$ of 0.3, which increases to 88% on 15L NRB, very dyspnoeic, RR 28/min, right-sided chest drain *in situ*, drained 50ml blood in the last hour (when unclamped) with no bubbling. Wound sites have a small amount of blood staining on the dressings.

C: BP 60/40mmHg, HR 120/min, sinus rhythm, visible JVP at the level of the ear lobe, quiet muffled heart sounds.
D: Drowsy, GCS 14: E-3, M-6, V-5. Blood sugar 5.5mmol/L.
E: Temperature 36.4°C.

What is the most likely cause of the deterioration?

a   Post-pneumonectomy syndrome.
b   Intracardiac shunting.
c   Bronchopleural fistula.
d   Acute haemothorax.
e   Cardiac herniation.

Question 13

You are asked to attend the ED urgently to help in the management of an unwell child. The patient is an 8-year-old girl with known brittle asthma. She had been at a barbeque with family when she became suddenly very wheezy. Mum has given her 10 puffs of salbutamol prior to bringing her to hospital. The ED team have administered salbutamol and ipratropium nebulisers (2.5mg and 250µg), 30mg oral prednisolone and an appropriate dose of intravenous magnesium. They are concerned as she remains very unwell.

On examination:

A: Maintaining own airway.
B: RR 45/min, shallow breaths, quiet chest on auscultation, using accessory muscles with intercostal recession, SpO_2 96% on 15L NRB. Unable to perform a peak flow and is struggling to talk in sentences. Venous blood gas: pH 7.35, pCO_2 6.1kPa.
C: HR 160/min, sinus rhythm, BP 80/40mmHg, cool peripherally.
D: Drowsy — rousable to voice.
E: Temperature 37.4°C.

What is the best next step in management?

a   IM adrenaline.
b   Broad-spectrum antibiotics.
c   Further dose of IV magnesium.
d   IV salbutamol bolus.
e   Aminophylline infusion.

● Question 14

You are doing the daily ICU review of a 24-year-old male patient who was admitted the night before with agitation, jaundice and hypotension. He has recently been travelling in India and there is a clinical suspicion that he has acute liver failure secondary to viral hepatitis. ICU admission was primarily for management of agitation, hypotension and low urine output. He has received 5L of crystalloid (0.9% saline) overnight but has continued to be hypotensive. Vasopressor support with noradrenaline has been commenced. The patient was intubated and ventilated overnight secondary to unmanageable agitation. Nursing staff report that despite high levels of sedative infusions, the patient remains 'light' and has developed sluggish pupillary responses.

On examination:

A: ETT 22cm at the lips, head in line, 30° head up and no tight tube ties.
B: RR 30/min, PS/CPAP — PEEP of 7.5cmH$_2$O, PS 10, SpO$_2$ 98% on an FiO$_2$ of 0.4, pH 7.28, PaCO$_2$ 4.4kPa, PaO$_2$ 11kPa, HCO$_3^-$ 14mmol/L, lactate 5.5mmol/L.
C: BP 100/60mmHg, HR 100/min, sinus rhythm, noradrenaline 0.3μg/kg/min, warm peripherally, oliguric, urine output 150ml in the last 12 hours.
D: Propofol 4mg/kg/hr, alfentanil 0.4mg/kg/hr, pupils equal, sluggish reaction to light, localising to pain and moving around in the bed despite sedation.
E: Temperature 36.2°C, icteric, abdomen soft and non-tender.

Blood test results from that morning are shown in Table 4.7.

Table 4.7. Blood test results.

Hb	130g/L	Na$^+$	145mmol/L
WCC	14 x 10^9/L	K$^+$	5.2mmol/L
Platelets	80 x 10^9/L	Urea	30.2mmol/L
PT	45 seconds	Creatinine	310μmol/L
APTT	38 seconds	ALT	800 IU/L
Fibrinogen	1.8g/L	Albumin	25g/L
		Bilirubin	250μmol/L
		Ammonia	270μmol/L

What is the best management of this patient's neurological status?

a   Paralyse and control ventilation.
b   Insert ICP bolt to monitor ICP.
c   Start CRRT.
d   Hypertonic saline bolus.
e   Actively cool the patient.

● Question 15

You are reviewing a 55-year-old patient who is on day 2 of their ICU stay who was admitted after becoming unwell during preparation for an outpatient gastroscopy. The patient has known critical aortic stenosis and was having a gastroscopy to investigate microcytic anaemia prior to a planned valve replacement surgery. There was no history of overt GI bleeding. Initial bloods showed an acute kidney injury and an ischaemic hepatitis, and a cardiac echo showed critical aortic stenosis with impaired LV function (EF of 15%; an ECHO from 1 month prior showed normal EF). The patient has become anuric overnight. The ICU registrar had commenced CRRT at a dose of 25ml/kg/hr with citrate anticoagulation at 10pm the preceding evening.

On examination:

A: Maintaining own airway.
B: RR 28/min, SpO$_2$ 98% on an FiO$_2$ of 0.5 HFNO, ABG as outlined in Table 4.8. Chest auscultation reveals bilateral crepitations and wheeze.
C: BP 100/75 mmHg, HR 85/min, sinus rhythm, cool peripherally, ejection systolic murmur, noradrenaline 0.3µg/kg/min.
D: GCS 14/15, M-6, V-4, E-4. PEARL.
E: Abdomen soft, tender palpable liver edge. Managing small amounts of oral diet. CRRT — CVVHD 25ml/kg/min dosage, achieved -200ml total balance since starting 12 hours ago. The nurses state they have had to increase the calcium dose twice since starting. Urine output 20ml over the last 12 hours.

The morning blood test results including an arterial blood gas are shown in Table 4.8.

Table 4.8. Blood test results.

Na$^+$	130mmol/L	PT	30 seconds	pH	7.08
K$^+$	5.4mmol/L	APTT	48 seconds	pCO$_2$	4.0kPa
Urea	16mmol/L	Fibrinogen	2.5g/L	pO$_2$	11.4kPa
Creatinine	350µmol/L			HCO$_3^-$	13mmol/L
ALT	1550 IU/L			BE	−16mmol/L
Albumin	38g/L			iCa^{2+}	1.0mmol/L
Bilirubin	185µmol/L			Lactate	8mmol/L
Ca^{2+}	2.7mmol/L				

What is the best option regarding ongoing management of the patient's CRRT?

a   Continue with the current regime and repeat at T:I calcium ratio in 6 hours.
b   De-escalate citrate anticoagulation and initially try CRRT with no anticoagulant.
c   Increase the dialysate rate.
d   Decrease blood flow rate.
e   De-escalate citrate anticoagulation and switch to heparin for anticoagulation.

● Question 16

You are reviewing a lady from the ED who has been admitted for high-flow nasal oxygen (HFNO). She is a 62-year-old woman who has a 3-day history of fever and lethargy. Over the last 24 hours she has developed a worsening dry cough and shortness of breath, along with diarrhoea and vomiting. The patient has a history of COPD and usually has several exacerbations over the summer months. The patient feels that high humidity levels make her breathing worse; consequently, for the past month she has used a dehumidifier next to her bed which initially did help.

SBA Paper 4: Questions

On examination:

A: Maintaining own airway.
B: Currently on CPAP 10cmH$_2$O, RR 30/min, previously SpO$_2$ 92% on an FiO$_2$ of 0.6 HFNO 50L/min, auscultation reveals crackles bi-basally, CXR shows patchy infiltrates at the bases (most predominant on the left side).
C: BP 130/80mmHg, no vasopressor, HR 60/min, sinus rhythm, warm peripherally, capillary refill 2 seconds, nil oedema.
D: Alert and orientated, speaking in short sentences as dyspnoeic. PEARL.
E: Temperature 38.4°C, abdomen soft, mildly tender.

The morning blood test results including an arterial blood gas are shown in Table 4.9.

Table 4.9. Blood test results.

Hb	135g/L	Na$^+$	130mmol/L	pH	7.36
WCC	15 x 10^9/L	K$^+$	4.5mmol/L	pO$_2$	10kPa
Platelets	160 x 10^9/L	Urea	8.4mmol/L	pCO$_2$	6.4kPa
CRP	140mg/L	Creatinine	100µmol/L	HCO$_3^-$	28mmol/L
PCT	4ng/ml	ALT	80 IU/L	BE	−4mmol/L
CK	500 U/L	Bilirubin	15µmol/L		
PO$_4^{3-}$	0.9mmol/L	AST	60 U/L		

What is the most likely causative infection?

a   *Mycoplasma pneumoniae*.
b   *Legionella pneumophila*.
c   *Streptococcus pneumoniae*.
d   *Haemophilus influenzae*.
e   Influenza A virus.

● Question 17

You are reviewing a critical care long-stay patient. The bedside nurse has asked you why this patient is taking much longer to wean than other critical care patients they have seen.

The patient is a 64-year-old man with alcohol dependency and diabetes as a result of chronic pancreatitis. He was admitted with an episode of pancreatitis 2 months ago and was intubated and ventilated on day 3 due to agitation. There have been two failed extubations due to agitation, and a percutaneous tracheostomy was inserted on day 12. The patient was initially started on decremental support weaning and managed to have his pressure support (PS) reduced to 12; however, on attempted further weaning he desaturated and became distressed. This pattern of failed weaning persisted over a period of weeks. Periods of sprint weaning have been tried in the last week, but the patient has not tolerated more than a few minutes of 0 PS. He has now been weaned off all his medications for agitation. Due to concerns regarding failure to wean, electrophysiology testing has been undertaken.

On examination:

A: Tracheostomy.
B: PS/CPAP 12/8 during the day, requires volume-controlled ventilation (VCV) overnight due to desaturation and apnoea episodes, SpO_2 98% on an FiO_2 of 0.24.
C: BP 150/80mmHg, no vasopressor, HR 90/min, sinus rhythm, warm peripherally.
D: PEARL. Eyes open spontaneously and he seems orientated, able to track with eye movements and can nod and shake his head. There is some attempt at mouthing words, and he is attempting to communicate using head movements. Power 1/5 proximal muscles, 2/5 hands and feet, no reflexes are elicited, sensation to light touch appears to be intact and proximal muscle groups appear visibly atrophied.
E: Temperature 36.3°C.

Nerve conduction studies are shown in Table 4.10.

SBA Paper 4: Questions

Table 4.10. Nerve conduction studies.

Sensory nerve action potential (SNAP)	Within the normal range
Compound motor action potentials (CMAP)	20% of the lower range of normal
Repetitive nerve stimulation	Normal
Direct muscle activation	Absent/reduced action potential excitability in multiple muscle groups

CSF study results are shown in Table 4.11.

Table 4.11. CSF study.

- Clear appearance
- Protein 0.3g/L
- WCC 4 cells/μL
- Glucose 3.5mmol/L

What is the most likely cause of his failure to wean?

a   Critical illness polyneuropathy.
b   Critical illness myopathy.
c   Myasthenia gravis.
d   Guillain-Barré syndrome.
e   Critical illness polyneuromyopathy.

● Question 18

You are asked to review a patient who was admitted 4 hours previously from the ED with a suspected diagnosis of diabetic ketoacidosis (DKA). The patient is a 55-year-old 80kg lady with type 2 diabetes, managed on metformin and dapagliflozin. The patient started with a 'chesty cough' 3 days ago, and then started to feel nauseous and unwell this morning, so attended the ED. The patient has received one bolus of fluid (1L of Hartmann's solution) due to hypotension and has then been on the standard fluid treatment regimen for DKA (currently a 2-hourly bag of 0.9% saline with potassium supplementation, with an additional 125ml/hr of 10% dextrose), and the patient is on a fixed-rate insulin infusion of 8 units per hour.

Venous blood gases and point-of-care (POC) tests are shown in Table 4.12.

Table 4.12. Blood gases and point-of-care (POC) test results.

	9.30 (on arrival)	10.30	11.30	12.30	13.30
pH	6.96	6.94	6.97	7.00	7.01
pCO_2 kPa	2.4	2.2	2.5	3.0	3.1
HCO_3^- mmol/L	5	5	5	8	8
Glucose mmol/L	14	15	14	12	10
Ketones mmol/L	6.5	6.6	6.4	5.8	5.5

What is the appropriate management based on the result of the latest blood gas?

a   Continue current management.
b   Increase insulin to 9 units/hr, continue current fluid regime.
c   Decrease insulin to 4 units/hr, continue current fluid regime.
d   Increase insulin to 9 units/hr and increase dextrose to 200ml/hr.
e   Decrease insulin to 4 units/hr and reduce dextrose to 50ml/hr.

● **Question 19**

You have been called, as part of the medical emergency team, to a patient on the labour ward. There is a woman who is having a tonic-clonic seizure. The lady is a 41-year-old P1G0 who is 38 weeks' gestation and has had an uneventful pregnancy so far. The lady was last seen at 36 weeks pregnant and has been feeling tired and achy; BP at this appointment was 135/75mmHg. The patient was due to be seen again by the midwife today for a further check-up, but she went into labour in the early hours. She attended the labour ward an hour ago and was already 6cm dilated. Her initial blood pressure was 160/85mmHg, and her urine was positive for protein +++; all other bloods have been sent but are still awaited. She had some low-dose oral labetalol 20 minutes after arrival but vomited shortly afterwards. Blood pressure taken just prior to the seizure was 180/90mmHg; the midwives were in the process of drawing up a labetalol infusion for this lady when she started to seize. She has had 15L NRB oxygen applied and is on her left side and is continuing to seize.

What is the most important immediate management for this patient?

a   Magnesium 2g IV bolus.
b   Labetalol infusion.
c   2mg IV lorazepam.
d   Immediate delivery of the baby.
e   Magnesium 4g IV followed by continuous infusion of 1g/hr.

Question 20

A 76-year-old man undergoes an emergency open AAA repair. He has a history of resistant hypertension on four agents (ramipril, candesartan, bendroflumethiazide and doxazocin), paroxysmal atrial fibrillation, intermittent claudication and is a smoker of 40 cigarettes a day.

Intra-operatively he required a suprarenal aortic cross-clamp and the estimated blood loss was 4L. He was transfused with a full major transfusion pack plus 1L cell salvaged blood. The operation was long and surgically complex, and the postoperative handover stated that the cross-clamp had to be reapplied several times. He was transferred to the ICU in the early hours of the morning intubated and ventilated. The nursing staff are concerned as he seems unstable with escalating noradrenaline requirements and the following parameters.

On examination:

A: ETT *in situ*.
B: SpO_2 90% on an FiO_2 of 0.4, PRVC 450ml x 18, PEEP of 8cmH$_2$O, Ppeak 22cmH$_2$O.

C: BP 110/60mmHg, noradrenaline 0.4µg/kg/min, HR 110/min AF, cool peripheries, moderate peripheral oedema, urine output 20–25ml/hr.
D: RASS −2 on propofol 25ml/hr and alfentanil 0.4mg/hr, PEARL size 3mm, cool feet with weak but palpable pulses.
E: Temperature 35.8°C (active warming ongoing), bruising to both flanks and around the umbilicus, abdomen distended and tender, bowels opened ++ in the last hour, IAP 18mmHg.

Blood test results including an arterial blood gas are shown in Table 4.13.

Table 4.13. Blood test results.

			On admission	Taken at review
Hb	80g/L	pH	7.35	7.28
Urea	10mmol/L	pCO_2	6.5kPa	6.0kPa
Creatinine	180µmol/L	HCO_3^-	22mmol/L	20mmol/L
		BE	−8mmol/L	−15mmol/L
		Lactate	3.5mmol/L	8mmol/L

What complication is most likely to be causing the current clinical picture?

a Cholesterol embolisation syndrome.
b Lower limb ischaemia.
c Ischaemic colitis.
d Abdominal compartment syndrome.
e Acute kidney injury.

● **Question 21**

Which of the following conditions is **not** associated with hypernatraemia?

a Cranial diabetes insipidus.
b Cerebral salt wasting.
c Nephrogenic diabetes insipidus.
d Hyperosmolar hyperglycaemic state.
e Conn's syndrome.

SBA Paper 4: Questions

● **Question 22**

Which of the following drugs could be used safely and without dose adjustment in a patient with myotonic dystrophy?

a   Morphine.
b   Suxamethonium.
c   Neostigmine.
d   Remifentanil.
e   Midazolam.

● **Question 23**

Which of the following are **not** caused by a human herpes virus (HHV)?

a   Infectious mononucleosis.
b   Rubella.
c   Eczema herpeticum.
d   Chickenpox.
e   Kaposi's sarcoma.

● **Question 24**

Which of the following ultrasound probes would be best suited to undertake transthoracic echocardiography (TTE)?

a   Phased array transducer with 3–5MHz frequency.
b   Microconvex curved array transducer with 5–8MHz frequency.
c   Linear array transducer with 6–13Hz frequency.
d   Large footprint curved array transducer with 2–5MHz frequency.
e   Phased array transducer with 5–10MHz frequency.

● **Question 25**

You are about to intubate a patient who is profoundly hypoxic from pneumonia, septic with a high vasopressor requirement (noradrenaline 0.45µg/kg/min) and has a significant acute kidney injury (creatinine 400µmol/L, K⁺ 5.9mmol/L). The patient is currently tolerating high-flow nasal oxygen at flow rates of 60L/min on an FiO₂ of 1.0 with an SpO₂ of 92%. You have a team assembled and are undertaking the team brief. What is the optimal induction regime for this patient?

a   Fentanyl 100µg, thiopentone 5mg/kg, suxamethonium 1.5mg/kg.
b   Ketamine 2mg/kg and rocuronium 1mg/kg.
c   Fentanyl 100µg, propofol 2mg/kg and rocuronium 0.6mg/kg.
d   Fentanyl 200µg, midazolam 4mg and atracurium 0.6mg/kg.
e   Fentanyl 100µg, ketamine 1mg/kg and rocuronium 1mg/kg.

● **Question 26**

Which of the following parameters would classify an adult patient as having a near-fatal asthma exacerbation?

a   PaCO₂ of 6.5kPa.
b   Hypotension.
c   Altered conscious level.
d   Silent chest.
e   PaO₂ <8kPa.

● **Question 27**

You are asked to review a patient in the ED who has presented unconscious following a presumed overdose. They were found surrounded by empty vodka and antifreeze bottles and had been expressing suicidal thoughts a few days prior to their admission. The blood gas shows a lactate of 10.5mmol/L. What type of lactic acidosis is this?

a   Type A.
b   Type B1.
c   Type B2.
d   Type B3.
e   Type C.

Question 28
You admit a patient to the ICU who has a diagnosis of acute alcoholic hepatitis. The hepatology registrar has asked you to work out if the patient would benefit from steroids. Which scoring system would you use to decide if the patient would benefit from steroids?

a   Lille score.
b   SOFA score.
c   Modified Maddrey Discriminant Function.
d   APACHE IV score.
e   MELD score.

Question 29
You receive a call from the microbiology lab to inform you that one of your patients has a positive blood culture. An aerobic Gram-positive coccus in chains which is catalase-negative and alpha-haemolytic has been grown. Which bacteria is this likely to be describing?

a   *Staphylococcus aureus.*
b   *Streptococcus pneumoniae.*
c   *Streptococcus pyogenes.*
d   *Enterococcus faecalis.*
e   *Neisseria meningitidis.*

Question 30
Which of the following represents the most common precipitant of Guillain-Barré syndrome (GBS)?

a   Immunisation.
b   *Campylobacter jejuni* infection.
c   *Cytomegalovirus* infection.
d   Varicella zoster virus infection.
e   HIV infection.

● **Question 31**

Which immunoglobulin is defined as: produced first in the immune response, 0.5–2g/L mean adult serum level, does not bind to mast cells or cross the placenta?

a IgA.
b IgD.
c IgE.
d IgG.
e IgM.

● **Question 32**

What blood product must be stored at room temperature and continuously agitated?

a Packed red blood cells.
b Platelets.
c Cryoprecipitate.
d Fresh frozen plasma.
e Human albumin solution.

● **Question 33**

You are called to assist with a lady on the labour ward who is Gravida 2 Para 2 and delivered 30 minutes ago with the placenta delivering 10 minutes later. The patient had an uneventful pregnancy and normal vaginal delivery. She now has active vaginal bleeding with an estimated blood loss of 800ml and is hypotensive and tachycardic. What is the most likely underlying cause of her blood loss?

a Retained tissue.
b Coagulopathy.
c Poor uterine tone.
d Genital tract trauma.
e Uterine rupture.

SBA Paper 4: Questions

Question 34

You are presenting a clinical trial at a journal club. The paper examines whether a drug reduces K^+ levels in patients with acute kidney injury who are not on CRRT. In the introduction, the paper states that it is a follow-up study to a trial that brought the drug to the market a few years ago. In this study the drug did reduce K^+ levels, but clinical experience over the last few years has been that the drug has no effect on potassium levels. The results of this new large randomized controlled trial demonstrate that the drug has no significant effect on K^+ levels. What statement can be made about the results from the first trial?

a   The null hypothesis was incorrectly accepted.
b   It is likely there was a type 1 error in the data.
c   It is likely there was a type 2 error in the data.
d   The results displayed a beta error.
e   There was no bias in the sampling.

Question 35

Which of the following is **not** a common cause of neonatal collapse?

a   Sepsis.
b   Intussusception.
c   Congenital heart disease.
d   Inborn errors of metabolism.
e   Non-accidental injury.

Question 36

You are asked to review a patient in the ED who has burns to the face and torso. The patient states that the burns are not as sore as they expected, and they are red, non-blanching and dry to the touch.

What kind of burn does this patient have?

a   Full-thickness burn.
b   Superficial partial-thickness burn.
c   Deep partial-thickness burn.
d   Superficial burn.
e   3rd degree burn.

● Question 37

A 25-year-old patient who was hit by a car and sustained a significant traumatic brain injury (TBI) is currently at day 56 of his ICU stay. He is on a slow tracheostomy wean. He is breathing spontaneously, and coughs on suctioning. He seems to have periods of being more awake during which he makes semi-purposeful movements (hand moves towards his face on coughing, increased movements when family speak to him) but is not obeying commands or visually tracking. Which of the following describes his neurology?

a   Coma.
b   Vegetative state.
c   Death (as diagnosed by neurological criteria).
d   Minimally conscious state.
e   Locked-in syndrome.

● Question 38

What is the most common complication of the administration of blood products?

a   Haemolytic transfusion reaction.
b   TACO (transfusion-associated circulatory overload).
c   FAHR (febrile, allergic and hypotensive reactions).
d   TRALI (transfusion-related acute lung injury).
e   Transfusion-transmitted infection.

SBA Paper 4: Questions

Question 39

The use of rasburicase in the prophylaxis of tumour lysis syndrome (TLS) prevents complications from which of the following?

a   Hyperkalaemia.
b   Hyperuricaemia.
c   Hyperphosphataemia.
d   Hypocalcaemia.
e   Hyperlipidaemia.

Question 40

You are involved in the management of an adult patient who is having a tonic-clonic seizure. The patient is not known to have epilepsy and has not taken any drugs to precipitate this. The patient has received buccal midazolam with the paramedics, is receiving 15L oxygen via a non-rebreathe mask and has had an IV cannula sited. On arrival to the ED the patient received a dose of IV lorazepam. They are continuing to have seizure activity. What is the next step in management?

a   Loading dose of levetiracetam.
b   Bolus of lorazepam.
c   RSI with propofol.
d   Loading dose of phenobarbital.
e   RSI with ketamine.

Question 41

Which of the following regarding Ebola is true?

a   It is an arbovirus.
b   Mortality for all strains is around 30%.
c   Ribavirin treatment reduces mortality.
d   It causes a viral haemorrhagic fever.
e   Relative bradycardia is typically seen in early infection.

Question 42

It is 3 a.m. and the nurse in charge of the ICU tells you that he has received a phone call from the microbiology lab to inform them that a patient in an open bay has grown *Candida auris* from a urine sample. There are no other cases of *C. auris* on the ICU. What, if anything, needs to be done about this from an infection control point of view?

a   Continue nursing the patient in the bay, with no additional barrier precautions or screening.
b   The patient should be moved to a cubicle, an apron and gloves should be used for patient contact, and all patients and staff in the bay need screening.
c   The patient should be moved to a cubicle, a long-sleeved gown and gloves used for contact, and all patients in the bay need screening.
d   All patients in the bay need moving to cubicles, a long-sleeved gown and gloves used for contact, the whole unit needs screening, and stop new admissions to the unit.
e   Continue nursing in the bay, a long-sleeved gown and gloves used for contact, with no additional screening needed.

Question 43

Which of the following antifungal agents acts via inhibition of the cell wall polysaccharide glucan?

a   Fluconazole.
b   Amphotericin.
c   Nystatin.
d   Flucytosine.
e   Anidulafungin.

Question 44

Which of the following is **not** associated with an increased risk of contrast-induced acute kidney injury?

a   Intra-arterial contrast administration.
b   Use of low-osmolar radiocontrast media.
c   eGFR <40ml/min/1.73m².
d   Age over 75.
e   Hypovolaemia.

● Question 45
Which of the following vitamins is fat-soluble?

a   Vitamin D.
b   Thiamine.
c   Vitamin C.
d   Folate.
e   Niacin.

● Question 46
Which of the following use a modified Stewart-Hamilton equation to calculate cardiac output?

a   Oesophageal Doppler.
b   The Fick method.
c   Arterial pressure waveform analysis.
d   Transthoracic electrical bioimpedance.
e   Transpulmonary thermodilution.

● Question 47
Which of the following would carry the most weight when undertaking Wells' scoring for suspected pulmonary embolus (PE)?

a   Haemoptysis.
b   Clinical features of deep vein thrombosis (DVT).
c   Previous DVT or PE.
d   Surgery in the previous 4 weeks.
e   Heart rate greater than 100.

Question 48

You are looking after a patient with ARDS and the consultant asks you to calculate the Murray score to see if they would be eligible for ECMO. The patient's respiratory parameters are as follows:

SpO_2 95% with a PaO_2 of 15 kPa on an FiO_2 of 1.0. The patient is ventilated on a pressure-regulated volume-controlled (PRVC) mode with a TV of 400ml, respiratory rate of 22/min and a PEEP of 10cm H_2O. Ppeak is 35cmH_2O, PPlateau is 30cmH_2O. The CT shows patchy infiltrates in both lower zones. What is the Murray score for the patient?

a   4.
b   3.5.
c   2.5.
d   5.
e   10.

Question 49

You are floating a pulmonary artery catheter (PAC) and the pressure reading on the screen is 25/10mmHg. Where is the pressure transducer currently sitting?

a   Right atrium.
b   Pulmonary artery wedge pressure.
c   Right ventricle.
d   Pulmonary artery.
e   Central venous pressure.

Question 50

You have taken a sample of ascitic fluid from a patient who has presented with confusion and is unable to give you any medical history. They have marked ascites on examination. The results of an ascitic tap are shown in Table 4.14.

Table 4.14. Results of an ascitic tap.

Ascitic results				Serum results	
Total protein	14g/L	Amylase	35 U/L	Amylase	85 U/L
Albumin	13g/L	Glucose	4.0mmol/L	Total protein	30g/L
WBC	252 cells/mm^3	LDH	100 IU/L	Albumin	28g/L
Neutrophils	200 cells/mm^3			Glucose	4.5mmol/L

What is the likely underlying diagnosis?

a   Pancreatitis.
b   Spontaneous bacterial peritonitis.
c   Secondary peritonitis.
d   Hepatic cirrhosis.
e   Bowel perforation.

Answer overview: Paper 4

Question:		Question:	
1	b	26	a
2	a	27	c
3	d	28	c
4	b	29	b
5	d	30	b
6	e	31	e
7	b	32	b
8	b	33	c
9	c	34	b
10	d	35	b
11	a	36	c
12	e	37	d
13	d	38	c
14	c	39	b
15	b	40	a
16	b	41	d
17	b	42	c
18	b	43	e
19	e	44	b
20	c	45	a
21	b	46	e
22	d	47	b
23	b	48	c
24	a	49	d
25	e	50	d

SBA Paper 4: Answers

Answer 1: b

The likely diagnosis here is propofol-related infusion syndrome (PRIS).

The pathophysiology of PRIS is not completely understood, but it is thought that propofol impairs the uptake and usage of free fatty acids and decouples oxidative phosphorylation. This affects cell substrate supply, hinders ATP generation and eventually leads to cell necrosis and death.

Prolonged high-dose propofol infusions (over 4mg/kg/hr for over 48 hours) may predispose to the development of PRIS. Additional risk factors include: young age (particularly paediatrics), inborn errors of metabolism, traumatic brain injury (due to high sedation requirements), and elevated catecholamine levels.

Clinical presentation is primarily with acidosis and profound cardiovascular impairment, notably myocardial dysfunction and hypotension. Depleted ATP stores and high free fatty acid levels may cause myocyte damage, antagonism of beta receptors and reduced sympathetic tone. Arrhythmias may be seen, including progressive bradycardia leading to asystole, new RBBB, Brugada-like ECG changes, VT, AF and SVT. Metabolically, a raised lactate and potassium, metabolic acidosis, high triglycerides and hyperthermia may be seen. Liver impairment can result either from congestion, lipid deposition within the liver or due to hypoperfusion. PRIS can cause damage to all muscle cells and results in a high CK, myoglobinuria and rhabdomyolysis.

Management of PRIS is primarily through early recognition, regular monitoring of triglycerides and CK and reducing or stopping propofol entirely (typically using midazolam as an alternative). If PRIS is already established, then stopping propofol is paramount, and cessation of any other lipid sources (e.g. TPN) should be considered. Providing organ support with vasopressors, inotropes, pacing and CRRT is often needed. In some cases, ECMO has been used with success. Providing carbohydrate in the form of a dextrose infusion may help to reduce lipolysis and provide an alternative energy substrate.

References

1. Loh N-HW, Nair P. Propofol infusion syndrome. *Contin Educ Anaesth Crit Care Pain* 2013; 13(6): 200–2.
2. Singh A, Anjankar AP. Propofol-related infusion syndrome: a clinical review. *Cureus* 2022; 14(10): e30383.

Answer 2: a

Patients who suffer burns due to fires and explosions are at risk of airway burns, especially if the face is affected. Burns with smoke inhalation represent a minority of burns presenting to hospital but are associated with high mortality. Smoke composition varies depending on the type of fire and so airway and lung injuries may result from heat (typically above the cords), and particulate matter in the airways or toxicity from inhaled compounds (e.g. cyanide and carbon monoxide).

Airway injury should be suspected if the fire is in an enclosed space, or the patient was unconscious during the incident. Clinical signs of airway and lung thermal injury include voice change, stridor, cough, burns to the lips, mouth or nose, hypoxia and a low GCS. If airway burns are suspected, the patient should be closely monitored and intubated early with an uncut tube if there is evidence of evolving airway burns and oedema. Early nasendoscopy to evaluate the airway injury may be used to help guide management.

Once the patient is intubated, they should undergo early bronchoscopy to facilitate therapeutic washout and clearance of particulate matter and grading of inhalational burn severity. Lung-protective ventilation should be used (range 4–8ml/kg, plateau pressure ≤30cmH$_2$O). The use of nebulised inhalational therapy is important in airway burns (but has a limited evidence base) but is not required immediately following intubation. Inhalational therapies typically include a combination of beta-2 agonists, heparin and N-acetylcysteine.

SBA Paper 4: Answers

Prophylactic antibiotics are not routinely indicated; however, close monitoring for secondary bacterial infection is required.

As the TBSA burn in this case is less than 15%, fluid resuscitation is not indicated. Management of these burns can be undertaken at a burns unit; however, burns greater than 25% TBSA with associated inhalational injury should be managed in a specialist burns centre.

References
1. Gill P, Martin RV. Smoke inhalation injury. *BJA Educ* 2015; 15(3): 143–8.
2. Devine MJ, Trainor DM. Critical care management of patients with severe burns and inhalational injury. *Anaesth Intensive Care Med* 2023; 24(7): 397–401.

Answer 3: d

Brainstem death testing (BSDT) is undertaken when a patient has an irreversible brain injury of known aetiology, with no potentially reversible causes for coma and apnoea. Exclusion criteria prior to testing include medications such as sedative agents and neuromuscular blockers as well as markedly abnormal blood electrolyte results. The acceptable ranges for testing are as follows (changes in the new 2025 form are in bold):

- Temperature **≥36°C**.
- Na$^+$ **125**–160mmol/L.
- K$^+$ >2.0mmol/L.
- PO$_4^{3-}$ 0.5–3.0mmol/L.
- Mg^{2+} 0.5–3.0mmol/L.
- Blood glucose 3.0–20.0mmol/L.

You should also be satisfied that 'no cardiovascular or respiratory disturbance is materially contributing to the observed coma or apnoea' and target normal parameters for blood pressure and oxygenation as is appropriate for the patient based on their medical history.

For the beginning of the apnoea test, the patient's PaCO$_2$ should be at least 5.3kPa and should be at or above their baseline (which may be significantly higher than this for those patients with chronic hypercapnic respiratory failure).

Please see page 247, Paper 3, Q34 for more information on BSDT.

References

1. Academy of Medical Royal Colleges (AoMRC) and Faculty of Intensive Care Medicine (FICM). Form for the diagnosis of death using neurological criteria, 2025. Available at: https://ficm.ac.uk/sites/ficm/files/documents/2024-12/Form%20for%20the%20Diagnosis%20of%20DNC%20-%20adults%20and%20children%20over%202%20years%20-%20January%202025.pdf.

Answer 4: b

The pleural fluid appearance and biochemistry combined with the initial microbiology findings of a known empyema-forming organism strongly suggests the presence of an empyema. From the clinical history it is evident this is a new empyema which has not previously been drained.

The British Thoracic Society guidance on the management of pleural infection advises the use of a fine-bore chest drain as first line, as this is associated with reduced post-procedural pain and no increase in hospital LOS or mortality. However, this guidance is ungraded and based on consensus opinion and there is limited evidence that directly compares the use of fine-bore to wide-bore chest drains in the management of empyema.

As this is the first presentation of empyema, a fine-bore chest drain should initially be sited. Should incomplete drainage or loculation of the pleural fluid develop, then consideration of a wide-bore surgical drain or a video-assisted thoracoscopic surgery (VATS) procedure is warranted.

A change of antibiotics alone is not appropriate in this case as the empyema requires drainage for management of the condition. As the causative organism is known, continuation of current therapy is not unreasonable with adjustments made according to sensitivity testing as required.

References

1. Roberts ME, Rahman NM, Maskell NA, *et al.* British Thoracic Society guideline for pleural disease. *Thorax* 2023; 78(Suppl 3): s1–42.

Answer 5: d

The clinical scenario is suggestive of *Pneumocystis jirovecii* pneumonia (PJP). Organisms of the *Pneumocystis* genus are ascomycetous fungi with cholesterol instead of ergosterol in the cell wall, which renders azole and polyene antifungals an ineffective treatment. PJP typically causes infection in immunosuppressed patients and can asymptomatically colonise immunocompetent patients.

Risk of infection is increased in the following groups: HIV infection, concomitant steroid use with another immunosuppressant, haematological malignancies, bone marrow and solid organ transplant recipients, immunosuppressant medication (e.g. anti-rejection, anti-TNF, purine analogue medications), primary immunodeficiency.

Patients typically present with shortness of breath and a dry cough. Exertion-induced hypoxia is characteristic of PJP. Imaging may initially be normal, but as the disease progresses patients usually develop bilateral widespread ground-glass infiltration originating from the hila outwards. Diagnosis is based on a clinical suspicion in combination with the presence of PJP on induced sputum or bronchoalveolar lavage (BAL) using immunofluorescence or PJP DNA on polymerase chain reaction (PCR).

The first-line antibiotic for treatment is co-trimoxazole (Septrin™) at a dose of 120mg/kg/day in 2–4 divided doses (typically 30mg/kg QDS). The addition of steroids (typically methylprednisolone 1–2mg/kg or prednisolone 40mg) has been shown to reduce mortality in HIV patients, with no clear evidence for use in non-HIV patients; however, they are widely used in patients with SpO_2 <92% or a PaO_2 <9.3kPa on room air. Alternative antimicrobials include pentamidine, clindamycin and primaquine or dapsone and atovaquone. Prophylaxis for PJP in high-risk patients is typically with 980mg a day of Septrin™.

In this clinical scenario, the patient is at risk of bacterial, atypical and PJP infection. Whilst the history and clinical findings suggest PJP, coverage for all possible infections would be appropriate until the causative organism is identified.

References

1. Carr A. Fungal infection. In: Bersten AD, Handy JM, Eds. *Oh's intensive care manual*, 8th ed. London: Elsevier; 2028: chapter 73: pp. 866–74.
2. Ramirez JA, Musher DM, Evans SE, *et al*. Treatment of community-acquired pneumonia in immunocompromised adults: a consensus statement regarding initial strategies. *Chest* 2020; 158(5): 1896–911.

3. www.uptodate.com. Epidemiology, clinical manifestations, and diagnosis of *Pneumocystis* pneumonia in patients without HIV. UpToDate, 2025. Available at: https://www.uptodate.com/contents/epidemiology-clinical-manifestations-and-diagnosis-of-pneumocystis-pneumonia-in-patients-without-hiv.

● Answer 6: e

There are many causes of acute weakness including pathology within the brain, spinal cord, peripheral nerves, neuromuscular junction (NMJ) or the muscles themselves.

Neurological causes can be divided into upper motor neurone (brain and descending tracts to the anterior horn of the spinal cord) and lower motor neurone (motor neurones within the spinal cord down to the neuromuscular junction). Upper motor neurone causes include: cerebrovascular accidents, intracranial masses (tumours, abscess), multiple sclerosis and spinal cord lesions.

Lower motor neurone (including NMJ) causes include Guillain-Barré syndrome, Lambert-Eaton syndrome, motor neuropathy, myasthenia gravis, motor neurone disease (upper and lower motor neurone signs).

Other causes include myositis, endocrine causes (adrenal insufficiency, hypothyroidism and hyperthyroidism, Cushing's syndrome), muscular dystrophies, medications (e.g. statins), toxins (e.g. alcohol).

The history and presentation in this case suggests myasthenia gravis. Myasthenia gravis is an autoimmune disease caused by autoantibodies to acetylcholine receptors at the neuromuscular junction. It is more common in women and peaks in young adulthood. In 70% of cases there is thymic abnormality, typically thymic hyperplasia. Older patients are more likely to have a thymoma.

Clinical presentation is of fatigable weakness (weakness increases the more the muscle is used), and most commonly ocular muscle involvement presenting as diplopia and ptosis. Bulbar muscle involvement and dysphagia are also commonly seen, along with proximal and trunk weakness affecting the upper limbs more than the lower limbs. There is no sensory or autonomic nerve involvement.

Lambert-Eaton syndrome is considered a myasthenic weakness but is due to anti-voltage-gated calcium channel antibodies, and often occurs as a paraneoplastic syndrome (classically small cell lung cancer). Autonomic involvement is common, and weakness typically affects the pelvic and thigh muscles with ocular and bulbar involvement being rare.

Diagnosis of myasthenia gravis is via the presence of one of the associated autoantibodies (nAChR, MuSK, lipoprotein receptor-related protein antibodies). A Tensilon test — assessment of power following administration of a short-acting acetylcholinesterase inhibitor such as edrophonium — can also be performed. Management is with anticholinesterase drugs (e.g. pyridostigmine), immunosuppression and thymectomy (if appropriate).

A myasthenic crisis is an acute worsening of myasthenic symptoms due to a number of triggers, including: infection, medication (in this case LRTI and erythromycin), pregnancy and surgery. These patients may require ICU admission and have a high risk of requiring intubation and ventilation due to respiratory muscle weakness and a high risk of aspiration due to bulbar dysfunction. Treatment of a myasthenic crisis may include the use of plasma exchange or IVIg therapy in addition to usual measures. For further information on precipitants see page 155, Paper 2, Q30.

References

1. Saxena M. Neuromuscular disorders. In: Bersten AD, Handy JM, Eds. *Oh's intensive care manual*, 8th ed. London: Elsevier; 2018: chapter 58: pp. 721–30.
2. Larson ST, Wilbur J. Muscle weakness in adults: evaluation and differential diagnosis. *Am Fam Physician* 2020; 101(2): 95–108.
3. www.uptodate.com. Clinical manifestations of myasthenia gravis. UpToDate, 2025. Available at: https://www.uptodate.com/contents/clinical-manifestations-of-myasthenia-gravis.

Answer 7: b

Metabolic alkalosis is commonly seen in critically ill patients. It results from a reduction in plasma hydrogen ion concentration, with a pH of >7.45 indicating an alkalaemia. It is possible to have an alkalosis without alkalaemia in patients with reduced hydrogen ion concentrations but a pH <7.45.

According to the Henderson-Hasselbalch theory, bicarbonate is not an independent determinant of pH, and instead bicarbonate concentrations fluctuate in response to changes in hydrogen ion and carbon dioxide concentration. The base excess quantifies the metabolic component of the acid-base state, and is the amount of acid or alkali required to bring the pH of blood back to 7.40 with a $PaCO_2$ of 5.2kPa. The standard base excess calculation includes an assumed Hb concentration.

The Stewart hypothesis of the acid-base balance is based on three variables independently influencing pH: the $PaCO_2$, the ATOT (total amount of weak acids in the plasma) and the strong ion difference (SID). Metabolic alkalosis can occur due to a decreased ATOT (decreased albumin) and increased SID. SID is the difference between the plasma concentration of fully dissociated cations (Na^+, K^+, Mg^{2+} Ca^{2+}) and anions (Cl^-, lactate, ketones, sulphate). In practice this is calculated as the difference between the Na^+ and the Cl^- with a normal value of 35mmol/L. Electrochemical neutrality must be maintained within the body; therefore, with a reduced SID (typically raised chloride) more H^+ ions are created by buffer systems to ensure an equal number of cations and anions. This increase in H^+ subsequently causes an acidosis. If there is an increased SID (high Na^+ or low Cl^-) then there is a deficit of anions and H^+ ions are absorbed by the buffer systems resulting in an alkalosis. The SID is typically made up of the HCO_3^- concentration plus the ATOT.

As albumin is the primary component of ATOT, hypoalbuminaemia results in an alkalosis, and HCO_3^- increases to maintain electrical neutrality. The renal response to low albumin is to retain chloride, with 1.4mmol/L of Cl^- retained for every 10g drop in total protein concentration resulting in a compensated alkalosis.

Frusemide administration may cause increased urinary losses of chloride without a significant increase in bicarbonate loss. The resulting alkalosis worsens with volume depletion, so if the patient is intravascularly depleted, Na^+ will increase, and in the case of frusemide coupled with reduced chloride, an increased SID and alkalosis are seen.

In the clinical scenario in question, whilst there is evidence of volume contraction with raised Na^+ that could be due to furosemide, the sudden change in GI output means that the alkalosis is much more likely to be due to new-onset significant hypochloraemia.

SBA Paper 4: Answers

References
1. Park M, Sidebotham D. Metabolic alkalosis and mixed acid-base disturbance in anaesthesia and critical care. *BJA Educ* 2023; 23(4): 128–35.
2. Tinawi M. Pathophysiology, evaluation, and management of metabolic alkalosis. *Cureus* 2021; 13(1): e12841.
3. Ghosh S. Acid base homeostasis: Stewart approach at the bedside. In: Malbrain ML, Wong A, Nasa P, Ghosh S, Eds. *Rational use of intravenous fluids in critically ill patients*. Cham: Springer; 2023: pp.153–65.

● Answer 8: b

There are a number of different causes of an elevated body temperature. Hyperthermia is an elevated body temperature with a normal thermoregulatory set temperature and distinct from fever, where the set point of the hypothalamus is increased to above 37°C resulting in temperatures above 37.7°C, with fever being the most common cause of elevated temperatures.

Body temperature varies throughout the day, but generally an elevated body temperature is considered to be >37.7°C and hyperpyrexia a temperature >41.5°C from either fever or hyperthermia.

The causes of hyperthermia include heat stroke, metabolic causes (e.g. hyperthyroidism), pharmacological agents that disrupt heat loss mechanisms and genetic abnormalities which result in heat-generating adverse drug reactions (e.g. malignant hyperthermia).

There are several possible causes of hyperthermia in the case in question; however, the rising CO_2 and rigidity strongly suggest a pharmacological toxidrome such as malignant hyperpyrexia (MH), serotonin syndrome, neuroleptic malignant syndrome, anticholinergic syndrome and MDMA overdose. Given that the patient is receiving general anaesthesia with a volatile agent, MH is highly likely.

MH is an autosomal dominant condition usually caused by a mutation in the ryanodine receptor RYR1. On exposure to a trigger (volatile anaesthetics or depolarizing muscle relaxants) the abnormal receptor releases excessive calcium into muscle cell cytosol resulting in sustained contraction of the muscle fibres. Initially this is aerobically powered, resulting in high CO_2 production, and subsequently anaerobic energy production takes over resulting in a metabolic acidosis. Onset of symptoms is within 2 hours of exposure, with a hypercarbia out of proportion to minute ventilation, sinus tachycardia, rapidly rising temperature and generalized muscular rigidity in 40% of cases.

Management includes cessation of the triggering agent (typically switch out to clean 'MH safe' anaesthetic machine and total intravenous anaesthesia) and administration of dantrolene (2.5mg/kg repeated every 5–10 minutes until response with a maximum initial dose of 10mg/kg). Active cooling measures and increased minute ventilation to manage hypercarbia should also be used.

Neuroleptic malignant syndrome (NMS) is a drug reaction to drugs that antagonize central dopamine transmission such as antipsychotics and typically happens within a month of starting the drug or dose increase. The central dopamine antagonism in the hypothalamus results in hyperthermia, and in other areas of the midbrain results in changes in mental status and the typical extrapyramidal symptoms (e.g. lead pipe rigidity, bradykinesia, tremors, tardive dyskinesia). Patients mount a high temperature over a longer period of time with onset over days to weeks and the temperature is below 42°C. Management includes cessation of the causative agent, sedation +/- paralysis which may reduce severity of the temperature, active cooling, and bromocriptine which reduces extrapyramidal symptoms and mortality. Dantrolene has no benefit in NMS. Serotonin syndrome results from excessive serotonin levels and occurs when multiple serotonergic agents have been used (SSRIs, SNRIs, MAOIs including linezolid, amphetamines, fentanyl, tramadol and ondansetron). It presents within 24 hours of receiving serotonergic agents and presents with altered mental state (agitation, delirium), autonomic stimulation (sweating, tachycardia, hyperthermia) and neuromuscular excitation (clonus, hyperreflexia). The Hunter criteria can be used to tell you if this is serotonin syndrome; if there is spontaneous clonus in the presence of a serotoninergic agent overdose or after the addition of a new agent, then the patient has serotonin syndrome. Treatment involves stopping any causative agents, active cooling, use of cyproheptadine (if enteral route available) or chlorpromazine. Although the patient is on an SSRI and has received additional serotonergic agents, the clinical onset is too rapid for serotonin syndrome and the rapid increase in carbon dioxide is not typical.

SBA Paper 4: Answers

References

1. Lam S, Strickland R. Thermal disorders. In: Bersten AD, Handy JM, Eds. *Oh's intensive care manual*, 8th ed. London: Elsevier; 2018: chapter 84: pp. 978–98.
2. www.uptodate.com. Pathophysiology and treatment of fever in adults. UpToDate, 2024. Available at: https://www.uptodate.com/contents/pathophysiology-and-treatment-of-fever-in-adults.
3. www.uptodate.com. Serotonin syndrome (serotonin toxicity). UpToDate, 2024. Available at: https://www.uptodate.com/contents/serotonin-syndrome-serotonin-toxicity.

Answer 9: c

This patient is presenting with a myxoedema crisis. There are signs of pre-existing hypothyroidism, and it is likely that she is having a myocardial infarction (MI) which has precipitated the crisis.

Myxoedema coma is the extreme end of hypothyroidism and has a mortality of between 30–60%. A myxoedemic crisis is thankfully rare and often presents without either myxoedema (non-pitting oedema) or coma in patients with longstanding unrecognised hypothyroidism who suffer an additional insult (such as infection, MI, surgery, trauma, hypothermia, hypoglycaemia).

Many of the features result from the underlying reduction in baseline metabolism secondary to reduced thyroid hormone levels, and affect the organ systems in different ways:

- Airway: goitre, vocal cord oedema and macroglossia.
- Respiratory: respiratory alkalosis due to reduced carbon dioxide production, diaphragmatic weakness and reduced exercise tolerance, reduced central sensitivity to hypoxia and hypercapnia (can result in a respiratory acidosis in response to a respiratory insult or reduction in GCS).
- Cardiovascular: reduced cardiac output with increased systemic vascular resistance leading to diastolic hypertension and heart failure, bradycardia and ECG changes (including prolonged QTc, small QRS complexes, non-specific ST and T wave changes and heart block).
- Neurological: personality changes, seizures and coma may all occur, generalised muscle weakness, hyponatraemia is common and can contribute to alterations in GCS.

- Other: weight gain, malabsorption, gut ileus, urinary retention, hypothermia, hypoglycaemia (due to reduced gluconeogenesis or concurrent adrenal insufficiency in Schmidt's syndrome).

Treatment is via thyroid hormone replacement and steroids (measure random cortisol prior to administering), along with treatment of any precipitating factor and supportive management as required. Replacement should be graduated to minimise the risk of myocardial ischaemia and arrhythmias.

References
1. Handy J, Li A. Thyroid emergencies. In: Bersten AD, Handy JM, Eds. *Oh's intensive care manual*, 8th ed. London: Elsevier; 2018: chapter 61: pp. 757–66.
2. www.uptodate.com. Myxedema coma. UpToDate, 2025. Available at: https://www.uptodate.com/contents/myxedema-coma.

● Answer 10: d

Autoimmune encephalitis is an increasingly recognised cause of encephalitis, mainly due to the availability of testing for the different causative autoantibodies rather than a change in underlying incidence. Many of these antibodies are associated with malignancy, and several have a high association with specific malignancies. In this clinical case the patient likely has an ovarian teratoma which is associated with anti-NMDA receptor antibody encephalitis.

The presentation of the encephalitis can vary dependent on the antibody in question, but in general, symptoms develop over a few days to weeks and include changes in cognition (disorientation, amnesia, confusion), seizures (focal or generalised), dysautonomia and behavioural changes/psychiatric symptoms (aggression, mood lability, hallucinations, sleep/wake cycle disturbance) and can cause pain due to peripheral nerve excitability. The presentation of anti-NDMA receptor antibody encephalitis is typically with an initial prodrome that may include headache and fever, then progresses to psychiatric symptoms (hallucinations, delusions, disorganised thinking, psychosis), with later symptoms including confusion, seizures and marked autonomic instability (which is often the reason for intensive care referral).

SBA Paper 4: Answers

A CT scan of the head is often unhelpful and likely to be normal, especially early on in the disease process. MRI scanning can be normal in the early stages but may show some abnormalities on FLAIR or contrast-enhancing sequences depending on the antibody in question. EEG findings again vary based on the causative autoantibody, and with the exception of the unique 'extreme delta brush' pattern found in anti-NDMA receptor antibody encephalitis, findings are likely to be suggestive rather than definitive. When autoimmune encephalitis is diagnosed, dependent on the antibody in question, further screening for malignancy may be indicated.

First-line treatment is with steroids, IVIg and plasmapheresis, with early neurological specialist referral vital. The main differential diagnosis is infective encephalitis, which may lead to a hesitancy to give immunosuppressant agents. In addition to antibody management, supportive management for any symptoms should be given, along with managing of any underlying malignancy if present.

References

1. Uy CE, Binks S, Irani SR. Autoimmune encephalitis: clinical spectrum and management. *Pract Neurol* 2021; 21(5): 412–23.
2. www.uptodate.com. Autoimmune (including paraneoplastic) encephalitis: clinical features and diagnosis. UpToDate, 2025. Available at: https://www.uptodate.com/contents/autoimmune-including-paraneoplastic-encephalitis-clinical-features-and-diagnosis.

Answer 11: a

Upper GI bleeding is commonly encountered on critical care, either as a presentation pathology (e.g. variceal bleeding) or as a consequence of other illness. Stress ulceration is a well-recognised complication of ICU stays with an incidence of around 8–45%. Rates have reduced from historical levels, in conjunction with routine use of prophylaxis with alkalinisation agents such as PPI medications. A large RCT comparing IV pantoprazole with placebo demonstrated a significant reduction in clinically important GI bleeds with PPI use but no significant differences in other outcomes including mortality.

There are several risk factors for clinically important GI bleeding in ICU. These were analysed in a systematic review which showed that factors consistently associated with increased risk of clinical important or overt GI bleeding (in studies with a moderate/low risk of bias) were coagulopathy, chronic liver disease and shock. Male gender and acute kidney injury were also shown to have an increased risk when all studies were included. Enteral nutrition has been shown to decrease the risk of GI bleeding. Recent studies have not suggested mechanical ventilation to be a predominant risk factor, which may be related to the widespread adoption of lung-protective ventilation strategies.

References
1. Cook D, Deane A, Lauzier F, et al. Stress ulcer prophylaxis during invasive mechanical ventilation. *N Engl J Med* 2024; 391(1): 9–20.
2. Granholm A, Zeng L, Dionne JC, et al. Predictors of gastrointestinal bleeding in adult ICU patients: a systematic review and meta-analysis. *Intensive Care Med* 2019; 45(10): 1347–59.
3. Simillis C, Shahnawaz R. Acute gastrointestinal bleeding. In: Bersten AD, Handy JM, Eds. *Oh's intensive care manual*, 8th ed. London: Elsevier; 2018: chapter 42: pp. 551–64.

Answer 12: e

Pneumonectomy is the surgical removal of an entire lung and carries a higher mortality rate than other lung resection surgeries, such as lobectomies and sleeve resection. Bronchial carcinoma is the most common indication for a pneumonectomy. Non-malignant indications include trauma with uncontrolled haemorrhage and infections (e.g. TB, fungal infection).

Routine surgery involves resection of the affected lung, with removal of the pulmonary artery up to the left atrium (intracardial pneumonectomy) or resection of the pleura, hemidiaphragm and hemipericardium (extrapleural pneumonectomy) are sometimes required. Patients are typically extubated at the end of the operation (as prolonged intubation increases the risk of bronchopleural fistula) and will often have a period of time in a high dependency area. There may or may not be a chest drain *in situ*, and this is initially left clamped to avoid mediastinal shift into the space. The drain is subsequently unclamped for a short period every hour to assess for bleeding.

There are several postoperative complications specific to pneumonectomy. Cardiac arrhythmias are commonly seen with 20–40% of patients developing AF, usually within 72 hours of surgery. Additional risk factors for new-onset AF are age over 65, male, right pneumonectomy, intracardiac pneumonectomy, coronary artery disease and hypertension.

SBA Paper 4: Answers

Post-pneumonectomy pulmonary oedema occurs in 2–5% and is associated with a mortality of over 50%. It is more common after a right-sided pneumonectomy and presents with shortness of breath and hypoxia, and occurs within 72 hours of surgery.

Post-pneumonectomy syndrome occurs due to extrinsic compression of the remaining mainstem bronchus and distal trachea following mediastinal shift and hyperinflation of the remaining lung. It typically occurs more than 6 months after surgery and is almost exclusive to patients undergoing right pneumonectomy. Symptoms include progressive shortness of breath, cough, inspiratory stridor and recurrent pneumonia.

Bronchopleural fistula is seen in 1.5% to 20% of patients and carries a significant associated mortality risk. It is more common in patients undergoing a right pneumonectomy due to poor blood supply of the right main bronchus and increased exposure of the stump compared to the left side. It can be early (within 2 weeks) presenting with cough, ongoing air leak from a chest drain, new air fluid level on CXR or later (after 2 weeks postop) with more non-specific signs.

Cardiac herniation (as described in this question) occurs when the heart herniates through the pericardial defect into the empty pleural space resulting in torsion of the heart. It is usually seen within 3 days of surgery presenting as sudden-onset shock, cyanosis, chest pain and signs of SVC obstruction. It is often precipitated by coughing, moving, vomiting or extubation. Treatment involves an immediate return to theatre to reposition the heart.

Intracardiac shunting is an uncommon complication of pneumonectomy and involves development of a right to left shunt through a patent foramen ovale or atrial septal defect (ASD). Symptoms include dyspnoea and platypnoea (worsening SOB on sitting or standing) occurring between 2 days and a year post-surgery.

References
1. Hackett S, Jones R, Kapila R. Anaesthesia for pneumonectomy. *BJA Educ* 2019; 19(9): 297–304.
2. www.uptodate.com. Sequelae and complications of pneumonectomy. UpToDate, 2025. Available at: https://www.uptodate.com/contents/sequelae-and-complications-of-pneumonectomy.

Answer 13: d

The British Thoracic Society (BTS)/Scottish Intercollegiate Guidelines Network (SIGN) have clear guidance on the assessment and management of asthma in children. An acute asthma attack is classified as follows:

- Moderate acute asthma: able to talk in sentences, SpO_2 ≥92%, PEF ≥50% best or predicted, in children aged 1–5 HR ≤140/min and RR ≤40/min, in children aged over 5 HR ≤125/min and RR ≤30/min.
- Acute severe asthma: unable to talk in complete sentences, or too breathless to feed, SpO_2 <92%, PEF 33–50% best or predicted, in children aged 1–5 HR >140/min and RR >40/min, in children aged over 5 HR >125/min and RR >30/min.
- Life-threatening asthma: clinical signs include exhaustion, hypotension, cyanosis, silent chest, poor respiratory effort and confusion. Measurements include PEF <33% best or predicted, O_2 sats <92%. Blood gas measurement should be considered from the ear lobe or a fingerprick, with a normal or raised $PaCO_2$ indicating worsening asthma.

Treatment:

- For moderate exacerbations: start with salbutamol via a spacer, repeated if needed, start with 2–4 puffs, can have up to 10 as needed.
- For severe: first line is nebulised salbutamol (O_2 driven) repeated every 10 minutes plus prednisolone (<2 years 10mg, 2–5 years 20mg, >5 years 30–40mg for 3 days); hydrocortisone can be used if unable to take oral medications. Oxygen should be given if SpO_2 <94%, aiming for 94–98%. If there is a poor response to the initial salbutamol nebuliser, ipratropium bromide should be added to the nebuliser (250μg with each 5mg of salbutamol every 30 minutes for up to 2 hours).
- Life-threatening: salbutamol and ipratropium nebulisers, repeating salbutamol every 10–15 minutes or continuous if able, ipratropium every 30 minutes; steroids as above. Oxygen therapy should be given aiming for O_2 sats 94–98%. The addition of $MgSO_4$ 150μg to each nebuliser in the first hour can be considered in hypoxic children, but this is not evidence-based. Second-line treatments include IV $MgSO_4$, salbutamol and aminophylline. Guidance suggests consideration of a

single IV dose of salbutamol (15µg/kg over 10 minutes) and/or a single dose of IV MgSO$_4$ (40mg/kg/day) in a child not responding to initial treatment. An infusion of salbutamol can be considered after the bolus in a PICU environment at a dose of 1–2µg/kg/min with regular measurement of the lactate. Aminophylline is not recommended in mild to moderate asthma attacks but may be considered as management for refractory severe asthma.
- Additional therapies: within the context of critical care, additional medications can be considered for those with a poor response to all the above, and these include ketamine, sevoflurane, ECMO and recombinant human DNA (these all have a no or poor evidence base). There is no role for routine antibiotic administration and they should only be prescribed if there are clear signs of bacterial infection.

The assessment and management of adults is discussed on page 48, Paper 1, Q15.

References

1. British Thoracic Society (BTS)/Scottish Intercollegiate Guidelines Network (SIGN). BTS/SIGN British guideline on the management of asthma — a national clinical guideline, SIGN 158, 2024. Available at: https://www.sign.ac.uk/media/2269/sign-158-2024-update-final.pdf.

Answer 14: c

Acute liver failure is associated with a high risk of mortality and the need for consideration of transplantation. Identification of the likely aetiology is important, as the outcomes and need for transplant consideration vary dependent on the underlying cause. For more information on the presentation and classification of ALF please see page 263, Paper 3, Q48.

Acute liver failure results in multi-organ involvement with a local and systemic inflammatory response to liver cell damage and presents with a SIRS-like response followed by a compensatory anti-inflammatory response (CARS) resulting in immune paresis and the risk of infections. The development of cerebral oedema is a significant complication and management strategies focus on the prevention and treatment of raised ICP.

Preventative management includes permitting spontaneous hyperventilation if the patient has been intubated. Higher grades of encephalopathy often necessitate invasive ventilation to manage airway protection or agitation. Lung-protective ventilation strategies should be employed with a target $PaCO_2$ of 4.5–5.5kPa; however, if the patient is spontaneously hyperventilating this may be tolerated rather than early institution of paralysis. Early initiation of CRRT can be considered in patients at high risk of developing cerebral oedema (oliguria, AKI, ammonia >200, high-grade encephalopathy, presence of SIRS). Maintenance of serum sodium in the range of 145–155mmol/L is recommended, with normal saline used for initial resuscitation and then hypertonic saline as an infusion to keep sodium in the target range. Routine active cooling is not recommended, with therapeutic hypothermia only used as a rescue therapy in established refractory raised ICP in patients awaiting transplantation within strict evidence-based protocols.

The use of ICP monitoring is decreasing, with no strong evidence that monitoring ICP improves outcomes coupled with the risk of fatal bleeding associated with ICP bolt insertion (1–4% risk of non-fatal bleeding, 1% risk of fatal bleeding). The insertion of ICP bolts is therefore only considered in patients with a very high risk of intracranial hypertension in specialised units familiar with their use in acute liver failure.

In cases of acute liver failure with established cerebral oedema, the interventions to consider include: bolus of mannitol or hypertonic saline, increasing CRRT dose and clearance of fluid, ensuring a CPP >60mmHg, deepening sedation to reduce cerebral metabolic rate, therapeutic hypothermia and therapeutic plasma exchange. The management of acute liver failure aside from prevention and management of cerebral hypertension and oedema includes the following:

- Circulation: target MAP of >65mmHg, if the patient is hypotensive despite effective fluid resuscitation; then vasopressor therapy is indicated with noradrenaline first-line and the addition of vasopressin if needed. Patients are at risk of relative adrenal insufficiency, so steroids (e.g. hydrocortisone 50mg QDS IV) should be administered if patients require a significant vasopressor dose. High-volume therapeutic plasma exchange, which is thought to help by removing vasoactive inflammatory cytokines, may be considered in specialist centres.

SBA Paper 4: Answers

- Renal: a large proportion (40–85%) of patients with ALF will have acute kidney injury. Earlier institution of CRRT in ALF patients should be considered in the presence of other indications such as high ammonia, sodium management and temperature control.
- Coagulation: there is reduced production of procoagulant and anticoagulant factors in ALF. In addition to standard laboratory coagulation tests (i.e. PT/APTT), point-of-care testing such as ROTEM® or TEG® can be used to guide management of coagulopathy. Routine correction of PT/INR with fresh frozen plasma is not routinely indicated as PT is a good marker of synthetic liver function. Platelets and fibrinogen levels are often better markers of bleeding risk and should be corrected for invasive procedures such as CVC or ICP monitor insertion, although discussion with the haematologists and neurosurgeons is also advised. If there is a significant bleeding episode, then correction of all clotting abnormalities is warranted in liaison with coagulation team advice.
- Nutrition: monitoring and correction of hypoglycaemia with low-volume high concentration glucose solution is recommended, to avoid administration of significant volumes of hypotonic fluid. Electrolyte derangement is common, and monitoring and correction of magnesium, calcium, potassium and phosphate is advised. Early initiation of enteral nutrition is beneficial, and prokinetics are often required. Post-pyloric feeding can be considered if absorption remains poor despite the use of prokinetics.

References

1. Aziz R, Price J, Agarwal B. Management of acute liver failure in intensive care. *BJA Educ* 2021; 21(3): 110–6.
2. Tujios S, Stravitz RT, Lee WM. Management of acute liver failure: update 2022. *Semin Liver Dis* 2022; 42(03): 362–78.

● Answer 15: b

There is an in-depth explanation on citrate overload and accumulation on page 42, Paper 1, Q11.

In this clinical scenario, the patient has multiple reasons for reduction in citrate metabolism, particularly impaired liver function and poor cardiac output. There are signs of citrate accumulation and toxicity but an ongoing need for CRRT. Given the significant coagulopathy the best option in this scenario is to de-escalate citrate anticoagulation and initially try CRRT with no anticoagulant. Consideration may be given to using prostacyclin or cautious heparin anticoagulation with close monitoring if circuit clotting occurs. Modified citrate regimes with altered post-filter ionised calcium targets and protocols are now used in some patients with acute liver impairment in specialised units.

References
1. Schneider AG, Journois D, Rimmelé T. Complications of regional citrate anticoagulation: accumulation or overload? *Crit Care* 2017; 21(1): 281.
2. Kidney Disease: Improving Global Outcomes (KDIGO). KDIGO clinical practice guideline for acute kidney injury, 2012. Available at: https://kdigo.org/wp-content/uploads/2016/10/KDIGO-2012-AKI-Guideline-English.pdf.

● Answer 16: b

Severe community-acquired pneumonia (CAP) is a common condition in critical care and is the most common cause of sepsis requiring ICU admission. Up to 10% of patients hospitalised with CAP are likely to need critical care. Pathogens may be typical, atypical, and viral, with the most common causative organism being *Streptococcus pneumoniae* (which is considered a 'typical' organism as it grows on routine culture media). The most common atypical pathogen (named as they will not grow on routine culture media) is *Legionella pneumophila*.

Legionnaires' disease is pneumonia caused by *Legionella pneumophila* (if infection only results in an isolated self-limiting fever it is termed Pontiac fever). *Legionella* bacteria are aerobic, Gram-negative intracellular bacilli. There are over 60 species in the family *Legionellaceae*, but *L. pneumophila* is the most common cause of human disease. Bacteria are found in water and soil and can contaminate water sources particularly those with warmer temperatures. Common reservoirs include water supplies for large facilities such as hospitals and hotels, and also hot tubs, birthing pools and humidifiers.

Clinical features start 2 to 10 days after exposure and include fever followed by cough (often dry) and shortness of breath. X-ray findings may be non-specific but are likely to show patchy infiltrates that may be unilateral or bilateral. Other symptoms include nausea, diarrhoea and vomiting. Blood tests often show hyponatraemia, mildly elevated transaminases, a CRP over 100mg/L and an elevated CPK. Phosphate levels may also be low. The combination of exposure to potentially contaminated water, elevated transaminases and hyponatraemia in a patient with known respiratory pathology makes *Legionella* infection the most likely answer.

Diagnosis is via several tests with urinary *Legionella* antigen the most rapid. However, this only detects *Legionella* serotype 1, hence a negative result does not fully exclude *Legionella* as a diagnosis. Polymerase chain reaction (PCR) testing of sputum has high diagnostic accuracy; however, obtaining a deep sputum culture can be difficult and the sensitivity for PCR from upper respiratory tract samples is low. Culture samples remain the gold standard, but the results may take 3–5 days to become available and the sensitivity of cultures is variable. They do have almost 100% specificity as colonisation of the airways with *Legionella* does not occur.

The management of severe *Legionella* pneumonia includes a beta-lactam and a macrolide (usually clarithromycin) with the macrolide being effective against *Legionella*. Once the diagnosis is established, a fluroquinolone such as levofloxacin or ciprofloxacin may be added.

References
1. bestpractice.bmj.com. *Legionella* infection — symptoms, diagnosis and treatment. BMJ Best Practice, 2024. Available at: https://bestpractice.bmj.com/topics/en-gb/414.
2. www.uptodate.com. Microbiology, epidemiology, and pathogenesis of *Legionella* infection. UpToDate, 2024. Available at: https://www.uptodate.com/contents/microbiology-epidemiology-and-pathogenesis-of-legionella-infection.
3. www.uptodate.com. Clinical manifestations and diagnosis of *Legionella* infection. UpToDate, 2025. Available at: https://www.uptodate.com/contents/clinical-manifestations-and-diagnosis-of-legionella-infection.
4. Morgan A, Glossop A. Severe community-acquired pneumonia. *BJA Educ* 2016; 16(5): 167–72.

● Answer 17: b

Critical illness weakness or ICU-acquired weakness (ICU-AW) is the most common cause of acute neuromuscular weakness in critical care patients. It presents as a symmetrical, bilateral flaccid weakness which occurs after a period of critical illness. There is often sparing of facial muscles. There are three subtypes: critical illness polyneuropathy (CIP), critical illness myopathy (CIM) and critical illness polyneuromyopathy (CINM) which is a combination of the first two. ICU-AW occurs in around 4–6% of patients, with CIM being the most common subtype.

Acute muscle wasting occurs within the first 72 hours of a critical illness and may continue with up to 2–3% muscle wastage per day of critical illness. As well as loss of muscle mass, the quality of muscle decreases with patchy myonecrosis, which may contribute to progression on to CIM. Inflammation associated with critical illness affects membrane excitability in several ways, including inactivation of voltage-gated sodium channels and deranged intracellular calcium homeostasis with altered contractility. Axonal degeneration may also occur due to microvascular impairment of the endoneurium, hyperglycaemia or axonal oedema. These factors amongst others contribute to CIP.

Electrophysiological investigation includes the use of nerve conduction studies (sensory nerve action potentials [SNAPs] and compound muscle action potentials [CMAPs]) and needle electromyography including measurement of motor unit action potentials (MUAPs).

CIP results in reduced amplitude on SNAPs and CMAPs with normal latency and velocity. Normal action potential excitability during direct muscle stimulation is seen; MUAPs are large and polyphasic in character. Axonal degeneration of sensory and motor nerves is seen, with normal creatine phosphokinase (CpK) levels and denervation atrophy on biopsy. A longer recovery time is seen with CIP than other forms of ICU-AW.

CIM results in preserved SNAPs (over 80% lower normal limit), reduced CMAPs (under 80% lower normal limit) and reduced or absent action potential excitability during direct muscle stimulation. Small short-duration, polyphasic MUAPs are typical. Abnormal spontaneous muscle activity results, with loss of thick filaments and mildly raised CpK levels. Recovery from CIM is usually good.

ICU-AW should be suspected in a patient without known neurological illness who is profoundly weak and struggling to wean off a ventilator with impaired sensation. Electrophysiological testing is the gold standard for diagnosis of ICU-AW but is not widely available.

References
1. Latronico N, Rasulo F, Eikermann M, Piva S. Illness weakness, polyneuropathy and myopathy: diagnosis, treatment, and long-term outcomes. *Crit Care* 2023; 27(1): 439.
2. Plaut T, Weiss L. Electrodiagnostic evaluation of critical illness neuropathy. StatPearls [Internet]; 2022. Available at: https://www.ncbi.nlm.nih.gov/books/NBK562270/.
3. Puthucheary Z. Intensive care unit-acquired weakness. In: Bersten AD, Handy JM, Eds. *Oh's intensive care manual*, 8th ed. London: Elsevier; 2018: chapter 57: pp. 706–20.

● Answer 18: b

Hyperglycaemic emergencies such as DKA and hyperosmolar hyperglycaemic state (HHS) are a frequent cause of critical care admission, and knowledge of when to admit and how to treat is paramount for an ICU doctor. Hospitals typically have their own DKA management guidelines; however, the Joint British Diabetes Societies have produced national guidelines for a number of diabetic care-related topics including DKA. Recent updates to guidance on DKA management include reduction of the IV insulin rate to 0.05 units/kg once blood glucose has dropped below 14mmol/L to reduce the risk of hypoglycaemia and hypokalaemia seen with higher rates of insulin administration.

DKA is diagnosed by the presence of the classic triad of: ketones over 3mmol/L in blood (or ++ or more in urine), pH less than 7.3 +/- bicarbonate under 15mmol/L and a blood glucose over 11.1 mmol/L; or markers of DKA with a known diagnosis of diabetes. Euglycemic DKA is increasingly seen in patients with type 1 diabetes, particularly those taking SGLT2 inhibitors. Although DKA typically presents in patients with type 1 diabetes, there is also a subset of ketosis-prone type 2 diabetics, most commonly patients of Afro-Caribbean or Hispanic descent.

Key priorities in DKA treatment are fluid resuscitation, electrolyte management and insulin therapy. Patients in DKA have deficits of both water and electrolytes, which may approximate to 100ml/kg of water, 7–10mmol/kg sodium and 3–5mmol/kg of chloride and potassium. The specific fluid management regimen implemented should follow local guidance but typically includes a bolus if the patient is haemodynamically unstable followed by 1L of fluid with added potassium over increasing time periods. More cautious regimes may be required in patients at risk of fluid overload. Normal saline (0.9%) is often preferred for ward-based fluid management as premade bags with potassium are readily available (whereas other crystalloids would need additional potassium adding introducing risk). Once the glucose level falls below 14mmol/L, 125ml/hr of 10% glucose should also be added.

Insulin therapy should start at 0.1 IU/kg as a fixed-rate infusion, with the aim of reducing blood ketones by 0.5mmol/L/hr. If blood ketones are not available, an increase in serum bicarbonate by 3mmol/L/hr or a decrease in the blood glucose by 3mmol/L/hr should be targeted. If a reduction in ketones (measured hourly) is not achieved, the hourly insulin rate should be increased by 1 unit per hour. If there is adequate improvement, the insulin rate should be reduced to 0.05 units/kg/hr to reduce the risk of hypoglycaemia once serum glucose is below 14mmol/L. Those patients on long-acting basal insulin should continue their usual dose, and newly presenting patients should be started on 0.25 units/kg SC once a day. Liaison with specialist diabetes physicians and care teams is recommended.

Critical care admission should be considered in patients with markers of severe DKA such as: ketones >6mmol/L, HCO_3^- <5mmol/L, pH <7.0, K^+ <3.5mmol/L on admission, GCS ≤12, SaO_2 <92% on air, SBP <90mmHg, HR >100 or <60 and anion gap >16. Critical care admission should also be considered in all patients who fail to improve or deteriorate despite starting DKA management.

In relation to electrolyte management, K^+ is the most critical to monitor and values should be kept between 4–5.5mmol/L. Other electrolytes including magnesium and phosphate should also be checked, although it is important to note that DKA treatment causes a drop in phosphate level which may not require supplementation if previously normal. If phosphate levels are low prior to treatment, then replacement should be considered.

Cerebral oedema, whilst still a risk in adult patients, is not commonly seen in adults but may occur in patients of low body weight, young adults, or in patients with other risk factors for cerebral oedema. This may require a slower fluid replacement rate.

References

1. Joint British Diabetes Societies for Inpatient Care. JBDS-IP. The management of diabetic ketoacidosis in adults, 2023. Available at: https://abcd.care/sites/default/files/site_uploads/JBDS_Guidelines_Current/JBDS_02_DKA_Guideline_with_QR_code_March_2023.pdf.
2. Umpierrez GE, Davis GM, ElSayed NA, *et al.* Hyperglycaemic crises in adults with diabetes: a consensus report. *Diabetologia* 2024; 67: 1455–79.

Answer 19: e

The definition and classification of pre-eclampsia is discussed in detail on page 59, Paper 1, Q25.

Pre-eclampsia without severe features tends to be managed by obstetric staff on the labour and postnatal wards and focuses mainly on blood pressure (BP) control. The first-line therapy for BP management in pre-eclampsia is oral labetalol; if this is poorly tolerated or BP control is insufficient, nifedipine and hydralazine are used with the aim of reducing BP to 135/85mmHg or less. If there are features of severe pre-eclampsia, delivery may be considered prior to 37 weeks' gestation.

Magnesium sulphate is the treatment of choice for eclamptic seizures and should be considered in patients with severe pre-eclampsia or patients with pre-eclampsia who are in critical care with delivery planned within 24 hours. Other antiepileptics such as benzodiazepines and phenytoin should not be used in this setting. Magnesium is primarily used to prevent the recurrence of seizures and has been shown to be more effective than alternative agents in this clinical setting. Magnesium is given as a loading dose of 4g over 5–15 minutes, followed by an infusion of 1g/hr for 24 hours or for 24 hours after the last seizure. If there is a further seizure, an additional bolus of 2–4g can be given. IV fluid should be limited to 80ml/hr unless there is evidence of ongoing fluid losses (such as bleeding). Delivery should be expedited, but seizures and hypertension should be managed in the immediate term. IV labetalol is recommended as repeated IV boluses or an infusion in patients with a SBP ≥160mmHg or DBP ≥110mmHg. If IV access is not immediately possible then immediate-release oral nifedipine can be used instead.

References

1. National Institute for Heath and Care Excellence (NICE), guideline NG133. Hypertension in pregnancy: diagnosis and management, 2019. Available at: https://www.nice.org.uk/guidance/ng133/chapter/Recommendations#management-of-pre-eclampsia.
2. www.uptodate.com. Preeclampsia with severe features: delaying delivery in pregnancies remote from term. UpToDate, 2025. Available at: https://www.uptodate.com/contents/preeclampsia-with-severe-features-delaying-delivery-in-pregnancies-remote-from-term.
3. bestpractice.bmj.com. Pre-eclampsia — symptoms, diagnosis and treatment. BMJ Best Practice, 2025. Available at: https://bestpractice.bmj.com/topics/en-gb/326.

● Answer 20: c

Abdominal aortic aneurysms (AAAs) are defined as a segmental full-thickness dilation of the aorta to >1.5 times its normal diameter of 2cm. In the UK there is population screening for men over 65 years old, and consideration for intervention once the aneurysm exceeds 5.5cm in diameter. Women are not routinely screened due to a lower incidence, but if found incidentally intervention is considered once the diameter is above 5cm.

Risk factors for the development of an AAA include age >65, male sex, smoking history, hypertension (HTN), COPD, presence of other vascular disease and family history. Risk factors for those with a known AAA suffering a rupture include: larger aneurysm size, faster rate of aneurysm expansion, age >60, female sex, HTN and smoking history. A ruptured AAA is almost always fatal without intervention and the options for management include open repair and endovascular aneurysm repair (EVAR). The choice of intervention is dependent on patient stability and suitability of anatomy for graft placement. EVAR can be performed under local anaesthetic, depending on the clinical status of the patient and their ability to tolerate the procedure.

Complications of both open repair and EVAR include abdominal compartment syndrome, ischaemic colitis, acute kidney injury and lower limb ischaemia (usually recognised at the end of surgery). Ischaemic colitis is much more common following ruptured AAA repair (compared to elective) and also after open repair (compared to EVAR). Symptoms include diarrhoea, abdominal pain and distension, rectal bleeding and rising lactate, and it is associated with significantly raised mortality. Acute kidney injury is common after ruptured AAA and is multifactorial; the use of iodine contrast during an

SBA Paper 4: Answers

EVAR may also contribute to renal injury. Complications specific to EVAR include endoleak (persistent blood flow within the aneurysm sac after EVAR), arterial injury (from vascular access site) and cholesterol embolization syndrome (disruption and embolization of a plaque in the aorta from the guidewires and graft causing a systemic autoimmune inflammatory process and end-organ damage).

References

1. Berry K, Gudgeon J, Taylor J. Anaesthesia for endovascular repair of ruptured abdominal aortic aneurysms. *BJA Educ* 2022; 22(6): 208–15.
2. www.uptodate.com. Management of symptomatic (non-ruptured) and ruptured abdominal aortic aneurysm. UpToDate, 2024. Available at: https://www.uptodate.com/contents/management-of-symptomatic-non-ruptured-and-ruptured-abdominal-aortic-aneurysm.

Answer 21: b

Hypernatraemia is defined as a serum sodium (Na^+) level >145mmol/L. It is most commonly due to a free water deficit but can also be due to excessive sodium load, which is typically iatrogenic following administration of Na^+- rich IV fluid (saline 0.9% or above and sodium bicarbonate). Symptoms occur once Na^+ rises above 155mmol/L and include restlessness, irritability, drowsiness, confusion, hyperreflexia and coma.

Causes of net free water loss include: insensible losses (burns, sweating), neurogenic and nephrogenic diabetes insipidus (DI)*, gastrointestinal losses (diarrhoea, enterocutaneous fistula, NG drainage), renal loss (loop diuretics, osmotic loss including HHS, polyuric phase of ATN, post-obstruction diuresis). Causes from sodium gain include: iatrogenic (saline, sodium bicarbonate, high sodium NG feed), primary hyperaldosteronism (Conn's syndrome) and Cushing's syndrome.

Urine osmolality is helpful in differentiating the likely causes of raised Na^+, with an osmolality of <300mOsmol/kg strongly suggestive of diabetes insipidus (DI) (the kidney is unable to concentrate the urine), 300–800mOsmol/kg suggestive of osmotic loss and >800mOsmol/kg due to free water deficit or sodium gain.

Management involves treatment of the underlying cause (e.g. desmopressin for cranial DI or cessation of the causative agent if iatrogenic) and fluid therapy to normalise Na⁺ levels. Raised Na⁺ should be reduced by no more than 12mmol/L/24 hours, with a maximum individual hourly decrease of 1mmol/L/hr, and Na⁺ levels checked every 2–3 hours until <150mmol/L. If the hypernatraemia is severe (>170mmol/L), then 0.9% saline should be used initially to prevent too rapid a Na⁺ decrease resulting in cerebral oedema. If Na⁺ is <170mmol/L, then significant volumes of hypotonic fluid solutions (5% dextrose, 0.45% saline) may be required.

* Diabetes insipidus is under the process of being renamed to better reflect the pathophysiology of the disease. The new name for cranial diabetes insipidus is arginine vasopressin deficiency (AVP-D) and for nephrogenic diabetes insipidus is arginine vasopressin resistance (AVP-R).

References

1. Yaqoob M, McCafferty K. Water balance, fluids and electrolytes. In: Kumar P, Clark M, Eds. *Kumar and Clark's clinical medicine*, 10th ed. London: Elsevier; 2020: chapter 9: pp. 168–202.
2. Bergmans DCJJ. Metabolic disorders: hypernatraemia. In: Waldmann C, Rhodes A, Soni N, Handy J. *Oxford desk reference: critical care*, 2nd ed. Oxford: Oxford University Press; 2019: chapter 25: pp. 457–8.
3. Levy MJ. Renaming cranial diabetes insipidus to AVP-deficiency. International Society of Endocrinology, 2025. Available at: https://www.isendo.org/renaming-cranial-diabetes-insipidus-to-avp-deficiency/.

● Answer 22: d

Myotonic dystrophy (MD) is an autosomal dominant disorder characterised as either type 1 or 2 depending on the genotypic abnormality. It is a multisystem disease that causes skeletal muscle weakness with myotonia (delayed muscle relaxation after contraction), cardiac conduction abnormalities, cataracts, frontal baldness, oesophageal dysfunction, mild cognitive impairment, glucose intolerance and low serum IgG.

Patients with MD may present to the ICU after routine surgery but may also present as a result of respiratory compromise secondary to infective or aspiration pneumonias. Therefore, knowledge of safe pharmacological management of these patients is important for an intensivist.

SBA Paper 4: Answers

MD patients may have significant but asymptomatic cardiac involvement, so an up-to-date ECHO may be useful in guiding care. They may also have cardiomyopathy or conduction defects and not infrequently require pacemaker insertion.

Patients are at risk of respiratory complications both from respiratory and oesophageal muscle weakness, but also due to an alteration of central respiratory drive and increased sensitivity to sedatives which can cause respiratory failure after general anaesthesia.

Following anaesthesia, patients with type 1 MD are at particular risk of complications and should avoid general anaesthesia where possible; patients with type 2 MD have a much lower risk of complications, which include postoperative pulmonary complications, a risk of cardiac arrhythmias and a risk of myotonias.

Myotonia can be triggered by cold, shivering and electrical stimulation, so the avoidance of a nerve stimulator is advised. Suxamethonium can lead to diffuse myotonia so should not be used in this patient group. Patients with MD have a higher sensitivity to non-depolarising muscle relaxants so smaller doses of shorter-acting agents are preferred. Reversal of neuromuscular blockade with neostigmine should be avoided as this can also precipitate myotonia; therefore, sugammadex reversal may be the best option. If sedative and anaesthetic agents cannot be avoided, the use of shorter-acting drugs such as propofol and remifentanil is preferential to longer-acting agents (such as benzodiazepines). Opiates carry a risk of respiratory depression, and regional techniques along with NSAIDs if appropriate are preferred. If opiates are used, then shorter-acting or smaller doses should be used.

References

1. Mangla C, Bais K, Yarmush J. Myotonic dystrophy and anesthetic challenges: a case report and review. *Case Rep Anesthesiol* 2019; 2019: 4282305.
2. www.uptodate.com. Myotonic dystrophy: treatment and prognosis. UpToDate, 2025. Available at: https://www.uptodate.com/contents/myotonic-dystrophy-treatment-and-prognosis.

Answer 23: b

The different types of herpes virus are discussed on page 156, Paper 2, Q31.

Herpes viruses can lead to a variety of clinical syndromes depending on the site of infection. Human herpes virus (HHV) 1 and 2 may cause 'cold sores', erythema multiforme and eczema herpeticum and other herpes simplex infections. HSV-1 tends to be responsible for herpes encephalitis and HSV-2 for genital herpes. Varicella zoster virus gives rise to chickenpox and shingles. *Cytomegalovirus* causes an infectious mononucleosis-like syndrome and hepatitis, and in the immunocompromised can cause pneumonitis and retinitis. HHV-6 is also known as 'sixth disease' and along with HSV-7 causes roseola infantum in children. Epstein-Barr virus causes infectious mononucleosis and can also lead to Burkitt's lymphoma and nasopharyngeal carcinoma. HHV-8 is associated with the development of Kaposi's sarcoma, particularly in the immunocompromised.

References

1. Barlow G, Irving W, Moss PJ. Infectious diseases. In: Kumar P, Clark M, Eds. In: *Kumar and Clark's clinical medicine*, 10th ed. London: Elsevier; 2020: chapter 20: pp. 488–582.
2. www.uptodate.com. Epidemiology, clinical manifestations, and diagnosis of herpes simplex virus type 1 infection. UpToDate, 2025. Available at: https://www.uptodate.com/contents/epidemiology-clinical-manifestations-and-diagnosis-of-herpes-simplex-virus-type-1-infection.

Answer 24: a

Ultrasound (US) scanners use high-frequency sound waves sent in pulses to create images based on the time and amount reflected back to the transducer from tissues. The transducer is the probe used on the body to acquire the images and contains a large number of tiny piezoelectric crystals. When electrical voltage is applied across the crystal it changes shape and emits ultrasound waves which pass through layers in the probe and focus the beam. This then passes into tissues and travels at different speeds depending on the tissue type. Some beams are reflected back to the probe when there is a change in speed between tissue types. The layout of the crystals and the frequency used dictates the kind of images that can be obtained.

Linear probes have the crystals arranged in a flat line and are typically higher frequency (6–13MHz). This produces good resolution of shallow structures but is less suited to imaging deeper structures (maximum depth around 6cm). These probes are typically used for vascular access and may also be used for superficial analysis of pleural sliding, the absence of which can indicate a pneumothorax.

Probes with a line of crystals mounted on a curve — creating a 'curved array' — are also known as curvilinear probes. This allows for a sector format image (a quarter circle with the point end at the skin expanding into a wider area of image capture to be visualised). These probes have a lower frequency (2–5MHz) which allows much greater depth of resolution (up to 30cm) and are typically used for abdominal ultrasound imaging. They may also be useful for imaging lung for pathology such as consolidation and pleural effusion.

A phased array transducer has a smaller square footprint with multiple rows of piezoelectric crystals which can switch independently between transmit and receive pulse sequences to produce a series of scan lines to form an image. These probes have a lower frequency (3–5MHz) allowing deeper image acquisition. These probes are primarily used for transthoracic echocardiography but can also be used for lung US (in a similar way to the curvilinear probes).

References

1. Wiersema U. Ultrasound in the intensive care unit. In: Bersten AD, Handy JM, Eds. *Oh's intensive care manual*, 8th ed. London: Elsevier; 2018: chapter 40: pp. 519–31.
2. Oates C. Physics and technology of ultrasound. In: Davey A, Diba A, Eds. *Ward's anaesthetic equipment*, 6th ed. London: Saunders, Elsevier; 2012: chapter 31: pp. 525–39.

Answer 25: e

The 4th National Audit Project of the Royal College of Anaesthetists (NAP4) reviewed major complications of airway management in the UK. It found that almost 20% of reported incidents occurred in intensive care, and a further 8% occurred in the emergency department (in the UK intubations in the emergency department are undertaken by anaesthetists or intensivists). Given there were an estimate of 2.9 million anaesthetics undertaken in theatre in that year, this study found that the risk of an adverse event in a patient undergoing emergency airway management in the ICU or ED is significantly higher compared to anaesthetics undertaken in a theatre environment.

The INTUBE study reported on major adverse events during the peri-intubation period on intensive care units across 29 countries and found that cardiovascular instability was the most common adverse event, occurring in 42% of patients, with 3% suffering a cardiac arrest. The range of induction agents used in this study was propofol, midazolam, etomidate and ketamine, with propofol the most frequently used agent and also the agent most commonly associated with cardiovascular collapse in post hoc analysis. First-pass intubation was associated with a significantly lower rate of major adverse events, as opposed to the need for two or more attempts.

It is difficult to recommend a single pharmacological approach for undertaking a modified rapid sequence induction in all ICU patients given the diversity of clinical situations encountered, and any technique will require a degree of individualisation. This patient is profoundly hypoxic, so rapid securing of the airway with either suxamethonium or rocuronium would be indicated. As they have an AKI with an already elevated potassium level, the use of suxamethonium would not be appropriate (as this may worsen hyperkalaemia leading to arrhythmias). Traditional induction doses of hypnotic agents (2mg/kg propofol, 5mg/kg of thiopentone and 2mg/kg of ketamine) are likely to aggravate the cardiovascular instability already seen as a result of sepsis. The addition of a short-acting opiate may reduce the dose of hypnotic agent with fentanyl often used due to its relatively cardiostable profile (alfentanil is a common alternative). Ketamine results in a lower mortality rate when compared to etomidate (and both have similar haemodynamic stability on induction). The induction dosage of ketamine IV is 1–2mg/kg, with the dosage for critically ill patients starting at 1mg/kg. The most important factor is to know the drugs you are using, and to titrate them in as needed and ensure you are prepared for likely haemodynamic compromise and manage this accordingly.

References

1. 4th National Audit Project of The Royal College of Anaesthetists and The Difficult Airway Society. Major complications of airway management in the United Kingdom, 2011. Available at: https://www.rcoa.ac.uk/sites/default/files/documents/2023-02/NAP4%20Full%20Report.pdf.

2. Russotto V, Myatra SN, Laffey JG, et al. Intubation practices and adverse peri-intubation events in critically ill patients from 29 countries. *JAMA* 2021; 325(12): 1164–72.
3. Russotto V, Tassistro E, Myatra SN. Peri-intubation cardiovascular collapse in patients who are critically ill: insights from the INTUBE study. *Am J Respir Crit Care Med* 2022; 206(4): 449–58.
4. Koroki T, Kotani Y, Yaguchi T, et al. Ketamine versus etomidate as an induction agent for tracheal intubation in critically ill adults: a Bayesian meta-analysis. *Crit Care* 2024; 28(1): 48.
5. Midega TD, Chaves RC de F, Ashihara C, et al. Ketamine use in critically ill patients: a narrative review. *Rev Bras Ter Intensiva* 2022; 34(2): 287–94.

● Answer 26: a

The severity of an asthma exacerbation is graded using peak expiratory flow (PEF), clinical observations, examination of the patient and blood gas analysis.

The British Thoracic Society (BTS) has clear guidance on the assessment and management of asthma in adults. The BTS classifies asthma severity as:

- Moderate acute asthma: increased symptoms, peak expiratory flow (PEF) 50–75% best or predicted, no features of severe asthma.
- Acute severe asthma: PEF 33–50%, RR ≥25/min, HR ≥110/min, unable to complete sentences in a single breath.
- Life-threatening asthma: clinical signs include decreased GCS, exhaustion, arrhythmias, hypotension, cyanosis, silent chest, poor respiratory effort. Measurements include PEF <33% best or predicted, O_2 sats <92%, PaO_2 <8kPa, 'normal' $PaCO_2$ 4.6–6kPa (as opposed to low in acute severe).
- Near fatal asthma: $PaCO_2$ >6kPa or need for mechanical ventilation, with high inflation pressures.

These are the severity categories used in the UK; slightly different criteria for each category may be used in other countries; in the US, exacerbations are graded as mild, moderate, severe and impending respiratory failure. In both categories an elevated $PaCO_2$ puts a patient in the most severe category.

References

1. British Thoracic Society(BTS)/Scottish Intercollegiate Guidelines Network (SIGN). BTS/SIGN British guideline on the management of asthma — a national clinical guideline, SIGN 158, 2024. Available at: https://www.sign.ac.uk/media/2269/sign-158-2024-update-final.pdf.
2. www.uptodate.com. Acute exacerbations of asthma in adults: emergency department and inpatient management. UpToDate, 2024. Available at: https://www.uptodate.com/contents/acute-exacerbations-of-asthma-in-adults-emergency-department-and-inpatient-management.

Answer 27: c

Hyperlactataemia is defined as a lactate concentration >2mmol/L.

During glycolysis glucose is metabolised to pyruvate (an intermediate metabolite) which in the presence of oxygen will enter the Krebs cycle. Under anaerobic conditions pyruvate is converted to lactate by lactate dehydrogenase. Pyruvate can also be produced via metabolism of alanine (an amino acid) and then converted to lactate as before. Lactate can also be metabolised via the pentose-5-phosphate pathway (mainly in red blood cells).

Lactate is produced in health at a rate of around 0.8mmol/kg/hr from skeletal muscle (40%), skin, brain, intestine and red blood cells. Lactate is then converted back to glucose predominantly by the liver (70% cleared via the Cori cycle) as well as back to pyruvate by the proximal tubule cells in the kidneys, skeletal and cardiac myocytes.

Hyperlactataemia has been classified by Cohen and Woods into two main subgroups: type A and type B:

- Type A: presence of tissue hypoxia, e.g. shock, severe hypoxaemia, severe anaemia, carbon monoxide poisoning.
- Type B: no significant tissue hypoxia, and is further subdivided based on cause:
  - B1: due to underlying disease such as sepsis, liver failure, malignancy, diabetes, phaeochromocytoma, thiamine deficiency;

- B2: due to drugs or toxins such as adrenaline, salbutamol, ethanol, methanol, ethylene glycol, salicylates among others;
- B3: due to rare inborn errors of metabolism such as G6PD deficiency, pyruvate carboxylase deficiency, deficiency of enzymes of oxidative phosphorylation.

Elevated lactate is often a combination of increased production and impaired clearance in critical illness and therefore patients may not fit neatly into any one of these categories. A lactate level of >5mmol/L in patients with a pH <7.35 or a base deficit >6 is associated with an 80% mortality.

Bacteria within the gut can produce D-lactate, an isomer of human lactate that cannot be produced or metabolised by human cells. In patients with mesenteric ischaemia there may be elevation in D-lactate from translocation of the D-lactate into the blood; however, this is not detected by standard lactate assays, so a separate assay is used. Elevated D-lactate may be used in the diagnosis of mesenteric ischaemia in patients too unwell to undergo CT scanning. Raised D-lactate levels can also be seen in short bowel syndrome, pancreatic insufficiency and in the presence of jejuno-ileal bypass, particularly after a large carbohydrate load.

References
1. Cosgrave DW, Higgins AM, Cooper J, Nichol AD. Hyperlactataemia in critical illness. In: Bersten AD, Handy JM, Eds. *Oh's intensive care manual*, 8th ed. London: Elsevier; 2018: chapter 19: pp. 171–7.
2. Phypers B, Pierce JT. Lactate physiology in health and disease. *Contin Educ Anaesth Crit Care Pain* 2006; 6(3): 128–32.

● Answer 28: c
Alcoholic hepatitis is a syndrome characterised by recent onset of jaundice (with or without other markers of liver decompensation) in a patient known to have ongoing significant alcohol consumption. The patient may not be currently drinking alcohol as it can occur days or weeks after cessation of alcohol consumption; however, a significant alcohol history and steatohepatitis must be present. It may be triggered by a large alcohol binge or by other factors such as sepsis, drug-induced liver injury or gallstones.

It presents with progressive jaundice associated with fevers (even without associated infection), malaise and weight loss. Bloods show an elevated bilirubin, neutrophilia and moderate elevation of transaminases with the AST 1.5–2 times higher than the ALT (this can be remembered with the phrase '**S**pirits are stronger than **L**ager'!).

Several prognostic models are employed to predict mortality, with two specifically used to identify patients who might benefit from treatment with steroids. Steroid use has been demonstrated in several studies to significantly improve survival in patients with severe alcoholic hepatitis; the cut-off values for steroid use are a score of ≥32 on the modified Maddrey Discriminant Function (most commonly used scoring system) and a score of ≥9 on the Glasgow Alcoholic Hepatitis Score (which identifies patients at the greatest risk of death without treatment). The Model for End-stage Liver Disease (MELD) score provides an indication of mortality risk, with scores >20 associated with an elevated 90-day mortality. The Lille model is calculated after 7 days of steroid treatment and is used to assess steroid response and the requirement for longer-term treatment.

For more information on physiological scoring systems see page 170, Paper 2, Q41.

References
1. European Association for the Study of the Liver; Thursz M, Gual A, Lackner C, *et al*. EASL clinical practice guidelines: management of alcohol-related liver disease. *J Hepatol* 2018; 69(1): 154–81.

 ## Answer 29: b

The most commonly used classification of bacteria is based on how their cell wall reacts to the Gram stain. Gram-positive organisms will appear purple/blue in colour, and Gram-negative organisms will appear pink/red. In addition to Gram staining, descriptions of the cell shape (cocci, bacilli or spirals) are also used to classify the bacteria, as well as the atmosphere in which they grow best (aerobic or anaerobic). These findings will help to guide antibiotic therapy even before full identification of the bacteria is achieved. Table 4.15 below summarises commonly encountered bacteria based on these three criteria.

Table 4.15. Classification of bacteria.

	Gram-positive (purple/blue)	Gram-negative (red/pink)
Aerobes		
Cocci	Clusters and catalase-positive: *Staphylococcus* Coagulase-positive: *Staphylococcus aureus* Coagulase-negative: *Staphylococcus epidermidis* Chains and catalase-negative: Alpha-haemolytic (partial haemolysis): *Streptococcus pneumoniae* and *viridans* Beta-haemolytic (complete haemolysis): Lancefield grouping (A-S), Group A *Streptococcus pyogenes*, Group B *Streptococcus agalactiae* Gamma-haemolytic (no haemolysis): *Enterococcus faecalis* and *faecium*	*Neisseria meningitidis* and *gonorrhoeae* Coccoid rods (very small rods that may appear like cocci): *Haemophilus influenzae* *Brucella* *Bordetella pertussis*
Bacilli/rods	Branching: *Nocardia* Non-branching spore-forming: *Bacillus anthracis* and *cereus* Non-branching clumps: *Corynebacterium diphtheriae* Listeria (small, tumbling motility, may be confused with various other bacteria)	Lactose fermenters: Fast: *Klebsiella*, *Escherichia coli*, *Enterobacter* Slow: *Citrobacter* and *Serratia* Lactose non-fermenters: Oxidase-positive: *Pseudomonas* Oxidase-negative: *Shigella*, *Salmonella*, *Proteus*
Anaerobes		
Cocci	Chains: *Peptococcus* and *Peptostreptococcus*	
Bacilli	Branching: *Actinomyces* Non-branching spore-forming: *Clostridia spp.* and *Clostridioides difficile*	*Fusobacterium* *Bacteroides*
Obligate intracellular organisms		*Chlamydia spp.* *Legionella* (aerobic)

Organisms that do not stain with the Gram stain include *Mycobacterium* and *Leptospira*, and the obligate intracellular organisms mentioned above.

References

1. www.uptodate.com. Approach to Gram stain and culture results in the microbiology laboratory. UpToDate, 2024. Available at: https://www.uptodate.com/contents/approach-to-gram-stain-and-culture-results-in-the-microbiology-laboratory.
2. www.uptodate.com. Anaerobic bacterial infections. UpToDate, 2024. Available at: https://www.uptodate.com/contents/anaerobic-bacterial-infections.

Answer 30: b

Around 70% of patients who develop Guillain-Barré syndrome (GBS) have suffered an infection in the preceding 2 to 6 weeks. Typically, molecules in the preceding infection are structurally similar to units of the peripheral nerve membrane, and the antibodies produced in response to the initial infection may then lead to GBS. This mechanism is thought to cause the AMAN (acute motor axonal neuropathy) and AMSAN (acute motor and sensory axonal neuropathy) variants of GBS. The aetiology of the AIDP (acute inflammatory demyelinating polyneuropathy) variant is less clear but is still thought to be immune-mediated. There are several different autoantibodies associated with GBS which are all associated with different clinical presentations (e.g. anti-GQ1B antibodies are associated with the Miller-Fisher syndrome variant).

Campylobacter jejuni is the most common predisposing infection, with up to 41% of patients showing evidence of recent infection and may be associated with a more severe clinical course. *Cytomegalovirus* accounts for a further 10–22% of cases. Other infections implicated in the development of GBS are influenza A, parainfluenza, hepatitis E, herpes viruses (VZV, Epstein-Barr), mumps, measles, HIV, Zika virus and *Mycoplasma*. There appeared to be a link between a flu vaccination in 1976 and an increase in GBS prevalence, but subsequent vaccinations do not appear to have been associated with a similar increase. Nonetheless, vaccination remains a potential cause of GBS, although influenza infection is seven times more likely to cause GBS than the flu vaccination. Other causes include surgery and trauma.

References

1. Saxena M. Neuromuscular disorders. In: Bersten AD, Handy JM, Eds. *Oh's intensive care manual*, 8th ed. London: Elsevier; 2018: chapter 58: pp. 721–30.
2. Nguyen TP, Taylor RS. Guillain-Barré syndrome. StatPearls [Internet]; 2023. Available at: https://www.ncbi.nlm.nih.gov/books/NBK532254/.

Answer 31: e

The human immune system is comprised of many cells and molecules and is subdivided into the innate immune system and the adaptive immune system. The innate immune system is present and functional from birth and provides the immediate immune response. It retains no memory of antigenic stimuli and has limited recognition of molecular patterns. It is comprised of several different white blood cell types (neutrophils, eosinophils, mast cells, basophils, monocytes) as well as organ-specific cells and soluble molecules such as complement, pentraxins (CRP), collectins and enzymes.

The adaptive immune system changes in response to encounters with pathogens and retains a memory. This response on the first encounter takes around 1–2 weeks and then 3–7 days on subsequent encounters. Cells within the innate immune system encounter pathogens and then pass on information to T lymphocytes within the adaptive immune system, enabling them to either remove the pathogen directly or to recruit B lymphocytes to produce antibodies against the pathogen. Mature B cells (known as plasma cells) secrete soluble immunoglobulins (also known as antibodies) in large quantities.

Immunoglobulins target, neutralise and remove pathogens and toxins from the blood and tissues via complement, phagocyte and mast cell activity (they bind to receptors on these cells to activate). Immunoglobulins are composed of four chains — two heavy and two light, which have constant regions (that dictate function) and variable regions (enable the antibody to bind to a specific antigen — a molecular structure that generates an immune response such as a protein, peptide, lipid or carbohydrate). The different functions of immunoglobulins can be divided into five main classes: M, G_{1-4}, A_{1-2}, D and E (Table 4.16).

Table 4.16. The different functions of immunoglobulins.

IgG	The dominant class of antibody with a mean adult serum level of around 8–16g/L. They have a γ heavy chain, a half-life of around 21 days and are the only antibody that can cross the placenta (by an active process) and provide immune activity in neonates. IgG is a smaller immunoglobulin and therefore penetrates tissues more easily.
IgM	The first produced in the immune response and have a mean adult serum level of 0.5–2g/L. They have a μ heavy chain and a half-life of approximately 10 days. This is the oldest class of immunoglobulin and is a very large molecule which penetrates tissue poorly. IgM has excellent complement activation, achieved via five complement binding sites.
IgA	Found in mucous membrane secretions (predominantly A_2, A_1 remains in the serum) and have a mean adult serum level of 1.4–4g/L. They have an α heavy chain and a half-life of approximately 6 days. These immunoglobulins have a secretory portion which prevents digestion in the intestinal and bronchial secretions.
IgE	Bind to mast cells and basophils and are responsible for the symptoms of an allergic reaction, as well as defence against nematode parasites. They are present in very small quantities within the serum with a mean adult serum level of 17–450ng/ml (where they predominantly act as a surface receptor). They have an ε heavy chain and a half-life of around 2 days.
IgD	Found on the surface membranes of B lymphocytes. They have a mean adult serum level of 0–0.4g/L, have a δ heavy chain and a half-life of around 3 days. They act as cell surface receptors on B lymphocytes and enable activation of these cells by the antigen.

References

1. Peakman M, Buckland M. Immunity. In: Kumar P, Clark M, Eds. *Kumar and Clark's clinical medicine*, 10th ed. London: Elsevier; 2020: chapter 3: pp. 39–68.

SBA Paper 4: Answers

2. Chapel H, Haeney M, Misbah S, Snowden N. Basic components: structure and function. In: *Essentials of clinical immunology*, 5th ed. Oxford: Wiley-Blackwell; 2006: chapter 1: pp. 1–32.

● Answer 32: b

Blood products are all initially derived from whole blood. There are several stages in the process to produce the different blood products. Whole blood first has an anticoagulant solution added (normally citrate), then agents to support red cell metabolism during processing and storage (usually glucose or adenine). It is then centrifuged via a heavy spin to create packed red blood cells (PRBCs) and platelet-poor plasma plus a buffy coat (white cells and platelets), or a light spin to create PRBCs and platelet-rich plasma.

The PRBCs are then stored at 2–6°C for up to 42 days. Once removed from refrigeration they should be administered fully within 4 hours, and if unused placed back into a fridge within 30 minutes; any longer mandates quarantining or discarding the cells based on local protocol. The blood must be administered through a CE-marked transfusion set. Priming the set with saline is not supported by the evidence or required.

Platelet-poor plasma from a heavy spin is rapidly frozen to −65°C and stored as fresh frozen plasma (FFP). It is stored at between −25 and −30°C for 24–36 months. This is defrosted prior to use and should be administered within 4 hours of issue. If delay is unavoidable, it can be stored for up to 24 hours at 2–6°C, or up to 120 hours at 2–6°C for use as part of the massive transfusion protocol.

FFP can undergo controlled thawing to precipitate a solution rich in higher-molecular-weight proteins — Factor VIIIc, vWF and fibrinogen — known as cryoprecipitate. It is subsequently refrozen for storage and is stored at between −25°C and −30°C for 24–36 months. It is then defrosted for use strictly within a 4-hour period and discarded if not used within this time.

Platelets are collected by two methods: use of a heavy spin of whole blood to create the buffy coat containing white cells and platelets, then a further light spin to separate the white cells from the platelets and provide a leucoreduced (not depleted) product from multiple donors; or via apheresis, where blood is collected, spun to remove the platelets, and then returned to the patient (using a continuous circuit and taking a few hours to collect). Once platelets are collected, they are stored in plasma with additive solution and need to be kept at 22°C with constant agitation. They can only be stored for a maximum of 5 days. No interruption to agitation should last more than 8 hours, and no more than 24 hours in total throughout the life span of the platelet unit.

A summary of product characteristics are shown in Table 4.17.

Table 4.17. Blood product characteristics.

Product	PRBC	FFP	Cryoprecipitate	Platelets
Storage temperature °C	2–6	−25 to −30	−25 to −30	20–24
Maximum time in storage	42 days	36 months	36 months	5 days
Time to administer once out of storage	4 hours	4 hours	4 hours	8 hours (if kept at temperature above)
Special points	Can be reissued if placed back in the fridge within 30 minutes	Can be kept at 2–6° post-defrosted for a period of time	Has to be used after defrosting	Needs continuous agitation in storage

Other products that can be derived from plasma include: albumin, factor VIII, Rh immunoglobulin, immunoglobulins and other clotting factor concentrates.

Leucodepletion of blood reduces the risk of alloimmunisation to human leucocyte antigens and is useful for patients who are likely to require multiple transfusions. Several methods are used to result in <5 x 10^6 white cells per unit: filtration within 48 hours of collection prior to storage, on demand within the lab after storage, or at the bedside using a specialised filter which removes the white cells during the transfusion.

SBA Paper 4: Answers

References

1. Basu D, Kulkarni R. Overview of blood components and their preparation. *Indian J Anaesth* 2014; 58(5): 529–37.
2. Robinson S, Harris A, Atkinson S, et al. The administration of blood components: a British Society for Haematology Guideline. *Transfus Med* 2018; 28(1): 3–21.
3. Murphy M, Pasi J, Roy N. Haematology. In: Kumar P, Clark M, Eds. *Kumar and Clark's clinical medicine*, 10th ed. London: Elsevier; 2020: chapter 16: pp. 319–78.

Answer 33: c

Major obstetric haemorrhage (MOH) is a significant cause of maternal morbidity and mortality. It is the leading cause of peripartum death worldwide, and the second most common direct cause of death in the UK.

Maternal haemorrhage is classified based on the stage of pregnancy during which it occurs and the severity of the bleed. Antepartum haemorrhage (APH) occurs from 24 weeks' gestation up to delivery of the foetus, primary postpartum haemorrhage (PPH) within 24 hours after delivery, and secondary PPH from 24 hours up to 12 weeks after delivery. The World Health Organization defines PPH as greater than 500ml blood loss. The Royal College of Obstetricians and Gynaecologists (UK) classify major PPH as moderate (1000–2000ml blood loss) or severe (≥2000ml).

A useful mnemonic for the causes of PPH is the four Ts — uterine a**T**ony, **T**rauma (to the genital tract), **T**hrombin (coagulopathy) and **T**issue (retained placenta). Of these, uterine atony is responsible for over 80% of PPH. Causes of APH are commonly due to placental problems such as placenta praevia and placental abruption, but uterine rupture and trauma/bleeding from other parts of the genital tract can also occur. Secondary PPH is predominantly caused by endometritis or retained products.

The management of MOH comprises multidisciplinary focus on resuscitation (delivered by senior members of the anaesthetic and obstetric teams), blood transfusion and management of the underlying condition. In PPH, this is likely to involve the use of uterotonics such as oxytocin (first line, given slowly to avoid vasodilation and hypotension), ergometrine (second line, IM or very slow IV to avoid hypertension) and prostaglandins (misoprostol or carboprost, not given IV and to be avoided in asthmatics). In pregnancy, the baseline fibrinogen level is higher, and therefore a fibrinogen >2g/L should be targeted with early use of fibrinogen concentrate of cryoprecipitate. Tranexamic acid is also indicated and a dose of 1g should be given within 3 hours of delivery, with a further 1g if bleeding continues after 30 minutes.

References
1.   Drew T, Carvalho JCA. Major obstetric haemorrhage. *BJA Educ* 2022; 22(6): 238–44.

 Answer 34: b
When a study is undertaken to answer a question which is formulated as a hypothesis, this is known as the null hypothesis and should be proved or disproved by the study (e.g. 'drug A is superior to drug B'). This null hypothesis states that there is no difference between the groups being tested and they are from the same population.

To answer this question, there must be enough data collected, as there will be some degree of error due to intrinsic variation in the samples. If this forms a large portion of the data, it may lead to an incorrect result. A power calculation defines the sample size needed in order to reveal a statistically significant difference should one exist and is usually set at 80–90% (a 10–20% chance of a false negative result). The sample size is dependent on a number of factors, but in general if there is a large, expected difference between the groups (i.e. you expect drug A to reduce mortality by 20%), then a smaller sample size to ensure a statistically significant result is required, and vice versa for smaller differences. An expected difference between the groups is required to undertake a power calculation, so an estimation of the likely population mean for each group is also required. This data may already be available from previous trials in the same population group, but often it isn't and thus the expected difference estimates may lead to inaccurate powering of studies.

Two main errors can occur in hypothesis testing:

- A type 1 error occurs when the null hypothesis is incorrectly rejected (so a difference is found where none exists). Clinically this can lead to an ineffective drug or intervention being used on a patient. The probability of a type 1 error is the α value, also known as the α error. It

is used to set the p value, and is typically 5% or 0.05, so that a statistically significant result is one that is less than 0.05.
- A type 2 error occurs when the null hypothesis is incorrectly accepted (so there is a difference in the population, but the data does not show this). Clinically this could lead to an effective drug or treatment not being used. The probability of a type 2 error is known as the β value or β error. It is used to calculate the desired power of a study — if a study is powered to detect a 20% β error, then the power is 1-β or 80% (there is an 80% chance that we will correctly reject the null hypothesis).

Errors may occur due to intrinsic variations in the samples (and this can normally be overcome by using the right sample size based on a power calculation) or by bias (a systematic or study design error). The different types of bias include selection bias (patient selection results in groups that are not comparable which can be overcome by randomisation), measurement bias, observer bias and equipment error (which can be overcome by blinding and using standardised measuring equipment/methods).

References
1. Spoors C, Kiff K. Statistics for the anaesthetist. In: Spoors C, Kiff K, Eds. *Training in anaesthesia: the essential curriculum*. Oxford: Oxford University Press; 2010: chapter 24: pp. 561–72.

Answer 35: b
A neonate is any child less than 28 days old or 44 weeks post-conceptual age. Sudden unexpected postnatal collapse (SUPC) is thankfully very rare but associated with significant morbidity and mortality.

The four main causes of neonatal collapse are: infections and sepsis, issues related to congenital heart disease, inborn errors of metabolism (always check the glucose!) and non-accidental injury (NAI). Although abdominal surgical conditions may also cause SUPC, intussusception is very unusual in this age group and is more common in older infants. The cause of SUPC is often unclear initially, so management is with general resuscitation and investigations to identify the underlying cause.

Patients are likely to need intubating. This should be done as an MDT with roles allocated and a checklist undertaken. Neonates are at risk of bradycardia so atropine should be drawn up and administered prior to intubation. Whilst 100% oxygen should be used initially, it should be titrated down as clinically able, particularly if there is a high suspicion of a patent ductus arteriosus dependent congenital heart problem. The addition of PEEP is often helpful.

Intravenous (IV) access should be secured promptly, with the umbilical vein utilised in those patients under 1 week old. If IV access is difficult to secure, the intraosseous (IO) route may be used. Signs of shock should be treated with fluid boluses in 5–10ml/kg aliquots, with an adrenaline infusion started once 40ml/kg total is reached (patients this age are often maximally vasoconstricted and the LV fails early so adrenaline is the inotrope of choice).

It is vital to check the glucose early and repeat regularly. Once intubated, ongoing sedation is often a morphine infusion alone but may vary with local practice. Full exposure and examination of the child and adequate warming via a resuscitaire with an overhead heat lamp or underbody heat pad should also be performed.

References

1. World Federation of Societies of Anaesthesiologists (WFSA) Resource Library. A practical guide for the management of the collapsed neonate — part 1 recognition and initial management, 2020. Available at: https://resources.wfsahq.org/atotw/a-practical-guide-for-the-management-of-the-collapsed-neonate-part-1-recognition-and-initial-management/.
2. Lal N, Varshney T. The collapsed newborn in the emergency department. *BJA Educ* 2018; 18(8): 254–8.

● Answer 36: c

Skin is composed of five layers of epidermis and two of dermis which sit on subcutaneous fat, connective tissue and muscle compartments. The deepest epidermal layer is continually dividing and migrating to the surface, resulting in regeneration every 2–3 weeks. The dermis layer contains nerves, blood vessels, exocrine glands and hair follicles. The top layer of the dermis provides support for the basal epidermal layer and therefore the epidermis cannot regenerate without this layer.

SBA Paper 4: Answers

Burn injuries are classified based on the aetiology (thermal, chemical, electrical, etc.), total body surface percentage involved and depth (see below).

Epidermal or superficial burns involve damage to the epidermis only. They present as simple erythema and are not included in calculations of body surface area involved. They may also be referred to as a first-degree burn (although this terminology is no longer used in the UK).

Superficial partial-thickness burns involve damage to the upper dermis, but the vascular and other deep dermal structures remain intact. They appear pale, pink and moist with blisters that form from fluid leak due to damaged blood vessels. They are very painful as nerve endings are exposed.

Deep partial-thickness burns affect a larger proportion of the deep dermal layer. The vascular plexus is coagulated by heat and only the deepest structures remain intact. They appear drier, red and non-blanching and they are less sensate. Partial-thickness burns (superficial and deep) can also be referred to as second-degree burns.

Full-thickness burns extend through the entire thickness of the dermis and may affect deeper structures. No dermal tissue remains intact in such cases. They appear waxy and white and may even look charred. They are not painful due to the destruction of the cutaneous nerves.

References
1. McCann C, Watson A, Barnes D. Major burns: Part 1. Epidemiology, pathophysiology and initial management. *BJA Educ* 2022; 22(3): 94–103.

● Answer 37: d

There are two components of consciousness: arousal and awareness. If there is a disruption of the relationship between arousal and awareness, a disorder of consciousness occurs. A fully conscious patient is defined as being awake with full awareness of themselves and their environment.

Assessment of conscious level is traditionally performed using the Glasgow Coma Scale (GCS), although this has some limitations in ICU patients. The

FOUR score is an alternative for intubated patients and contains four criteria (each with a maximum of 4 points): eye response, motor response of upper extremities, brainstem reflexes and respiration pattern.

Coma is defined as absent wakefulness and awareness lasting more than 6 hours. It has many different causes, including traumatic brain injury, metabolic derangement, toxins and cerebral infection.

A patient in a vegetative state will demonstrate wakefulness but no awareness and preserved capacity for spontaneous or stimulated induced arousal (such as sleep-wake cycles). They will display reflexive behaviour only. Spontaneous limb movements may occur but not to command. It is typically seen in patients previously in a coma who are more awake but have extensive damage to both cerebral hemispheres with a relatively preserved brainstem. When this lasts longer than 4 weeks it is termed a persistent vegetative state.

A minimally conscious state comprises wakefulness with minimal awareness. Affected patients have severely altered consciousness with minimal but discernible behavioural evidence of self and environment awareness. They may respond to external stimuli but not reproducibly and do not obey commands.

Several coma-like syndromes are also recognised and include: locked-in syndrome (where there is complete paralysis below the third cranial nerve and the patient may have preserved consciousness and cognition but can only communicate via eye movements), catatonia (patients are awake but mute with decreased motor activity and fixed posture secondary to psychiatric illness) and akinetic mutism (caused by bilateral frontal lobe lesions or hydrocephalus; patients are awake but completely immobile and silent).

References

1. White H, Ventakesh B. Disorders of consciousness. In: Bersten AD, Handy JM, Eds. *Oh's intensive care manual,* 8th ed. London: Elsevier; 2018: chapter 49: pp. 629–42.

SBA Paper 4: Answers

● Answer 38: c

In the UK every year, a Serious Hazards of Transfusion (SHOT) report is published which documents all reported complications associated with blood product use. The absolute risk of death from being transfused a blood product is 1 in every 58,000 components and the risk of harm is five times that. The leading cause of transfusion-related death is pulmonary complications which result in over 75% of the deaths reported in July 2024. Platelets are the most likely component to cause a reaction.

There are several different hazards of transfusion:

- Febrile, allergic and hypotensive reactions (FAHRs) can occur up to 24 hours following a transfusion of blood products where there is no other obvious cause for the symptoms. This category is the most common transfusion reaction with 336 episodes recorded in 2023, of which 119 caused major morbidity (but no deaths). Most reactions occurred following red blood cell administration with platelets second, likely due to the fact that many more red blood cells are transfused. Febrile and allergic reactions are categorised as mild, moderate or severe based on the symptoms and signs, with a mild febrile reaction being a temperature over 38°C (with a rise of 1–2° from baseline) but no other features. A severe allergic reaction would be anaphylaxis. Mild reactions are not reportable to SHOT, so it is likely that the number of FAHR reactions are higher than those in the report. Hypotensive reactions are either moderate or severe, with moderate being a drop in BP without signs of shock, and severe being hypotension with signs of shock.
- Pulmonary complications include transfusion-associated circulatory overload (TACO) and non-TACO. TACO is an acute or worsening respiratory compromise or pulmonary oedema during or up to 12 hours after, that is not explained by the patient's underlying condition (SHOT reporting will accept up to 24 hours post-transfusion). An assessment should be made regarding the patient's fluid balance and risk of circulatory overload when prescribing blood products, and consideration given to the concomitant use of diuretics. Non-TACO pulmonary complications include transfusion-related acute lung injury (TRALI), TACO-TRALI (where elements of both exist) and pulmonary

complications not classified as either TACO or TRALI. The diagnosis of TRALI is based on the presence of an acute-onset hypoxaemia (sats <90%) with bilateral changes on imaging and no left atrial hypertension, onset within 6 hours of transfusion and with no alternative risk factors for ARDS.
- Haemolytic transfusion reactions present with fever, a fall in haemoglobin, a rise in bilirubin and LDH and a positive direct antiglobulin test. They generally occur within 24 hours of transfusion (but sometimes can present over 24 hours after). All reported cases in the 2023 report followed red blood cell transfusion.
- Transfusion-transmitted infections (TTIs) are defined as evidence in the recipient of an infection after transfusion with no evidence prior to this, and one of the components received came from a donor with the same infection. The meticulous screening processes used in the donation process make these unusual, and in the 2023 report only two cases were confirmed (one malaria and one hepatitis A infection). Data from 1996 onwards in the UK showed a total of 89 TTIs, with 45 of these from platelet transfusions.

References

1. Soutar R, McSporran W, Tomlinson T, *et al*. Guideline on the investigation and management of acute transfusion reactions. *Br J Haematol* 2023; 201(5): 832–44.
2. Narayan S, Editor, on behalf of the Serious Hazards of Transfusion (SHOT) Steering Group. The 2023 annual SHOT Report; 2024. Available at: https://www.shotuk.org/wp-content/uploads/myimages/Annual-SHOT-Report-2023-V1.2.pdf.

Answer 39: b

Information on the presentation and management of tumour lysis syndrome can be found on page 127, Paper 2, Q10.

Rasburicase catalyses the formation of allantoin (which is water-soluble) from uric acid resulting in a rapid reduction in uric acid levels. It is used in the prevention and management of hyperuricaemia to prevent acute kidney injury. All the other electrolyte abnormalities may occur in the context of tumour lysis syndrome, although hyperlipidaemia does not.

SBA Paper 4: Answers

References

1. Wigmore T, Gruber P. Implications of solid tumours for intensive care. In: Bersten AD, Handy JM, Eds. *Oh's intensive care manual*, 8th ed. London: Elsevier; 2018: chapter 46: pp. 601–7.

● Answer 40: a

When seizure activity lasts more than 5 minutes it is termed status epilepticus (SE). Continuous seizure activity for more than 30 minutes is associated with a risk of long-term consequences and neuronal death. If seizures continue despite first- and second-line therapy this is termed refractory SE and usually requires a general anaesthetic. This occurs in approximately one in five patients with SE and carries a worse prognosis. SE can be convulsive (tonic-clonic) or non-convulsive (coma with EEG evidence of seizure activity but no visible movements).

Most patients with SE are not known epileptics and it is often secondary to central nervous system or system illness (such as encephalitis, stroke, tumours, metabolic disturbances). It also occurs less commonly in patients with pre-existing epilepsy.

The management of seizures should initially be with supportive care — assess and manage the airway as required, high-flow oxygen, monitoring, obtaining IV access and assessment of blood sugar.

First-line treatment for SE is with benzodiazepines: buccal midazolam, rectal diazepam or IV lorazepam may all be used. If there is ongoing seizure activity 5 minutes after the first dose, a repeat dose of benzodiazepine can be given. The main inhibitory mechanism in the brain is GABA receptor-mediated; with prolonged seizure activity there is a reduction in GABA receptor activity, therefore, only two doses of benzodiazepines are recommended, prior to moving onto second-line treatments. If there is no response to two doses of benzodiazepines then a second-line agent such as levetiracetam (Keppra®), phenytoin or sodium valproate should be given. NICE guidelines state that Keppra® may be quicker to administer and have fewer adverse effects but doesn't specifically state this is the preferred option. If there is no response to one second-line treatment then consideration should be given to the use of an additional one, but only after expert guidance is sought.

In refractory SE, the patient is likely to need a general anaesthetic to control the seizures. Propofol or thiopental are reasonable options for induction due to their anticonvulsant properties. An alternative to general anaesthesia is phenobarbital; however, it is likely at this point the patient will require a definitive airway so a general anaesthetic and intubation will be performed in addition. Ketamine may be used as an adjunct if seizures are still difficult to control despite the measure outlined above. It is thought that NMDA receptor activation plays an important role in refractory seizures, so NMDA receptor antagonists such as ketamine can be useful for refractory or super refractory SE (SE beyond 24 hours of anaesthetic therapy).

References

1. National Institute for Health and Care Excellence (NICE), guideline NG217. Epilepsies in children, young people and adults, 2022. Available at: https://www.nice.org.uk/guidance/ng217/resources/epilepsies-in-children-young-people-and-adults-pdf-66143780239813.
2. Opdam H. Status epilepticus. In: Bersten AD, Handy JM, Eds. *Oh's intensive care manual*, 8th ed. London: Elsevier; 2018: chapter 50: pp. 643–50.

● Answer 41: d

Viral haemorrhagic fever is a clinical syndrome associated with haemorrhagic manifestations caused by a range of different viruses. Some of the viruses causing viral haemorrhagic fever are arboviruses: zoonotic viruses transmitted through the bites of insects, typically mosquitoes and ticks. Examples of viral haemorrhagic fevers are: yellow fever, hantavirus, Lassa fever, Marburg and Ebola.

Yellow fever is caused by a *Flavivirus* (an arbovirus) and has a wide spectrum of illness severity. An immunisation is available for travel to endemic areas (Africa and equatorial South America). Mild infection presents similarly to influenza, whereas severe disease has three distinct phases: initially a high fever of 39–40°C for 4–5 days with headache, arthralgia and a relative bradycardia are seen. Patients then appear to recover and are then relatively well for a few days before deteriorating with returning fever, jaundice, hepatomegaly and gastrointestinal bleeding all frequently encountered. In severe disease the haemorrhage may lead to shock, coma and death. Management is supportive.

SBA Paper 4: Answers

Marburg and Ebola are both caused by the *Filoviridae* virus family and are named after the area in which they first appeared. The natural reservoir of the virus is unknown but as filoviruses are zoonotic it is thought that fruit bats may be the natural host. The illness begins with high fever, myalgia and severe headache and on the fifth day a maculopapular rash starts on the face and may spread to the rest of the body. Diarrhoea is profuse, and from day seven, haematemesis, melaena and haemoptysis may all be seen. In Ebola, chest pain and dry cough are prominent. The *Ebolavirus* has five species which have different mortality rates ranging from 40% up to 90%. Treatment is mainly symptomatic but there are some experimental therapies being trialled, including monoclonal antibodies and remdesivir.

References

1. Barlow G, Irving W, Moss PJ. Infectious diseases. In: Kumar P, Clark M, Eds. *Kumar and Clark's clinical medicine*, 10th ed. London: Elsevier; 2020: chapter 20: pp. 513–21.

Answer 42: c

Candida auris is a highly transmissible emerging fungal pathogen that is resistant to a number of antifungal agents. It may be present as a coloniser but can also cause invasive candidal infections, which carry a high mortality rate if multidrug-resistant. There are different types of *C. auris* based on where they were first isolated. *C. auris* is commonly resistant to fluconazole (with resistance to other azoles also frequently seen) and around a third are amphotericin-resistant, leaving only echinocandins as treatment options. Some strains have demonstrated echinocandin resistance, meaning there are no available antifungal treatment options.

In addition to its drug resistance, *C. auris* has a high heat resistance and can tolerate high salt concentrations. It has been found to be able to survive for 7 days on general surfaces and up to 14 days on plastic devices. Patients can become colonised within 4 hours of exposure and high dependency areas are at higher risk for transmission. Identification of *C. auris* using traditional lab methods is challenging, and being misidentified as a different candida frequently occurs. The most reliable method is via matrix-assisted laser desorption/ionisation time-of-flight (MALDI-TOF) mass spectrometry, which may not be available in all laboratories.

Scrupulous infection control measures are key, preventing nosocomial spread of a known case of *C. auris*. As transmission may occur from both infected and colonised patients the management is the same for both groups. Affected patients should be cared for in a single room with contact precautions. PPE with a long-sleeved gown and gloves and a face shield (if there is a risk of bodily fluid exposure) should be used for the patient or surrounding equipment contact. Equipment in the room should be single use for that patient, and the room terminally cleaned once the patient leaves. Not all disinfection products are effective against *C. auris* so discussion with your local infection control team is vital.

Patients who have been in contact or may have shared equipment with an affected patient (e.g. all patients in an open bay) will require screening with skin swabs as directed by local infection control policy. These patients will need repeated swabs and only deemed clear when two negative swabs taken at least a week apart without antifungal treatment are recorded.

If there is evidence of nosocomial transmission of *C. auris* within an ICU, then screening of all patients on the unit should take place, with cohorting of affected and non-infected patients vital. New admissions to the unit should be minimised until the transmission route and source are identified and managed, and staff may also need to be screened if no patient source is ascertained.

References

1. GOV.UK. Candida auris: laboratory investigation, management and infection prevention and control (draft). Available at: https://www.gov.uk/government/consultations/candida-auris-update-to-management-guidance/candida-auris-laboratory-investigation-management-and-infection-prevention-and-control-draft.
2. Aldejohann AM, Wiese-Posselt M, Gastmeier P, Kurzai O. Expert recommendations for prevention and management of *Candida auris* transmission. *Mycoses* 2022; 65(6): 590–8.
3. Jones CR, Neill C, Borman AM, *et al*. The laboratory investigation, management, and infection prevention and control of *Candida auris*: a narrative review to inform the 2024 national guidance update in England. *J Med Microbiol* 2024; 73(5): 001820.

SBA Paper 4: Answers

● Answer 43: e

There are three main classes of antifungal drugs:

- Polyene antifungals interact with sterols in the fungal membrane, causing an increase in membrane permeability and damage to the organism. Polyenes include nystatin (which is not absorbed through mucous membranes so is used topically, orally or as a pessary), amphotericin (a potent but nephrotoxic IV polyene often given in its liposomal form to reduce toxicity) and flucytosine (given in combination with amphotericin for cryptococcal meningitis and severe systemic candidiasis).
- Azole antifungals inhibit fungal sterol synthesis resulting in a damaged cell wall. There are two main groups: imidazoles (such as ketoconazole, clotrimazole and miconazole) which are only used topically due to the risk of liver damage with systemic use and triazoles (such as fluconazole, voriconazole and posaconazole). All triazoles may cause QT prolongation, inhibition of CYP P450 enzymes and hepatotoxicity. Fluconazole has good enteral absorption and CNS penetration, and is used for mucosal, systemic and CNS infections. Many non-albicans *Candida* are intrinsically resistant to fluconazole, and *C. albicans* can also develop resistance. Voriconazole has a broad spectrum of activity including *Candida*, *Cryptococcus* and *Aspergillus* infections.
- Echinocandin antifungals act by inhibiting the cell wall polysaccharide glucan. Caspofungin is used for invasive candidiasis and aspergillosis and as an empirical treatment for fungal infections in neutropenic patients. Anidulafungin is used for invasive candidiasis.

References

1. Barlow G, Irving W, Moss PJ. Infectious diseases. In: Kumar P, Clark M, Eds. *Kumar and Clark's clinical medicine*, 10th ed. London: Elsevier; 2020: chapter 20: pp. 559–63.
2. Joint Formulary Committee. British National Formulary, 2024. Available at: https://bnf.nice.org.uk/.

● Answer 44: b

Contrast-induced acute kidney injury (CI-AKI) is defined as a rise in serum creatinine of 25% from a patient's baseline within 48 hours of a radiological procedure with contrast. In a small number of patients, however, the creatinine may not peak until up to 5 days after contrast.

The main patients at risk of CI-AKI are those with pre-existing chronic kidney disease (CKD), particularly with an eGFR of <40ml/min/1.73m^2 and coexistent diabetes mellitus. Other patient-related risk factors include heart failure, renal transplantation, age >75, hypovolaemia at the time of contrast administration (particularly in combination with recent NSAID use), and concurrent ACE inhibitor use.

The type, volume and site of contrast administration can also affect the incidence of CI-AKI. Older contrast agents are more ionic and hyperosmolar compared with newer agents and are more nephrotoxic. Low- and iso-osmolar agents are now routinely used and associated with a lower risk of CI-AKI. The risk of CI-AKI increases in line with the dose administered with doses under 125ml tending to be safer, but doses as small as 20ml may still be problematic in patients with diabetic nephropathy. Interventional procedures with intra-arterial contrast administration (such as coronary angioplasty) are associated with the highest risk of CI-AKI, whereas intravenous contrast administration for diagnostic imaging has a much lower risk.

The prevention of CI-AKI can be attempted via identification and correction of modifiable risk factors where possible (stopping nephrotoxic drugs, correction of hypovolaemia, use of low- or iso-osmolar contrast agents, only undertaking necessary scans/scanning without contrast). A patient's individual level of risk can be evaluated (for example, with the Mehran Risk Score) and if deemed intermediate or high risk, the use of pre-hydration is supported. Several different agents have been used in pre-scan protocols, including 0.9% saline, N-acetylcysteine and sodium bicarbonate. Several studies have compared these different regimes with no single approach demonstrated to be superior, so 0.9% saline pre-hydration is frequently used as it is safe, inexpensive and readily available.

References

1. Kidney Disease: Improving Global Outcomes (KDIGO). KDIGO clinical practice guideline for acute kidney injury, 2012. Available at: https://kdigo.org/wp-content/uploads/2016/10/KDIGO-2012-AKI-Guideline-English.pdf.

2. www.uptodate.com. Prevention of contrast-induced acute kidney injury associated with computed tomography. UpToDate, 2024. Available at: https://www.uptodate.com/contents/prevention-of-contrast-induced-acute-kidney-injury-associated-with-computed-tomography.
3. Faggioni M, Mehran R. Preventing contrast-induced renal failure: a guide. *Interv Cardiol* 2016; 11(2): 98–104.
4. Weisbord SD, Gallagher M, Jneid H, *et al.* Outcomes after angiography with sodium bicarbonate and acetylcysteine. *N Engl J Med* 2018; 378(7): 603–14.
5. Nijssen EC, Rennenberg RJ, Nelemans PJ, *et al.* Prophylactic hydration to protect renal function from intravascular iodinated contrast material in patients at high risk of contrast-induced nephropathy (AMACING): a prospective, randomised, phase 3, controlled, open-label, non-inferiority trial. *Lancet* 2017; 389(10076): 1312–22.

● Answer 45: a

In 1913, Casimir Funk proposed the concept of vital amines or 'vitamins' after observing that rice hulk protected chickens against beriberi (it was later discovered that rice hulk contained thiamine). By the mid-20th century all the main vitamins had been isolated and synthesised. Recommended daily allowances of these vitamins were agreed with the aim of preventing deficiency diseases.

General vitamin deficiency is commonly associated with malnutrition, whereas deficiencies of specific vitamins tend to be associated with certain medical problems (e.g. vitamin D deficiency in renal disease, vitamin B12 and folate in small bowel disease). Vitamins can be divided based on structure into fat-soluble or water-soluble. Fat-soluble vitamins include A, D, E and K. Toxicity may occur with fat-soluble vitamins.

Vitamin A is found in oily fish, dairy and eggs, and margarine is often fortified with vitamin A. It is important for retinal function, and deficiency can lead to night blindness and complete visual loss in severe cases.

Vitamin D is found in oily fish and eggs, and many foods are fortified with vitamin D. It is important for many processes but particularly for bone mineralisation, and deficiency can lead to rickets (in children) or osteomalacia (any age group).

Vitamin E is found in plant oils, animal fats, seeds and nuts. It acts as an antioxidant and contributes to membrane stability. Deficiency results in ataxia and haemolytic anaemia in premature infants.

Vitamin K is found in green vegetables, liver, cheese and kiwi fruit. It is a co-factor in the production of clotting factors II, VII, IX and X as well as proteins within coagulation and bone formation pathways. Deficiency leads to bleeding disorders and may be linked to osteoporosis.

The remaining vitamins are water-soluble and include B1 (thiamine), B2 (riboflavin), niacin, B6 (pyridoxine), B12 (cobalamin), folate and vitamin C (ascorbic acid).

For more information on vitamin B1 deficiency please see page 160, Paper 2, Q33.

References
1. Marinos E, Lanham-New S, Kok K. Nutrition. In: Kumar P, Clark M, Eds. *Kumar and Clark's clinical medicine*, 10th ed. London: Elsevier; 2020: chapter 33: pp. 1236–42.
2. Mozaffarian D, Rosenberg I, Uauy R. History of modern nutrition science — implications for current research, dietary guidelines, and food policy. *BMJ* 2018; 361: k2392.

Answer 46: e

There are several different methods used for measuring cardiac output in intensive care patients. These can be subcategorised according to how invasive they are (invasive, semi-invasive, non-invasive), or by what they are primarily measuring (cardiac output or stroke volume).

Those measuring cardiac output include:

- Fick method, which is based on the premise that the amount of a substance taken up by an organ per unit time is a product of the arteriovenous difference in concentration of the substance and the blood flow to that organ. The equation is rearranged such that the blood flow (or cardiac output) is equal to the oxygen uptake from the lungs divided by the difference between the mixed venous O_2 concentration (from pulmonary artery catheter) and the arterial O_2

SBA Paper 4: Answers

concentration. The indirect Fick method uses CO_2 excretion instead and requires partial rebreathing of CO_2 to calculate. Although the Fick method was the historical gold standard, it is rarely used clinically today.

- Thermodilution uses a bolus of cold water (0–4°C) injected into either a pulmonary arterial catheter or a central line. The change in temperature of the blood is then measured (either further along the pulmonary artery catheter or by an arterial line sited in the femoral or brachial artery) and the mean decrease in temperature is inversely proportional to the cardiac output. This is calculated using a modification of the Stewart-Hamilton equation. Indicator dilution may also be used in this manner, with a dye or marker such as lithium injected into a peripheral vein and then measured at a sensor attached to an arterial line. Techniques that measure remotely from the injection site are termed transpulmonary, as the indicator travels through the heart and pulmonary circulation and can be used to calculate additional values such as extravascular lung water. Indicator or thermodilution techniques are used to calibrate cardiac output monitors used in arterial pressure waveform analysis.

Those measuring stroke volume include:

- Arterial pressure waveform analysis is derived by two different methods although both aim to utilise the arterial waveform to calculate the stroke volume which is then multiplied by the heart rate to provide a measure of cardiac output. Pulse contour analysis uses the area under the curve to calculate stroke volume. This requires an easily detectable dicrotic notch and the arterial line waveform, so arterial lines need to be sited in the femoral or brachial artery. Pulse index continuous cardiac output (PiCCO) monitors utilise this method. The alternative is pulse power analysis which converts the pressure signal into a volume signal to determine stroke volume. The algorithm used is not based on the waveform morphology so is less impacted by factors such as damping and can be used with a peripherally sited arterial line (such as a radial). This is the mechanism used In LiDCO monitors.
- Doppler measurement may also be used to assess stroke volume. An in-depth description of oesophageal Doppler monitoring is provided on page 261, Paper 3, Q47. The Doppler technique can also be used

transcutaneously using parasternal (transpulmonary) and suprasternal (transaortic) windows.
- Thoracic electrical bioimpedance and bioreactance can be measured via electrodes on the chest wall. Alternating currents (high frequency, very low amplitude) are passed through the thorax and changes in thoracic bioimpedance throughout the cardiac cycle provide an estimate of stroke volume. It is one of the only truly non-invasive cardiac monitors, but prone to inaccuracies in critical care due to factors such as motion artefact, electrical interference, change in tissue water content and dysrhythmias.

References

1. Sturgess D, Watts R. Haemodynamic monitoring. In: Bersten AD, Handy JM, Eds. *Oh's intensive care manual*, 8th ed. London: Elsevier; 2018: chapter 16: pp. 134–49.
2. Kong R, Vetrugno L. Cardiac output monitoring. In: Davey A, Diba A, Eds. *Ward's anaesthetic equipment*, 6th ed. London: Saunders, Elsevier; 2012: chapter 16: pp. 351–68.

Answer 47: b

The Wells' scoring system is used to estimate the clinical probability of a pulmonary embolus (PE) and can help guide clinicians as to whether imaging modalities are indicated. It should be used alongside the clinical history and examination and is not designed for use in critical care patients due to the inherent complexity and raised probability of thromboembolic events in this patient cohort.

The Wells score is calculated as follows:

- Clinical signs and symptoms of a deep vein thrombosis (DVT) — 3 points.
- PE is the likely diagnosis — 3 points.
- Heart rate >100 — 1.5 points.
- Immobilisation for at least 3 days OR surgery in the last 4 weeks — 1.5 points.
- Previous objectively diagnosed PE or DVT — 1.5 points.
- Haemoptysis — 1 point.
- Malignancy (receiving treatment within the last 6 months or palliative) — 1 point.

<2 points: patient is at low risk of PE (1.3% incidence) — use D-dimer or the Pulmonary Embolism Rule-out Criteria (PERC) score to rule out PE.
2-6 points: patient is at moderate risk of PE (16.2% incidence) — D-dimer +/- CTPA.
>6 points: patient is at high risk of PE (37.5% incidence) — CTPA only (no D-dimer).

The Pulmonary Embolism Severity Index (PESI) is a scoring system that is used to predict likely mortality from PE based on the following factors: age, sex, comorbid conditions (cancer, heart failure, COPD), clinical findings (pulse, BP, RR, temperature, GCS, saturations). It is often used to decide whether it is safe to manage someone at home, but a score putting patients at high or very high risk (mortality up to 25%) can be used as an indicator that the patient may benefit from higher levels of care.

References
1. MDCalc. Wells' Criteria for Pulmonary Embolism. Available at: https://www.mdcalc.com/calc/115/wells-criteria-pulmonary-embolism#next-steps.
2. MDCalc. Pulmonary Embolism Severity Index (PESI). Available at: https://www.mdcalc.com/calc/1304/pulmonary-embolism-severity-index-pesi.

Answer 48: c

Extracorporeal membrane oxygenation (ECMO) is a therapy used in selected patients with severe ARDS. The Faculty of Intensive Care Medicine (FICM) guidance states that ECMO should only be used in patients with severe ARDS (defined as a Murray score of ≥3 or a pH of <7.2 due to uncompensated hypercapnia) with a weakly recommended GRADE rating (Grading of Recommendations Assessment, Development and Evaluation) in support of this. The literature review undertaken for these recommendations included one major trial — the CESAR study — as the only other applicable trial data is from 1979 (when routine use of lung-protective ventilation was not a standard of care and results were therefore not applicable to contemporary practice). CESAR randomised 180 patients with severe ARDS to receive either ECMO or standard care. Of the 90 in the ECMO group, only 76% received ECMO. There was a significant decrease in mortality in the ECMO group, all of whom were managed at the ECMO centre even if they did not receive ECMO. The Murray score is used to assess the severity of ARDS and define if the patient is eligible for referral and consideration of ECMO. The score is the total of the below divided by four, with a maximum score of 4 and a trigger for referral being ≥3 (Table 4.18). Patients with a score of ≥2.5 (as with the patient in the question) who are deteriorating rapidly should also be considered for ECMO.

Table 4.18. The Murray score.

Criteria/score	0	1	2	3	4
P:F in kPa	≥40	30–39.9	23.3–29.9	**13.3–23.2**	<13.3
PEEP (cmH$_2$O)	≤5	6–8	**9–11**	11–14	≥15
Compliance (ml/cmH$_2$O)	≥80	60–79	40–59	**20–39**	≤19
CXR quadrants infiltrated	0	1	**2**	3	4

Compliance is calculated using tidal volume/driving pressure (PPlateau – PEEP).

References

1. Peek GJ, Clemens F, Elbourne D, *et al*. CESAR: conventional ventilatory support vs extracorporeal membrane oxygenation for severe adult respiratory failure. *BMC Health Serv Res* 2006; 6(1): 163.
2. The Faculty of Intensive Care Medicine. Guidelines on the management of acute respiratory distress syndrome, 2018. Available at: https://ficm.ac.uk/sites/ficm/files/documents/2021-10/Guidelines_on_the_Management_of_Acute_Respiratory_Distress_Syndrome.pdf.
3. www.rbht.nhs.uk. ECMO referrals and transfer pathway. Royal Brompton & Harefield hospitals. Available at: https://www.rbht.nhs.uk/our-services/clinical_support/critical-care-and-anaesthesia/ecmo-and-severe-respiratory-failure-service/ecmo-referrals-and-transfer-pathway.

● Answer 49: d

The pulmonary artery catheter (PAC, also known as a Swan-Ganz catheter) is a large-gauge multi-lumen catheter that is 110cm in length and is inserted via an introducer sheath into the internal jugular, subclavian or femoral veins. It has several proximal ports to enable fluid administration or administration of cold water for thermodilution cardiac output measurement. At the tip there is a balloon that is inflated (normally around 1.5ml of air) once the catheter is within the right atrium, and with constant pressure transducing from the port it is slowly advanced until it reaches the pulmonary artery. At this point a pulmonary artery wedge pressure (which approximates to left ventricular end-diastolic pressure) is measured and the balloon is then deflated.

The pressure wave seen as the balloon is advanced indicates its location (Figure 4.1). It begins with a CVP trace (1), then a right atrial trace (which is identical to the CVP trace), with a mean pressure between 0 and 6mmHg. In the right ventricle (2) a systolic pressure of between 15 and 25mmHg is seen and a diastolic pressure of 0 to 8mmHg. On moving into the pulmonary artery (3), the systolic pressure is in the same range as the right ventricle, but there is an increase in the diastolic pressure to a range of 8 to 15mmHg, with a mean pressure in health of 10–20mmHg. The balloon then continues to be advanced until it wedges (typically in a medium-sized pulmonary artery). At this position there will then be a pressure of around 6 to 15mmHg, and this is termed the pulmonary artery wedge or occlusion pressure (4). Once this

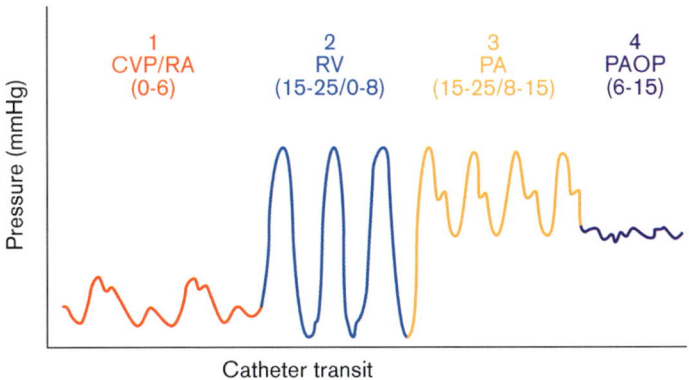

Figure 4.1. Pulmonary artery catheter waveforms.

measurement is noted, the balloon should then be deflated to avoid ischaemia, and the trace should return to a pulmonary arterial trace; if it does not then the catheter should be withdrawn until this is re-established.

Pulmonary artery catheters are now infrequently used in critical care due to the emergence of other cardiac output monitors which are less invasive and associated with fewer complications. The complications encountered with insertion and maintenance of a PAC include perforation of the pulmonary artery, air embolism, arrhythmias, conduction defects, valvular damage, knotting of the catheter, thrombosis, pulmonary infarction, infection.

References
1. Sturgess D, Watts R. Haemodynamic monitoring. In: Bersten AD, Handy JM, Eds. *Oh's intensive care manual*, 8th ed. London: Elsevier; 2018: chapter 16: pp. 134–49.
2. Kong R, Vetrugno L. Cardiac output monitoring. In: Davey A, Diba A, Eds. *Ward's anaesthetic equipment*, 6th ed. London: Saunders, Elsevier; 2012: chapter 16: pp. 351–68.

● Answer 50: d

Ascites is an accumulation of fluid in the peritoneal cavity. The most common cause of ascites is hepatic cirrhosis leading to portal hypertension. The International Club of Ascites defines ascites as:

- Uncomplicated: ascites which is not infected or associated with hepatorenal syndrome and can be graded as mild (only detectable on ultrasound), moderate (causing moderate bilateral abdominal distention) and large (marked abdominal distention).
- Refractory: ascites that cannot be prevented with medical treatment after initial therapeutic paracentesis and is either diuretic-resistant or diuretic-intractable (unable to use an effective diuretic dose due to side effects).

Analysis of the ascitic fluid can help with diagnosis and cause of the ascites, and identification of other intra-abdominal pathology. Analysis can include some or all the following:

- Protein/albumin: total protein >30g/L indicates that the fluid is an exudate, and below this figure, a transudate. The serum ascites albumin gradient (SAAG) is more commonly used and is calculated by subtracting the ascitic fluid albumin from the serum value taken on the same day. A result above 11g/L (or 1.1g/dL) is found in patients with portal hypertension from all causes (primarily liver disease including portal vein thrombosis and liver metastasis, but also from heart failure or constrictive pericarditis). SAAG measurements below 11g/L are caused by conditions such as pancreatitis, nephrotic syndrome, peritoneal TB and carcinomatosis. In patients with a raised SAAG, cardiac causes can be differentiated from hepatic causes if the total protein is above 25g/L (in hepatic ascites the total protein is typically <25g/L).

- Cell count: a neutrophil count above 250 cells/mm^3 is diagnostic for bacterial peritonitis. If the sample is very blood-stained then a correction must be performed (one white cell is subtracted for every 750 red blood cells, and one neutrophil subtracted for every 250 red blood cells) to provide a corrected neutrophil count. A raised white cell count is present in both spontaneous bacterial peritonitis and secondary bacterial peritonitis. Runyon's criteria can be used to identify patients with secondary bacterial peritonitis with a neutrophil count of >250 cells/mm^3 and two out of three of the following: total protein >10g/L, glucose <2.8mmol/L and LDH greater than the upper limit of normal for serum.
- Amylase: the normal level in uncomplicated ascites is approximately 40% of serum levels. This will increase in bowel perforation or pancreatitis, and the ratio of ascitic:serum amylase levels may reach 6:1 in pancreatitis (with normal being 0.4).
- Glucose: ascitic fluid glucose is usually similar to serum levels; however, it can be lower in TB, malignancy and bowel perforation and significantly reduced in secondary bacterial peritonitis.

References

1. Aithal GP, Palaniyappan N, China L, *et al*. Guidelines on the management of ascites in cirrhosis. *Gut* 2021; 70(1): 9–29.
2. www.uptodate.com. Evaluation of adults with ascites. UpToDate, 2024. Available at: https://www.uptodate.com/contents/evaluation-of-adults-with-ascites.

SBA Paper 5: Questions

Question 1

You are called to assist with a patient in the ED, who has come in with a suspected overdose and low GCS. The ED registrar tells you that the patient was found surrounded by a variety of empty tablet packets, including diazepam, codeine, amitriptyline and paracetamol.

Observations on your assessment are as follows:

A: Tolerating nasal airway.
B: Sats 98% on an FiO_2 of 0.5, RR 10/min.
C: BP 100/60mmHg, HR 130/min, ECG shows a sinus tachycardia, QRS 120ms, QTc 490ms.
D: GCS 6 (E-1, V-1, M-4), pupils size 7 bilaterally and reactive, glucose 5.8mmol/L.
E: Temperature 36.0°C, skin feels hot and dry.

You decide that the patient needs intubating and ask for them to have a fluid bolus of 500ml lactated Ringer's solution (Hartmann's solution), prior to undertaking intubation. You have completed a safety check list prior to a rapid sequence induction, when you note that the patient has gone into ventricular tachycardia (VT) with a pulse.

What is the best management of the pulsed VT?

a   300mg IV amiodarone.
b   DC cardioversion.
c   100ml IV 8.4% sodium bicarbonate ($NaHCO_3$).
d   1 unit/kg IV insulin, followed by an insulin infusion supplemented with 10% dextrose.
e   2g IV magnesium sulphate.

● Question 2

You are working on the cardiac intensive care unit and are asked to review a patient due to concerns regarding their pacemaker. You are informed that a similar issue happened overnight and one of the settings was altered, which had made things better, with only intermittent periods of bradycardia. However, there is now a persistent lower heart rate with hypotension, and consequent rise in noradrenaline requirements. The patient had a mitral valve repair 3 days ago and has atrial and ventricular epicardial pacing wires *in situ* set to a rate of 80. The monitor shows that the heart rate is 40. You ask for a 12-lead ECG; the rhythm strip shows a 2:1 heart block with an atrial rate of 80 and a QRS complex following alternate p waves, but with pacing spikes after every p wave. You review the pacemaker and note it is set at a rate of 80/min in DDD mode, the atrial sensing light is flashing with every p wave, but the ventricular sensing light is not flashing with each QRS complex.

What is the most likely underlying problem?

a   Maturation of the ventricular wire.
b   Ventricular wire displacement.
c   Atrial wire displacement.
d   Atrial wire maturation.
e   Pacemaker malfunction.

● Question 3

You are asked to review a patient in the ED who was found at home in her bed, unconscious and unrousable, by her daughter. The patient is 75 years old and has a history of hypothyroidism, type 2 DM (on metformin and empagliflozin), ischaemic heart disease and hypertension. The patient is normally independent at home and needs help with shopping. Her daughter last saw her 2 days previously; she was complaining of a slight cough but was otherwise well. She has been in the ED for 90 minutes and has received a bolus of 500ml of 0.9% saline, and now has an infusion running at 1000ml/hr. You have been asked to review the patient, as the lady remains drowsy.

On examination:

A: Maintaining own airway.
B: Sats 94% on an FiO_2 of 0.5, RR 18/min, crepitations at the right base on auscultation.
C: BP 100/60mmHg, HR 95/min, sinus rhythm, increased skin turgor, dry mucous membranes, urine output 100ml in the last hour, overall fluid balance 1400ml positive.
D: GCS 10 (E-2, V-3, M-5), PEARL.
E: Temperature 35.5°C, abdomen soft and non-tender.

The results of blood tests (including arterial blood gases) taken on arrival and at 1 hour are shown in Table 5.1.

Table 5.1. Blood test results.

	On admission	After 1 hour of treatment
pH	7.31	7.32
pCO_2	6.3kPa	6.1kPa
pO_2	9.0kPa	9.5kPa
HCO_3^-	18mmol/L	19mmol/L
Ketones	0.9mmol/L	0.8mmol/L
Glucose	55mmol/L	50mmol/L
Na^+	155mmol/L	156mmol/L
K^+	5.5mmol/L	5.1mmol/L
Urea	10mmol/L	10mmol/L

What should be the treatment over the next hour?

a   Increase rate of 0.9% saline.
b   0.5 units/kg insulin infusion, continue same infusion of 0.9% saline.
c   Continue current rate of fluids with 0.9% saline plus 40mmol KCl.
d   Continue current rate of fluids with 0.45% saline plus 40mmol KCl.
e   0.1units/kg/hr insulin infusion, continue same infusion of 0.9% saline.

● Question 4

You are on a night shift covering the neurosurgical ICU when you are called to review a patient. The patient is a 56-year-old lady, who is normally fit and well. She presented to a local district general hospital with a thunderclap headache and confusion at 4pm. A CT scan and angiogram showed a subarachnoid bleed, classified as Fisher grade III, with a posterior communicating artery aneurysm. She was transferred to the tertiary hospital and underwent radiological coiling at 6pm. She was stable after the procedure, with a GCS of 14, and was admitted to the neurosurgical high dependency unit for observation. She received a dose of nimodipine at 8pm and some paracetamol for a headache, but no other medications have been administered. The nursing staff report it was difficult to get her to take medication, as she seemed a little drowsier than she had been immediately post-procedure. They are concerned that she is getting progressively more drowsy.

Examination is as follows on your review:

A: Patient snoring, nasal airway inserted which is well tolerated.
B: Sats 99% on an FiO_2 of 0.4, RR 18/min, chest is clear.
C: BP 130/70mmHg, HR 70/min, warm peripherally and well perfused, urine output 40ml/hr.
D: GCS 8 (E-2, V-2, M-4), pupils size 2 PEARL, downward gaze, no localising neurology.
E: Temperature 36.8°C.

Which of the following represents the complication of subarachnoid haemorrhage, that is most likely to be causing the symptoms in this patient?

a   Rebleed.
b   Vasospasm.
c   Hyponatraemia secondary to cerebral salt wasting.
d   Seizures.
e   Hydrocephalus.

● Question 5

You are asked to review a lady in the ED of a district general hospital, for consideration of admission to critical care. She is a 59-year-old lady who has presented with breathlessness and pleuritic chest pain 1 week after having had surgical fixation of an ankle fracture, sustained 2 days prior to surgery. She hasn't taken the apixaban she was prescribed post-op, because she has lost the tablets. She has a history of gastro-oesophageal reflux disease (GORD) and takes regular omeprazole. She has no previous history of venous thromboembolic disease. The closest cardiothoracic centre with interventional radiology capabilities is a 30-minute ambulance transfer away.

On examination:

A: Maintaining her own airway.
B: Sats of 95% on an FiO_2 of 0.4, RR of 24/min, PaO_2 of 9.3kPa, $PaCO_2$ of 4.5kPa, lactate 1.8mmol/L.
C: BP 100/60mmHg, HR 110/min, sinus rhythm, warm peripherally with no oedema.
D: Alert and orientated, complaining of severe pleuritic chest pain.
E: The whole of her right leg is swollen.

Investigations undertaken are shown in Table 5.2.

Table 5.2. Investigations.	
CT pulmonary angiogram (CTPA)	Large right-sided pulmonary embolus with evidence of right heart strain
Bedside ECHO	Evidence of right ventricular strain, with dilatation of the RV and some flattening of the intraventricular septum
Troponin I	160ng/L (upper limit for the assay is 20ng/L)

What should be the first-line treatment for this patient?

a   Thrombolysis.
b   Surgical embolectomy.
c   Inferior vena cava filter insertion.
d   Treatment dose of low-molecular-weight heparin.
e   Percutaneous catheter-guided treatment.

● Question 6

You are working on the cardiac intensive care unit when you are called to a patient who, 3 hours earlier, had returned to theatre after an aortic valve replacement. The nursing staff are concerned as the patient is hypotensive.

On examination:

A: ETT.
B: Sats 92% on an FiO_2 of 0.5, PRVC Vt 500ml x 18, PEEP of 8cmH$_2$O.
C: BP 70/40mmHg, HR 95/min, sinus rhythm, cool peripherally, nil in mediastinal drains (last emptied 40 minutes ago), quiet heart sounds, CVP 22mmHg, noradrenaline 0.4µg/kg/min — increased from 0.2µg/kg/min over the last hour.
D: Sedated on propofol and alfentanil, PEARL.
E: Temperature 36.5°C, urine output 5ml for this hour (30ml hour prior).

Arterial blood gases and cardiac output monitoring for the past few hours are shown in Table 5.3.

Table 5.3. Blood gases and cardiac output monitoring.

	Post-op	2 hours ago	Current
pH	7.36	7.35	7.28
pCO_2	5.5kPa	5.4kPa	6.0kPa
pO_2	10.5kPa	10.4kPa	9.5kPa
HCO_3^-	22mmol/L	20mmol/L	18mmol/L
Lactate	2.0mmol/L	2.2mmol/L	4.5mmol/L
CVP	5mmHg	8mmHg	22mmHg
Cardiac index (CI)	3L/min	2.8L/min	1.8L/min
Stroke volume variation (SVV)	5%	8%	15%

What is the best management of this patient's hypotension?

a   Resternotomy.
b   Vasopressin infusion.
c   Dobutamine infusion.
d   Bolus of fluid.
e   Percutaneous pericardiocentesis.

● Question 7

You are reviewing a patient who has just been admitted to the ICU from the ED with urosepsis. The patient is a 74-year-old man with a history of HTN (on ramipril), previous NSTEMI and GORD (on omeprazole). He had been in the ED for 4 hours and had received 3L of fluid but remained hypotensive and was admitted for vasopressor support. An arterial line shows his blood pressure has been approximately 100/50mmHg, on 5mg/hr of metaraminol. During your admission review you notice he has gone into fast atrial fibrillation (AF).

On examination:

A: Maintain own airway.
B: Sats 99% on an FiO_2 of 0.3, RR 22/min, chest clear on auscultation.
C: BP 90/50mmHg on 6mg/hr metaraminol, HR 135/min, AF with no ischaemic changes on 12-lead ECG, cool peripheries, capillary refill time (CRT) 4 seconds, 20ml dark urine in a recently inserted catheter bag.
D: Alert and orientated, no pain.
E: Temperature 38.7°C, abdomen soft, suprapubic tenderness on palpation.

What is the best initial management for this patient's arrhythmia?

a   300mg bolus of amiodarone.
b   500µg bolus of digoxin.
c   50mg PO atenolol.
d   500ml bolus of Hartmann's.
e   Synchronised DC cardioversion.

Question 8

You are reviewing a 22-year-old polytrauma patient on the ICU. Thirty-six hours previously the patient fell off his mountain bike, sustaining the following injuries: small traumatic subarachnoid haemorrhage with small frontal lobe contusion, rib fractures 3–8 on the right side with an associated small haemopneumothorax, no abdominal injuries, a pelvic fracture and a right-sided mid-shaft femoral fracture. A chest drain was inserted in the ED and a full major transfusion pack of blood products was administered. He was then immediately transferred to theatre where he had fixation of his pelvis and femur, requiring a further 2 units of red blood cells and an adult dose of FFP intra-operatively. He was transferred to critical care and was subsequently extubated onto low-flow oxygen. During the night (24 hours post-injury) his oxygen requirement escalated; a repeat CXR showed no pneumothorax and patchy consolidation on the right side.

You are now reviewing the patient on day two post-injury. The nurses are concerned as he seems to have become confused this morning; they also commented that a blood gas sample looks unusual.

On examination:

A: Maintaining own airway.
B: Sats 95% on an FiO_2 of 0.8 on HFNO 50L, RR 28/min, bilateral crackles to midzones, chest drain minimal output, swinging not bubbling, PaO_2 of 8.5kPa on ABG.
C: BP 90/50mmHg unsupported, HR 110/min, warm peripherally, mild peripheral oedema, urine output 30ml in the last hour.
D: GCS 13 (E-3, V-4, M-6), PEARL, no focal neurology.
E: Temperature 38.2°C, abdomen soft non-tender, non-blanching rash on the anterior chest wall and neck.

You are concerned about the change in his clinical picture, so you order a CT head and chest and send off some blood tests. The results are shown in Table 5.4.

SBA Paper 5: Questions

Table 5.4. Blood test results and CT scan report.

Hb	85g/L	PT	20 seconds
WCC	15 x 10^9/L	APTT	35 seconds
Platelets	65 x 10^9/L	Fibrinogen	1.8g/L
		Creatinine	180µmol/L
CT scan report	CT head — SAH unchanged, small amount of oedema at the site of contusion, otherwise nil new		
	CT chest — bilateral patchy ground-glass changes throughout the lung fields, 'crazy paving' pattern of septal thickening, no residual haemopneumothorax, chest drain tip sat in the apex, rib fractures as per previous scan		

Which of the following best explains the clinical picture?

a   Transfusion-related acute lung injury.
b   Pulmonary contusion.
c   Fat embolus syndrome.
d   Neurogenic pulmonary oedema.
e   Acute respiratory distress syndrome.

● Question 9

You are asked to review a patient on the ward for consideration of admission to critical care for renal replacement therapy. The patient is 17 years old and normally fit and well and was admitted the day before with nausea and vomiting, lethargy and easy bruising. The only other history is that around a week ago he had a 'tummy bug' after eating a sausage, that he thinks was not well cooked. He developed vomiting and blood-stained diarrhoea, a stool culture taken by the GP at the time grew an *E. coli* but the patient recovered without antibiotics. He was taking regular ibuprofen and paracetamol for about a week due to the abdominal pain. On arrival to hospital, he was found to be in acute renal failure, but was still passing urine; however, over the last few hours he has been anuric with a rising potassium. The team have done an extended renal work-up.

Blood test results are shown in Table 5.5.

Table 5.5. Blood test results.

Hb	90g/L	Na$^+$	138mmol/L
WCC	15 x 10^9/L	K$^+$	6.1mmol/L
Platelets	33 x 10^9/L	Creatinine	450µmol/L
Blood film	Schistocytes	Urea	28mmol/L
ADAMTS13 activity	70%	Haptoglobin	Undetectable
Complement	C3 and C4 within normal range	Urinalysis	Blood 1+ Protein 1+ Cells only seen, no cell casts

What is the most likely cause of his renal impairment?

a   Shiga toxin haemolytic uraemic syndrome.
b   Atypical haemolytic uraemic syndrome.
c   Acute tubular necrosis.
d   Thrombotic thrombocytopenic purpura.
e   Acute interstitial nephritis.

● Question 10

A 54-year-lady with a past medical history of type II diabetes on metformin presents to the ED with a swollen painful leg. She went over on her ankle in the garden 4 days ago and had been managing to walk on it, but it has been getting worse over the last few days. An X-ray of the ankle shows no bony injury but some significant soft tissue swelling, and she is hypotensive despite 2L of fluid over the past hour. The ED registrar states that she initially responded to fluid but is now deteriorating again and has spreading erythema and increasing pain in her leg. In addition to IV fluid therapy, she has received 15mg of morphine, Tazocin® and clindamycin IV.

On examination:

A: Maintaining her own airway.
B: Sats 95% on an FiO_2 of 0.5, RR 24/min, chest clear on auscultation.
C: BP 85/40mmHg, HR 110/min, cool peripheries, CRT 4 seconds.
D: Slightly muddled, PEARL, blood glucose 16mmol/L, severe pain in right leg.
E: Temperature 38.2°C, right leg red and swollen from the knee downwards with redness spreading 1cm beyond the demarcation line drawn on admission to the ED.

Blood test results including an arterial blood gas are shown in Table 5.6.

Table 5.6. Blood test results.

Hb	110g/L	Na^+	135mmol/L	pH	7.30
WCC	26 x 10^9/L	K^+	5.4mmol/L	pO_2	9kPa
Platelets	180 x 10^9/L	Creatinine	160µmol/L	pCO_2	5.6kPa
Neutrophils	22 x 10^9/L	Urea	12mmol/L	HCO_3^-	17mmol/L
CRP	240mg/L			Lactate	3.5mmol/L

What is the treatment priority?

a IVIg.
b Change antibiotics to meropenem and vancomycin.
c Insertion of central line.
d Hyperbaric oxygen therapy.
e Surgical debridement.

  Question 11

A 65-year-old man with a history of alcohol excess presents to the ED with severe epigastric pain radiating into his back. He states that this has developed over the last 24 hours and is associated with occasional vomiting. You have been asked to review him, as despite 3L of fluid, he is hypotensive with a new oxygen requirement and severe pain. A CT scan of his abdomen has been requested but not performed.

On examination:

A: Maintaining own airway.
B: Sats 94% on an FiO_2 of 0.6, RR 24/min, quiet bases on auscultation, CXR shows a bilateral raised hemidiaphragm with a small effusion on the left-hand side.
C: BP 90/60mmHg, HR 105/min, cool peripherally, CRT 3 seconds, minimal peripheral oedema.
D: Alert and orientated, in obvious discomfort despite 20mg of morphine.
E: Temperature 38.2°C, abdomen distended and tender, no evidence of shifting dullness.

All blood results including an arterial blood gas are shown in Table 5.7.

Table 5.7. Blood test results.

Hb	122g/L	Na^+	130mmol/L	pH	7.32
WCC	16 x 10^9/L	K^+	5.2mmol/L	pCO_2	4.5kPa
Neutrophils	14 x 10^9/L	Creatinine	140µmol/L	pO_2	10kPa
Platelets	155 x 10^9/L	Urea	11mmol/L	BE	−5mmol/L
ALT	50 IU/L	Blood urea nitrogen (BUN)	12mmol/L	HCO_3^-	18mmol/L
ALP	100 IU/L			Lactate	2.1mmol/L
Amylase	3000 U/L	Bilirubin	10µmol/L	Glucose	15mmol/L
		Albumin	30g/L		

Which of the following severity assessment scores could be calculated with the currently available information?

a   Revised Atlanta classification.
b   Bedside Index of Severity in Acute Pancreatitis (BISAP).
c   Balthazar score.
d   Glasgow-Imrie score.
e   Ranson score.

Question 12

A 55-year-old lady with a history of diabetes is admitted to the ICU with community-acquired pneumonia. She is subsequently intubated and ventilated, requiring vasopressors via a central line and is receiving IV co-amoxiclav as antibiotic therapy. You notice a reducing urine output and worsening acidosis so repeat blood tests including U&Es and a clotting screen are requested. Her renal function tests are stable, but you are subsequently informed that the clotting is abnormal, and some additional tests have been added for you to review. You are also told that her sputum sample has grown MRSA. You go back and review the patient; there is no signs of active bleeding, but the nursing staff have said that her line sites are a little oozy.

The blood test results are shown in Table 5.8.

Table 5.8. Blood test results.

Hb	98g/L	PT	20 seconds
WCC	24×10^9/L	International Normalised Ratio (INR)	1.9
Neutrophils	22×10^9/L	APTT	45 seconds
Platelets	78×10^9/L	Fibrinogen	0.9g/L
		Fibrin degradation products	45mg/L (normal range <10mg/L)

What is the best management of this patient's coagulopathy?

a   Cryoprecipitate.
b   Fresh frozen plasma (FFP).
c   Urgent discussion with microbiology regarding a change in antibiotic therapy.
d   Platelet transfusion.
e   Unfractionated heparin infusion.

Question 13

A 25-year-old 48kg lady with no previous past medical history presents to the ED with a suspected mixed overdose of diazepam, codeine and alcohol. After

2 hours of supportive treatment in the ED, her GCS is reduced and not improving and she has a BP of 80/40mmHg despite receiving 3L of 0.9% saline.

On examination:

A: Tolerating nasal airway.
B: Sats 99% on an FiO_2 of 0.3, RR 12/min, chest clear.
C: BP 80/40mmHg, HR 60/min, warm peripherally, CRT <2 seconds.
D: GCS 9 (M-4, E-2, S-3), PEARL size 4 bilaterally.
E: Abdomen soft, catheterised, urine output 500ml over 2 hours.

Her arterial blood gas results are show in Table 5.9.

Table 5.9. Arterial blood gas results.

pH	7.28	Na^+	136mmol/L
pO_2	15kPa	Cl^-	115mmol/L
pCO_2	6.0kPa	Lactate	1.0mmol/L
HCO_3^-	20mmol/L		

What is the most likely primary cause of the acidosis?

a   Unmeasured anions.
b   Reduced strong ion difference.
c   Respiratory acidosis.
d   Increased strong ion difference.
e   Lactic acidosis.

● **Question 14**

You are reviewing a 65-year-old polytrauma patient who fell from a ladder whilst cleaning his gutters. His past medical history includes mild COPD and hypertension. A summary of his injuries is as follows:

- Scalp laceration which has been sutured; no intracranial or neck injury.
- Fractured 4th to 12th ribs on the left with multiple flail segments, underlying contusions, left-sided intercostal drain for haemopneumothorax.
- Grade 2 splenic laceration which is being conservatively managed.
- Left-sided humoral fracture — open reduction and internal fixation (ORIF) already undertaken.

He is on day 5 of his admission and had a failed extubation yesterday due to increased oxygen requirements and pain issues despite having a working epidural. He is now reintubated and in a spontaneous breathing mode with an FiO_2 of 0.4, PS of 10cmH$_2$O and PEEP of 5cmH$_2$O, generating tidal volumes of around 7ml/kg. On these settings he has O_2 saturations of 98% and a PaO_2 of 10.4kPa.

What represents the most appropriate next step in his management?

a   Switch to a plain epidural, add in PCA and attempt extubation.
b   Increase PEEP and no sedation hold today.
c   Surgical discussion and consideration of rib fixation.
d   Tracheostomy for likely prolonged weaning.
e   Sedation hold but no reattempt at extubation.

Question 15

You are reviewing a patient who is on day 4 following an out-of-hospital cardiac arrest (OOHCA). He had an initial downtime of 40 minutes, then following return of spontaneous circulation (ROSC), underwent primary PCI and stenting of his left anterior descending and left circumflex arteries. He was then admitted to the ICU for standard post-arrest care for the next 72 hours. A CT scan of his brain performed at the time of admission to hospital showed loss of grey/white matter differentiation consistent with hypoxic brain injury. On a sedation hold on day 3, status myoclonus resistant to clonazepam was observed. The handover from the night team is that he had a period of instability overnight and then his pupils became fixed and unreactive at 6am. A repeat CT head scan was performed which showed worsening of the initial radiological changes. Given these findings, his sedation (propofol and alfentanil) was stopped to allow neurological assessment.

What is the most appropriate next step in this patient's management?

a   Undertake BSDT from midday today.
b   Continue sedation hold to allow further assessment of neurology.
c   EEG to rule out status epilepticus.
d   Continue with best supportive care and undertake BSDT the following day.
e   Perform four-vessel CT angiography.

● Question 16

You are working in a district general hospital and are asked to attend the ED to assist with the transfer of a patient for a CT scan. The patient is a 66-year-old man with a history of hypertension and AF on warfarin. He had complained of a headache and some dizziness to his husband that morning. He later became confused and sleepy so was brought to the ED where he became agitated. You were called to assist with sedation for a CT scan although on review you learn that he had become more settled again and had his imaging performed.

The CT scan shows an intracranial haemorrhage in the right cerebellum with a small amount of blood in the 4th ventricle but no hydrocephalus. The hospital you are working in has an acute stroke unit but no neurosurgical capability.

On examination:

A: Maintaining own airway.
B: 98% sats on an FiO_2 of 0.28, RR 15/min, chest clear.
C: BP 165/85mmHg, HR 85/min, AF, warm peripherally, CRT <2 seconds, point-of-care INR 2.3.
D: GCS 9 (E-2, V-2, M-5), PEARL size 3, blood glucose 4.8mmol/L.
E: Temperature 36.5°C.

What is the next treatment priority?

a   Prothrombin complex concentrate.
b   Immediate transfer to a neurosurgical centre.
c   10mg vitamin K.
d   Labetalol infusion aiming for a blood pressure of 120–140mmHg.
e   Intubation and ventilation.

● Question 17

You are reviewing a 65-year-old lady with a history of COPD who was originally admitted with a community-acquired pneumonia 13 days ago. She was intubated and ventilated on day 2 for a combination of respiratory failure and possible anaphylaxis to the co-amoxiclav she was receiving. She grew *Pseudomonas* in her sputum and had her antibiotics changed to ciprofloxacin. She had a tracheostomy inserted on day 10 following two failed extubation attempts and is currently undertaking a slow respiratory wean. She started with loose stools 3 days ago and a stool sample was *C. difficile* glutamate dehydrogenase (GDH)-positive. A second sample is pending for *C. difficile* toxins A and B. She has been on oral vancomycin for the last 3 days.

The bedside nurse restarted sedation overnight due to agitation and pain, and the patient is now also needing vasopressor therapy. The patient's abdomen appears more distended.

On examination:

A: Tracheostomy size 8.
B: Sats 94% on an FiO_2 of 0.5, RR 25/min, quiet bases.
C: BP 90/50mmHg on 0.4µg/kg/min of noradrenaline, HR 110/min, cool peripheries, CRT 4 seconds, urine output 20ml/hr.
D: Sedated on propofol 20ml/hr and alfentanil 0.3µg/kg/min. PEARL.
E: Temperature 39.2°C, abdomen very distended and tympanic, tender on palpation and the patient grimaces and localises, ongoing loose watery stools, around 6–7 per day.

Blood test results from today including an arterial blood gas are shown in Table 5.10 (result from the previous day in brackets).

Table 5.10. Blood test results.

Hb	105g/L	pH	7.30
WCC	28 x 10⁹/L (14 x 10⁹/L)	pCO_2	4.0kPa
Platelets	260 x 10⁹/L	pO_2	9.1kPa
Na⁺	140mmol/L	BE	−5mmol/L
K⁺	5.0mmol/L	HCO_3^-	18mmol/L
Creatinine	160µmol/L (110µmol/L)	Lactate	3mmol/L
Urea	14mmol/L	Enzyme immunoassay for *C. diff* toxin A+B	Positive for A and B

What is the most appropriate next management step for this patient?

a   IVIg.
b   Vancomycin enemas and oral fidaxomicin.
c   CT abdomen and surgical referral.
d   Faecal transplant.
e   Bezlotoxumab.

● Question 18

A patient is admitted to the ICU after a percutaneous coronary intervention (PCI) to the right coronary artery. They have a central line and arterial line *in situ* and cardiac output monitoring via a LiDCO system (pulse power analysis). The patient presented with complete heart block which resolved following successful revascularisation. The patient required intubation and ventilation during the PCI due to agitation.

On examination:

A: ETT.
B: Sats 98% on an FiO_2 of 0.4, ventilator settings: volume-controlled ventilation, Vt 420ml (6ml/kg) x 20 breaths/min, PEEP of 12cmH₂O, chest clear.
C: BP 90/60mmHg, HR 80/min, sinus rhythm, warm peripheries, mild peripheral oedema, CRT <2 seconds, CVP 13mmHg, CO 3.5L/min,

SBA Paper 5: Questions

Systemic Vascular Resistance Index (SVRI) 2000 dynes/sec/cm^5/m^2. Bedside ECHO shows an enlarged RV which is poorly contractile but a well contracting LV.
D: Sedated on propofol 15ml/hr and alfentanil 0.2μg/kg/min.
E: Abdomen soft, 1cm liver edge palpated, apyrexial.

What is the best next step in the management of this patient?

a   Reduce PEEP to 5cmH$_2$O.
b   500ml fluid bolus.
c   Start milrinone.
d   40mg IV frusemide.
e   Start noradrenaline.

● Question 19

You are asked to review a 57-year-old patient on the haematology oncology ward who has a fever, abdominal pain, vomiting and diarrhoea. He finished a course of induction chemotherapy with cytarabine and daunorubicin for acute myeloid leukaemia 10 days ago. A CT scan of his abdomen shows inflammatory stranding in the mesenteric fat surrounding the ileum, bowel wall thickening in the terminal ileum and caecum, and atelectasis at their lung bases.

On examination:

A: Maintaining own airway.
B: Sats 98% on an FiO$_2$ of 0.5, RR 24/min, quiet bases on auscultation, no added sounds.
C: BP 85/50mmHg, HR 110/min, warm peripherally, CRT 3 seconds, no peripheral oedema.
D: Alert and orientated, PEARL.
E: Temperature 38.8°C, right-sided abdominal tenderness on palpation with mild distension, no rashes.

Blood test results from blood taken on admission are shown in Table 5.11.

Table 5.11. Blood test results.

Hb	82g/L	Na$^+$	140mmol/L
WCC	110 x 10^9/L, 90% blast cells	K$^+$ Creatinine	5.0mmol/L 140μmol/L
Neutrophils	0.3 x 10^9/L	Urea	6.5mmol/L
Platelets	85 x 10^9/L	PO$_4^{3-}$	1.4mmol/L

What is the likely diagnosis?

a Tumour lysis syndrome.
b Typhlitis.
c Leukostasis.
d Graft vs. host disease.
e Appendicitis.

● Question 20

You are reviewing a 62-year-old man with COPD who has been admitted to the ICU for non-invasive ventilation (NIV). In the last year he has needed six courses of steroids for exacerbations (normally he only needs one or two per year) which he ascribes to the worsening damp in his house. He presented with acute shortness of breath with cough productive of blood-stained sputum which is not usual for him. He suffered from tuberculosis as a boy but tells you that he was given the 'all clear' in his 20s. A sputum sample has already been sent off to the labs for testing, and several blood tests and a high-resolution CT chest are pending.

On examination:

A: Maintaining own airway.
B: SpO$_2$ 90% on an FiO$_2$ of 0.6, NIV 18/7.5 cmH$_2$O achieving a Vt of 400ml, RR 26/min, coarse creps right mid zone and left lower zone on auscultation.
C: BP 140/75mmHg, HR 85/min, sinus rhythm, warm peripherally.
D: Alert and orientated.
E: Temperature 37.8°C.

Investigation results available so far are shown in Table 5.12.

Table 5.12. Blood test results and CT report.

Hb	140g/L	Na$^+$	138mmol/L
WCC	14 x 10^9/L	K$^+$	4.8mmol/L
Neutrophils	12 x10^9/L	Creatinine	100µmol/L
Eosinophils	0.4 x 10^9/L	Urea	8.5mmol/L
Platelets	260 x 10^9/L	Anti-neutrophil cytoplasmic antibody	Negative
CRP	140mg/L	Sputum beta-d glucan	Positive
CT thorax		Multiple small nodules in the right middle lobe and left lower lobe exhibiting a halo sign, left base nodule 2cm in diameter with cavitation, ground-glass opacity throughout the left lower and right middle lobe	

What is the most likely diagnosis?

a   Tuberculosis.
b   Invasive aspergillosis.
c   PVL *Staphylococcus*.
d   Vasculitis.
e   Allergic bronchopulmonary aspergillosis.

● Question 21

Which of the following signs or symptoms during a spontaneous breathing trial (SBT) would indicate a failed trial?

a   Increase in SBP from 140mmHg to 160mmHg.
b   PaO$_2$ 10kPa on an FiO$_2$ of 0.35 at the end of the SBT.
c   Increase in HR from 70/min to 100/min.
d   Comfortable and settled at the end of the SBT.
e   RR of 25/min at the end of the SBT.

● **Question 22**

Which of the following laws is used to measure oxygen saturation levels with a pulse oximeter?

a   Beer's law.
b   Henry's law.
c   Charles' law.
d   Dalton's law.
e   Fick's law.

● **Question 23**

Which of the following would **not** be an indication for urgent or expedited chest drain insertion?

a   Pneumothorax 2cm maximum depth in a 60-year-old patient with severe COPD.
b   Spontaneous pneumothorax 4cm maximum depth in an asymptomatic patient.
c   Pleural effusion with a pH of 7.15 on pleural aspirate testing.
d   Symptomatic bilateral pneumothorax.
e   Symptomatic hemopneumothorax.

● **Question 24**

Which of the following is used to assess the energy expenditure of a ventilated ICU patient?

a   MUST score.
b   NUTRIC score.
c   Indirect calorimetry.
d   Body Mass Index (BMI).
e   Middle upper arm circumference (MUAC).

SBA Paper 5: Questions

● **Question 25**

Which of the following is an example of quantitative continuous data?

a   Blood type.
b   Heparin-induced thrombocytopaenia score.
c   Gender.
d   Number of children a patient has.
e   Body Mass Index (BMI).

● **Question 26**

Which of the following findings on blood and urine testing would **not** be consistent with a diagnosis of rhabdomyolysis?

a   Hyperuricaemia.
b   Creatine kinase 20,000 U/L.
c   Hyperkalaemia.
d   Hypercalcaemia.
e   Urine dipstick positive for blood.

● **Question 27**

Which of the following anticoagulants acts via inhibition of factor Xa to prevent factor Xa from cleaving prothrombin to thrombin?

a   Warfarin.
b   Fondaparinux.
c   Rivaroxaban.
d   Dabigatran.
e   Unfractionated heparin.

● **Question 28**

Which of the following medications is associated with the highest risk of constipation?

a   Alfentanil.
b   Omeprazole.
c   Propofol.
d   Low-molecular-weight heparin.
e   Paracetamol.

● **Question 29**

Which of the following is correct regarding lagophthalmos (incomplete eyelid closure)?

a   Grade 0 lagophthalmos requires regular lubrication to the eye.
b   Any corneal exposure would be classed as grade 1 lagophthalmos.
c   Lubrication and taping of the eyelids are advised in grade 1 lagophthalmos.
d   In grade 0 lagophthalmos the eyelid is completely closed.
e   Any conjunctival exposure without corneal exposure would be classed as grade 2 lagophthalmos.

● **Question 30**

Which Vaughan-Williams class of antiarrhythmic drugs does amiodarone fall into?

a   Class II.
b   Class III.
c   Class Ia.
d   Class Ib.
e   Class IV.

SBA Paper 5: Questions

● Question 31
In which of the following patients is enteral nutrition via a nasogastric tube **not** indicated?

a   Day 0 patient intubated and ventilated for pneumonia, minimal vasopressor requirements.
b   Day 2 patient with pancreatitis, intubated and ventilated for agitation.
c   Day 1 patient with urosepsis, BP controlled on 0.3μg/kg/min of noradrenaline, on CPAP overnight for obstructive sleep apnoea.
d   Day 1 patient who is still intubated and ventilated after an emergency ruptured abdominal aortic aneurysm.
e   Day 0 patient who is receiving targeted temperature management after an out-of-hospital cardiac arrest.

● Question 32
Which of the following is the most significant risk factor for the development of invasive candidiasis?

a   Central venous catheter.
b   Urinary catheter.
c   Mechanical ventilation.
d   Total parenteral nutrition.
e   Prolonged antibiotic use (≥7 days).

● Question 33
You are treating a patient with suspected encephalitis. An MRI scan shows involvement of the temporal lobe. What is the most likely aetiology?

a   *Neisseria meningitides*.
b   Herpes simplex virus.
c   Anti-NMDA receptor antibody encephalitis.
d   West Nile virus.
e   *Toxoplasma gondii*.

Question 34
What is the best management option for delirium in an ICU patient with a diagnosis of acute alcoholic hepatitis and significantly abnormal liver function tests?

a   Lorazepam.
b   Quetiapine.
c   Clonidine infusion.
d   Chlordiazepoxide.
e   Haloperidol.

Question 35
In which of the following conditions is IV magnesium sulphate **not** indicated?

a   Acute severe asthma.
b   Atrial fibrillation.
c   Status epilepticus.
d   Torsade de pointes.
e   Neuroprotection of neonate in preterm labour.

Question 36
With regards to human immunodeficiency virus (HIV) and acquired immunodeficiency syndrome (AIDS), which of the following is correct?

a   HIV2 is associated with faster progression to AIDS compared to HIV1.
b   Advanced HIV disease is defined in persons living with HIV with a CD4 cell count of <200 cells/mm^3 or presenting with a WHO stage 3/4 AIDS-defining illness.
c   Once a patient has transitioned into AIDS the diagnosis is permanent.
d   HIV is a DNA virus.
e   Primary HIV infection is the commonest cause of patients with HIV being admitted to critical care.

SBA Paper 5: Questions

● **Question 37**

According to the Resuscitation Council UK Advanced Life Support (ALS) guidelines what is the first-line treatment for a patient with complete heart block associated with chest pain and hypotension?

a   Isoprenaline infusion.
b   Adrenaline infusion.
c   Transcutaneous pacing.
d   Glucagon bolus.
e   Atropine bolus.

● **Question 38**

What type of cardiomyopathy is most likely in a 55-year-old female patient with a history of alcohol excess?

a   Arrhythmogenic right ventricular cardiomyopathy.
b   Hypertrophic cardiomyopathy.
c   Dilated cardiomyopathy.
d   Restrictive cardiomyopathy.
e   Peripartum cardiomyopathy.

● **Question 39**

You are required to undertake a transfer for a ventilated patient from your district general hospital to a tertiary hospital 30 minutes away. The patient is on a portable ventilator which uses 2L/minute driving flow, and the patient is on an FiO_2 of 0.5, Vt 500ml, RR 20/min. How much oxygen should you have available for the transfer?

a   360L.
b   420L.
c   720L.
d   210L.
e   300L.

Question 40

A 50kg patient has come to critical care from the emergency theatre with a laparotomy wound soaker catheter *in situ*. The anaesthetist has not had time to load the system with local anaesthetic. You wish to perform a sedation hold and hopefully extubate the patient. Which of the following would be the maximum safe dose of local anaesthetic you could administer for this patient?

a   25ml 0.5% bupivacaine.
b   20ml 0.25% bupivacaine.
c   10ml 1% lignocaine.
d   40ml 0.25% bupivacaine.
e   10ml 0.5% bupivacaine.

Question 41

Which of the following is true with regard to acute coronary syndrome?

a   A patient presenting with NSTEMI who is unstable should have PCI within 24 hours.
b   Unstable angina is associated with a troponin rise.
c   A patient with a STEMI 30 minutes from a PCI-capable hospital should be thrombolysed.
d   All patients presenting with ACS should be loaded with aspirin and clopidogrel.
e   A patient who presents with typical ischaemic chest pain but dies prior to troponin being measured, has had a type 2 MI.

Question 42

You are called down to assist with a patient in the ED who has presented with pleuritic chest pain and shortness of breath, having recently returned from holiday in Australia. They now have a blood pressure of 70mmHg systolic. Which classification of shock is most likely?

a   Distributive.
b   Cardiogenic.
c   Hypovolaemic.
d   Neurogenic.
e   Obstructive.

● Question 43

You receive a call from an anaesthetist asking if they can have a postoperative bed for an 80-year-old patient, having an elective laparotomy for bowel and single-segment liver resection for cancer. The request is on the basis of the patient's cardiopulmonary exercise testing result. Which of the following results would trigger consideration of a critical care bed postoperatively?

a   Peak VO_2 30ml/kg/min.
b   Anaerobic threshold 10ml/kg/min.
c   Peak VO_2 65% of predicted.
d   Patient only achieved 85% of predicted work.
e   HR increased to 135/min during the CPET.

● Question 44

You are reviewing a patient on the ward who is known to have Child-Pugh C liver disease, secondary to alcohol excess. They have come in generally unwell with suspected spontaneous bacterial peritonitis and have been started on broad-spectrum antibiotics. The patient's creatinine was 60μmol/L a week ago and is now 230μmol/L and they are oliguric. Serum albumin is 24g/L. You suspect hepatorenal syndrome and acute kidney injury (HRS-AKI). Which of the following would be the first-line treatment for this condition?

a   Terlipressin.
b   Albumin.
c   Octreotide and midodrine.
d   Transjugular intrahepatic portosystemic shunt.
e   Liver transplantation.

● **Question 45**

Which of the following indications for renal replacement therapy in an acutely unwell patient would intermittent haemodialysis be indicated, in preference to haemofiltration?

a   Uraemia.
b   Acidosis.
c   Lithium toxicity.
d   Hyperkalaemia.
e   Fluid overload.

● **Question 46**

By which mechanism is MRSA resistant to methicillin?

a   Production of beta-lactamase.
b   Outer membrane acting as a barrier.
c   Plasmid-mediated gene transfer.
d   Alteration of penicillin-binding protein.
e   Spontaneous gene transfer.

● **Question 47**

You are called to a patient on the unit who has just received a dose of amoxicillin and is now profoundly wheezy, hypotensive and has a widespread urticarial rash. The nurse has given the patient his EpiPen, put on 15L of oxygen and has started a bolus of IV fluid. You get to him around 5 minutes after the first adrenaline dose. What is the most appropriate management at this point in time in a patient with ongoing hypotension and respiratory distress?

a   100mg IV hydrocortisone.
b   10mg IV chloramphenicol.
c   50µg IV adrenaline.
d   500µg IV adrenaline.
e   Start an adrenaline infusion.

Question 48

A patient you have been looking after has been accepted for donation after circulatory death (DCD), after a decision for withdrawal of life-sustaining treatment (WOLST) has been made. You know the case well and have extensively liaised with the patient's family. You undertake WOLST for this patient in the anaesthetic room of the emergency theatre. WOLST proceeds and the patient dies within 10 minutes and goes on to donate their kidneys. What Maastricht classification would this patient be?

a   Category 1.
b   Category 2.
c   Category 3.
d   Category 4.
e   Category 5.

 Question 49

You are called to assist with a patient who has come into the ED after spraying some pesticide on his garden that he found in the back of his dad's shed. He did not wear any personal protective equipment. He has presented with profuse vomiting, diarrhoea and salivation and on examination his heart rate is 30 bpm and his pupils are pinpoint. He has been stripped and washed, is on 15L NRB oxygen and IV access has just been achieved. What should be the next step in management?

a   Pralidoxime.
b   Fomepizole.
c   Hydroxocobalamin.
d   Naloxone.
e   Atropine.

Question 50

The secretion of which of the following hormones is increased in a patient with hypercalcaemia?

a   Parathyroid hormone.
b   Cortisol.
c   1,25-dihydroxycholecalciferol.
d   Calcitonin.
e   Thyroid hormone.

Answer overview: Paper 5

Question:			Question:	
1	c		26	d
2	a		27	c
3	c		28	a
4	e		29	d
5	d		30	b
6	a		31	c
7	d		32	e
8	c		33	b
9	a		34	a
10	e		35	c
11	b		36	b
12	c		37	e
13	b		38	c
14	c		39	b
15	d		40	d
16	a		41	a
17	c		42	e
18	a		43	b
19	b		44	b
20	b		45	c
21	c		46	d
22	a		47	c
23	b		48	c
24	c		49	e
25	e		50	d

5 SBA Paper 5: Answers

● Answer 1: c

Tricyclic antidepressant (TCA) poisoning can cause toxicity via several mechanisms, anticholinergic effects (antimuscarinic activity similar to atropine), cardiac sodium channel blockade and alpha-1 adrenergic receptor blockade. Anticholinergic effects can cause a sinus tachycardia, confusion, drowsiness, dilated pupils, hot dry skin and urinary retention. In cases of severe toxicity this can progress to seizures, coma and respiratory depression. Sodium channel blockade is responsible for most of the ECG changes seen, with prolongation of the PR, QRS and QT intervals, and atrioventricular block. The QRS prolongation can lead to ventricular arrhythmias. TCA poisoning can also cause a serotonin syndrome, especially if taken in combination with other serotonergic drugs (for more information on this and other hyperthermia syndromes see page 311, Paper 4, Q8). In the patient described, there is a predominance of features suggestive of significant TCA poisoning.

The management of tricyclic overdose depends on the severity of the poisoning, and treatment of additional toxins which may have been concurrently taken:

- Cardiac toxicity: analysis of the QRS complex is key; above 100ms is associated with an increased risk of arrhythmias and a 26% chance of seizures; above 160ms and there is a 50% chance of ventricular arrhythmias. According to TOXBASE, a prolonged QRS of ≥160ms, VT or cardiac arrest should be treated with 100ml 8.4% $NaHCO_3$, a QRS of 120–160ms should be treated with 50ml 8.4% $NaHCO_3$; however, other sources have recommended the use of $NaHCO_3$ for anyone with a QRS

of over 100ms. NaHCO$_3$ should be administered via a large cannula or central vein, and the potassium should be monitored as it will cause a reduction in the serum K$^+$ levels. In arrhythmias refractory to NaHCO$_3$, magnesium can be used, particularly if there is significant QTc prolongation. An alternative for refractory arrhythmias would be lignocaine. Amiodarone should be avoided as it will further prolong the QTc. Other Na$^+$ channel blocking agents, e.g. procainamide and flecainide (Vaughan Williams class IA and IC), should also be avoided as they have a similar effect to TCAs.
- Hypotension: should be managed with IV fluids; vasopressor therapy can be used if refractory to other treatment. Noradrenaline is the preferred initial agent; adrenaline should not be used as a first-line therapy, as it may cause worsening hypotension due to beta-receptor agonism only (given there is alpha-receptor blockade by the tricyclics). In refractory cases, treatments include hypertonic saline and high-dose insulin therapy, for improving severe impairment of myocardial contractility.
- Seizures: should be treated with benzodiazepines, as the mechanism of seizure activity is via GABA-A receptor inhibition; second-line management is typically with general anaesthesia. Antiepileptic agents, such as levetiracetam, can also be used. In the event of a mixed overdose with benzodiazepines, flumazenil should not be used as it can lower the seizure threshold. Agitation and delirium are also primarily managed with benzodiazepines, and reasonably high doses may be required; if refractory to this, then haloperidol or ketamine can be used.

References

1. www.toxbase.org. TOXBASE — the primary clinical toxicology database of the National Poisons Information Service. Poisons-index-A-Z/a-products/amitriptyline. Available at: https://www.toxbase.org.
2. www.uptodate.com. Tricyclic antidepressant poisoning. UpToDate, 2024. Available at: https://www.uptodate.com/contents/tricyclic-antidepressant-poisoning.

Answer 2: a

Temporary pacing wires can either be transvenous, transoesophageal or epicardial. Transvenous pacing is typically used when a patient needs urgently pacing as a temporary measure, prior to insertion of a temporary permanent or permanent pacemaker.

Following cardiac surgery, a patient may have epicardial pacing wires inserted if they are at high risk of being pacing-dependent, or likely to have a period of conduction abnormalities. Risk factors for this include valvular surgery, advancing age, poor left ventricular (LV) function, structural heart disease, diabetes, preoperative beta-blocker or digoxin use and a history of arrhythmias. Leads can be unipolar, with an electrode in the heart and one at the skin, or bipolar with two electrodes a small distance apart in the heart (smaller electrical potential required). The leads are typically placed on the right atrium (and brought out of the skin to the right of the sternum), and on the diaphragmatic side of the right ventricle (with the wires brought out to the left of the sternum).

The modes available depend on which wires are *in situ* and utilise a three-letter code — chamber paced, chamber sensed and response to sensing.

There are three main settings on the pacemaker box:

- The rate (heart rate you wish the patient to have).
- The sensitivity.
- The output.

The setting dials lie adjacent to the port into which the wires are plugged. There are two lights per port: one for sensing, one for output.

Pacemaker check:

- Turn down the rate until an intrinsic rhythm appears (which may not occur if patients are pacing-dependent), monitor the blood pressure closely and do not reduce the rate further if there is cardiovascular instability.
- Check the sensitivity (each lead needs to be done separately). Sensitivity is the minimum current that the pacemaker can detect, with a lower number indicating greater sensitivity. The sensitivity at which the pacemaker starts to register is called the sensitivity threshold; the number is usually set at half the threshold to ensure detection of smaller signals and to ensure the pacemaker will continue to sense even if less current can get to the electrode (e.g. due to lead fibrosis or maturation). A sensitivity number that is too low means that the

electrode may interpret electrical signals distant to the electrode such as R/T waves in the case of an atrial lead, and subsequently inappropriately inhibit a pacing output. A sensitivity number which is too high may mean that the lead does not sense correctly and hence may pace inappropriately, for example, a ventricular lead not sensing an R wave and consequently delivering a pacing output potentially resulting in an R on T phenomenon.
- Check the output (if the patient has an intrinsic rhythm). The output is the current (in mA) that is delivered during a pacing output. This number is checked by setting the pacemaker rate above the intrinsic rate and slowly turning down the output until there is a pacemaker spike without an associated QRS complex. The output is then slowly turned up again until there is mechanical capture with each pacing spike and this figure is called the capture threshold. The output is then set at 2–3 times this value to minimise the risk of a pacing output not being associated with mechanical capture.

There are a few problems that can be encountered with temporary epicardial pacing wires:

- Failure to pace: the pacemaker is set to deliver output, but no spikes are seen. This could be because the wires have migrated away from the myocardium or are not properly inserted into the pacemaker box. It could also be due to a problem with the pacemaker, or it could be that the sensitivity threshold is set too low — such that it is inappropriately inhibiting an output because it is interpreting a distant signal.
- Failure to capture (the issue we are seeing in the scenario): the pacemaker is producing an output that creates a pacing spike on the ECG, but without associated mechanical capture (contraction of the atria or ventricles), meaning that the output is not high enough. A common cause of this is wire maturation — there is an inflammatory response to the wires, which causes fibrosis around them, and after 3–4 days this can result in failure to capture. This can be overcome by increasing the output, but this can produce more inflammatory reaction and fibrosis so continual increase in the output is not a viable solution (if the patient is pacing-dependent at this point they will likely need a permanent system inserted). This can also occur with an ischaemic myocardium or electrolyte abnormalities — particularly hyperkalaemia.

- Pacemaker-induced tachycardia (uncommon): this only occurs in VDD or DDD pacing and is when the sensing is set too low. The pacemaker interprets a ventricular pacing spike as an endogenous p wave leading to another pacing spike creating a continuous cycle which is only stopped if the atrial lead is removed, or the pacemaker is switched to an asynchronous mode.

References

1. Waqanivavalagi SWFR. Temporary pacing following cardiac surgery — a reference guide for surgical teams. *J Cardiothorac Surg* 2024; 19(1): 115.
2. Reade MC. Temporary epicardial pacing after cardiac surgery: a practical review. Part 1: general considerations in the management of epicardial pacing. *Anaesthesia* 2007; 62(3): 264–71.
3. Reade MC. Temporary epicardial pacing after cardiac surgery: a practical review. Part 2: selection of epicardial pacing modes and troubleshooting. *Anaesthesia* 2007; 62(4): 364–73.
4. Safavi-Naeini P, Saeed M. Pacemaker troubleshooting: common clinical scenarios. *Tex Heart Inst J* 2016; 43(5): 415–8.

Answer 3: c

The hyperosmolar hyperglycaemic state (HHS) occurs less frequently than diabetic ketoacidosis (DKA) but is associated with a high mortality rate. It is characterised by a combination of severe hyperglycaemia (>30mmol/L), hyperosmolality and significant free water loss/dehydration in the absence of significant ketosis (serum ketones ≤3mmol/L) or acidosis (pH >7.3). Fluid losses can be between 100–220ml/kg (up to 22L for 100kg patients) and K^+ losses 4–6mmol/kg. It can occur in patients with type 1 or type 2 diabetes, but more commonly in older adults with type 2 diabetes. In HHS, there is a small amount of insulin secretion that minimises ketone production but does not prevent hyperglycaemia. A mixed picture of both DKA and HHS can be seen — and this is present in around a third of hyperglycaemia presentations. The morbidity and mortality in HHS are due to an association with vascular events such as myocardial infarction (MI), stroke or arterial thrombus, and also the neurological complications such as cerebral oedema and central pontine myelinolysis (CPM) due to rapid changes in osmolality.

HHS typically develops over days resulting in severe dehydration and metabolic disturbances. The main precipitants are chest and urinary infections (in 30–60% of patients); other causes include acute cerebrovascular events, MI, surgery, pancreatitis and medications.

Indications for discussion with critical care and consideration of admission include: osmolality >350mOsmol/kg, Na⁺ >160mmol/L, pH <7.1, K⁺ <3.5mmol/L or >6mmol/L on admission, GCS <12, oxygen saturations <92% on air, SBP <90mmHg, heart rate <60/min or >100/min, urine output <0.5ml/kg/hr, AKI, hypothermia, or a macrovascular event.

The goals of treatment in HHS are to replace fluid and electrolyte losses, normalise the osmolality (at around 3–8mOsmol/kg an hour) and normalise the blood glucose. This can be done initially with fluid correction only, and insulin should only be started once the patient has received enough fluid to correct their dehydration (typically a positive balance of at least 2–3L). Refer to your hospital's local guideline for detailed management.

Management in the first hour: treat the underlying cause. Fluids: 0.9% saline 1000ml/hr, with fluid boluses as needed if BP is <90mmHg. Insulin should only be commenced within the first hour if the patient has ketonaemia; either that falls into the category of: DKA (ketones >3mmol/L and pH <7.3; mixed DKA and HHS, dose of 0.1units/kg/hr of insulin; or ketonaemia without acidosis (ketones of 1–3mmol/L and pH >7.3), dose of 0.5units/kg/hr of insulin.

Investigations should be conducted on arrival and hourly for the first 6 hours: serum osmolality (measured directly or estimated using the formula [(2 x Na⁺) + glucose + urea]), venous plasma blood glucose, venous blood gas, urea and electrolytes, capillary blood ketones. In addition, on arrival, the patient should have other investigations to try and establish an underlying precipitant (e.g. blood cultures, ECG, CXR, etc.).

Management from 60 minutes to 6 hours: treat the underlying cause. Ongoing fluid therapy to achieve a decrease in osmolality of 3–8mOsmol/kg/hr and glucose of 5mmol/L/hr. Aim for a fluid balance of around 3L positive by 6 hours. Aim for a serum potassium of 3.5–5mmol/L and a glucose of 10–15mmol after initial correction. Insulin should only be started once fluid replacement is adequate and the glucose concentrations have plateaued (with the exception of the criteria stated above). Insulin should be given at a dose of 0.5mmol/kg/hr as an infusion.

SBA Paper 5: Answers

Management past 6 hours: ongoing fluid replacement as needed, aiming for a positive fluid balance of 3–6L by 12 hours, estimate the likely total fluid losses and aim to replace these by 24 hours.

The complete resolution of biochemistry may not be seen for several days, during which time appropriate thromboprophylaxis should be prescribed due to the high risk of thromboembolic events.

The patient in the question has an initial estimated osmolality of 375mOsmol/kg, and on repeat an hour later has an estimated osmolality of 372mOsmol/kg; this represents an acceptable rate of reduction, with a drop in glucose of 5mmol/L. There are not enough data points yet to say if the glucose level has plateaued; the K^+ level is in the range that needs replacement. The correct option is to continue the current rate of fluid with potassium added in. Hyperglycaemia causes a measuring error with sodium, such that the serum level measured is lower than the true serum level (dilutional or translocational hyperosmolar hyponatraemia). The true serum Na^+ can be calculated using the following formula:

Corrected sodium Na^+ = measured sodium $[Na^+]$ + [Glucose – 5.6] x 0.288 (all in mmol/L).

References
1. Joint British Diabetes Societies for Inpatient Care. The management of hyperosmolar hyperglycaemic state (HHS) in adults, 2022. Available at: https://abcd.care/sites/default/files/site_uploads/JBDS_Guidelines_Current/JBDS_06_The_Management_of_Hyperosmolar_Hyperglycaemic_State_HHS_%20in_Adults_FINAL_0.pdf.
2. Umpierrez GE, Davis GM, ElSayed NA, et al. Hyperglycaemic crises in adults with diabetes: a consensus report. *Diabetologia* 2024; 67(8): 1455–79.
3. MDCalc. Sodium correction for hyperglycemia. Available at: https://www.mdcalc.com/calc/50/sodium-correction-hyperglycemia#evidence.

● Answer 4: e
Subarachnoid haemorrhages (SAHs) are most frequently caused by rupture of a saccular aneurysm, which are acquired rather than congenital. Around 20% of subarachnoid haemorrhages are non-aneurysmal and include causes such as trauma, vascular malformations and intracranial arterial dissection. Most aneurysms do not rupture; the biggest risk factors for an aneurysmal rupture are hypertension, cigarette smoking and family history. Most SAHs occur

without an identifiable trigger, but in some an acute elevation in blood pressure secondary to caffeine, physical exertion or sudden sympathetic stimulation (being startled or angered) may be associated.

Radiological and clinical grading systems for SAH are discussed on page 74, Paper 1, Q40.

Treatment of an aneurysmal SAH is either by endovascular coiling undertaken in an interventional radiology suite, or by open surgical clipping of the aneurysm. Management of the aneurysm is ideally done as soon as possible after the initial bleed, and ideally within 24 hours to limit the risk of rebleeding. Aside from aneurysm management, care of SAH patients focuses on the prevention of complications (notably with the use of nimodipine for the prevention of vasospasm).

There are several complications that can occur after SAH:

- Rebleeding (of aneurysm) — 4–14% risk in the first 23 hours, maximal risk at 2–12 hours. There is a higher risk for rebleeding with larger aneurysm size, higher grade of SAH, longer time to treating aneurysm, high blood pressure and incomplete treatment of aneurysm.
- Vasospasm and delayed cerebral ischaemia (DCI) — typically occurs at between days 4–14, and in around 30% of patients. Not all DCI is caused by vasospasm, but it is the most common cause. More information can be found on page 173, Paper 2, Q44.
- Elevated intracranial pressure (ICP) and hydrocephalus — raised ICP can occur in around half of SAH patients, and a common cause is hydrocephalus. Hydrocephalus affects up to 30% of patients with SAH, secondary to obstruction of CSF flow by blood in the ventricles and usually presents within hours of the initial bleed. It presents with a progressive deterioration in GCS and in some, ocular signs are seen such as constricted pupils, downward eye deviation or restricted up gaze. Management is primarily with CSF diversion, via an external ventricular drain or lumbar drain.
- Hyponatraemia — this develops in up to 30% of patients with SAH. It is mediated by hypothalamic injury and has two distinct mechanisms:
  - syndrome of inappropriate antidiuretic hormone secretion (SIADH) (most common form, euvolaemia, treatment often with hypertonic saline, takes days to weeks to develop);

- cerebral salt wasting (high urine output with high urinary sodium leading to a hyponatraemic, hypovolaemic patient, treated with isotonic fluid administration and fludrocortisone if struggling to maintain euvolaemia).
- Seizures — new seizures occur in 8–15% of patients with SAH; if they occur prior to aneurysm treatment they can be a sign of rebleeding. Most seizures are tonic-clonic. Non-convulsive status epilepticus can be seen post-SAH but is unusual and is typically a cause of failure for neurology improvement.
- Cardiopulmonary complications — these complications can manifest including pulmonary oedema which occurs in around 23% of patients and cardiac arrhythmias in around 35%.

References

1. Marcolini E, Hine J. Approach to the diagnosis and management of subarachnoid hemorrhage. *West J Emerg Med* 2019; 20(2): 203–11.
2. www.uptodate.com. Aneurysmal subarachnoid hemorrhage: epidemiology, pathogenesis, and risk factors. UpToDate, 2025. Available at: https://www.uptodate.com/contents/aneurysmal-subarachnoid-hemorrhage-epidemiology-pathogenesis-and-risk-factors.
3. www.uptodate.com. Aneurysmal subarachnoid hemorrhage: treatment and prognosis. UpToDate, 2025. Available at: https://www.uptodate.com/contents/aneurysmal-subarachnoid-hemorrhage-treatment-and-prognosis.

Answer 5: d

Globally, venous thromboembolism (VTE) is the third most frequent cardiovascular syndrome, behind MI and stroke. The biggest risk factors for the development of VTE include lower limb fracture, hip or knee replacement surgery, major trauma, MI or hospitalisation for heart failure (in the previous 3 months), previous VTE and spinal cord injury.

In 2019, the European Society of Cardiology in collaboration with the European Respiratory Society released new guidelines for the diagnosis and management of PE. This guideline clarified the definitions of pulmonary embolus (PE) severity as follows:

- High risk is PE with one of the following three markers of haemodynamic instability: cardiac arrest, obstructive shock (SBP

<90mmHg or vasopressors to achieve SBP >90mmHg with adequate filling plus evidence of end-organ hypoperfusion) or persistent hypotension (SBP <90mmHg, or SBP drop ≥40mmHg lasting over 15 minutes not caused by an alternate pathology, e.g. sepsis, arrhythmia).
- Intermediate risk PE is subdivided into two categories — high and low:
  - intermediate high risk: elevated troponin plus evidence of right ventricular (RV) dysfunction, elevated N-terminal portion of brain natriuretic peptide (NT-proBNP), CTPA signs including elevated RV/LV end-diastolic ratio and intraventricular septal bowing, ECHO signs including hypokinesis of the RV free wall and a straight intraventricular septum;
  - intermediate low risk: raised troponin or signs of RV dysfunction (not both and may have neither). PE Severity Index (PESI) scoring of over class II.
- Low risk: absence of RV dysfunction and a PESI score of class II or below.

The American Heart Association uses a different classification system:

- Massive PE: BP <90mmHg systolic (or 40mmHg below normal) for >15 minutes or cardiac arrest.
- Submassive PE: RV dysfunction (CT/ECHO), thrombus in RV, raised troponin, BNP >90ng/L, ECG changes.

PEs that don't meet either of the above criteria are non-massive or low-risk PE.

Treatment:

- High-risk PE: thrombolysis is indicated and significantly reduces mortality, compared to anticoagulation alone. Heparin should be given immediately on suspicion of a diagnosis of PE prior to thrombolysis. NICE recommends unfractionated heparin in this scenario. If the patient is in a centre that can provide surgical embolectomy or catheter-guided treatment, these are also indicated for high-risk PE, and for consideration in patients who are unstable despite thrombolytic therapy. Catheter-guided thrombolysis is associated with a lower bleeding risk compared to standard thrombolysis. If a patient

has an absolute contraindication to anticoagulation, then an IVC filter would be indicated (or if the patient has recurrent PE despite adequate anticoagulation).
- Intermediate high-risk PE: the evidence for thrombolysis in this group is still not clear. It does reduce morbidity from the PE but significantly increases bleeding risk, including intracerebral bleeds. These patients should be started on treatment dose low-molecular-weight heparin (LMWH) and can be considered for further treatment if they become more unstable. There is some evidence for half-dose thrombolysis in this group, and the PEITHO-3 study hopes to answer this question (results are expected at the end of 2025).
- Intermediate low-risk PE: anticoagulation alone (either LMWH or a novel oral anticoagulant non-vitamin K antagonist oral anticoagulant [NOAC]).

Treat for 4–6 weeks if the cause is temporary, 3 months for first idiopathic PE and 6 months for others.

References
1. Leidi A, Bex S, Righini M, et al. Risk stratification in patients with acute pulmonary embolism: current evidence and perspectives. *J Clin Med* 2022; 11(9): 2533.
2. Konstantinides SV, Meyer G, Becattini C, et al. 2019 ESC guidelines for the diagnosis and management of acute pulmonary embolism developed in collaboration with the European Respiratory Society (ERS). *Eur Heart J* 2020; 41(4): 543–603.
3. Schulman S, Konstantinides S, Hu Y, Tang LV. Venous thromboembolic diseases: diagnosis, management and thrombophilia testing: observations on NICE guideline [NG158]. *Thromb Haemost* 2020; 120(08): 1143–6.

Answer 6: a

Cardiac tamponade after cardiac surgery is uncommon, but when it does occur requires prompt identification and management to prevent cardiorespiratory arrest. If it occurs within the first 7 days postoperatively it is considered an acute postoperative cardiac tamponade, and if after 7 days then it is a late postoperative cardiac tamponade and carries a higher mortality rate.

Cardiac tamponade after cardiac surgery can have one of two mechanisms. If there is a gradual increase in pericardial fluid, the pericardial sac can stretch to accommodate. The increased pressure is equally distributed around the heart and so the lower pressure right heart is affected first; this is the same physiology as for a medical tamponade and is less likely to be the cause in an acute postoperative cardiac tamponade. More commonly, tamponade arises from a blood clot within the pericardial space that may only compress one part of the heart, or a rapid bleed into the pericardial space. A small volume of blood (around 150–200ml) would be enough to impact cardiac filling as the pericardium would not have enough time to expand and adapt. Therefore, the classical signs of a tamponade such as pulsus paradoxus may not be present, and it may be more challenging to pick up on transthoracic cardiac ECHO. Transoesophageal ECHO is better at picking up tamponade, and there needs to be the presence of a collection of fluid/clot with features of cardiovascular consequences such as compression of one or more cardiac chambers.

Findings in a postoperative patient that would be concerning for the presence of cardiac tamponade include: falling blood pressure or rising vasopressor requirement, rising lactate, signs of poor peripheral perfusion (low urine output, deteriorating GCS), rising CVP, reduced or no output from pericardial drains (though ongoing bleeding from drains does not rule it out), pulsus paradoxus in spontaneously ventilated patients, reverse pulsus paradoxus in ventilated patients (increase in BP during inspiration and decrease on expiration).

The management of a patient is dependent upon how stable or unstable the patient is. Sometimes slight manipulation of the drains by the surgeons will allow the blood to drain and remedy the problem. If the patient is rapidly deteriorating or unstable, peri-arrest or has suffered a cardiac arrest, then they will need an urgent resternotomy to open up the pericardial sac and relieve the tamponade. This can be undertaken either on the ICU or in theatre, depending on the stability of the patient. Pericardiocentesis has no place in the management of postoperative tamponade as the collections are small and may be localised and consist of clotted blood.

References

1. Carmona P, Mateo E, Casanovas I, *et al.* Management of cardiac tamponade after cardiac surgery. *J Cardiothorac Vasc Anesth* 2012; 26(2): 302–11.
2. Rosser J, Schwarz L, Gomersall C. Cardiac intensive care: beyond BASIC. Early complications. Department of Anaesthesia and Intensive Care, The Chinese University of Hong Kong; 2018: pp. 79–98.

Answer 7: d

Atrial fibrillation (AF) is the most common arrhythmia in patients in intensive care, and approximately 14% of patients will have it at some point during their critical illness. As well as having the potential to cause haemodynamic instability and cause thromboembolic events, critically ill patients experiencing new-onset AF will have longer ICU lengths of stay, increased lengths of mechanical ventilation and increased in-hospital mortality.

The management of AF in critical care is not clear-cut, and the large number of guidelines on the management of AF in the community and in stable patients are not necessarily applicable to the critically unwell patient cohort. Anticoagulation may fail to prevent strokes, and electrical and chemical cardioversion is often unsuccessful during critical illness. There is an absence of high-quality studies looking at the treatment for AF in critical care, but there was a systematic narrative review of the current evidence undertaken in 2020.

AF is often precipitated by the underlying illness and treatment of that will help to manage the rate and may result in cardioversion; for example, fluid resuscitation and correction of electrolyte imbalances particularly potassium and magnesium. In some cases, AF will be a primary arrhythmia (particularly after cardiac surgery), when rate or rhythm control of the AF should be the initial therapeutic goal.

AF management is divided into rate or rhythm control (cardioversion). Multiple studies have not demonstrated a preferential approach, aside from patients with LV dysfunction in whom rhythm control has a reduced mortality when compared to rate control.

Treatment options include:

- Amiodarone: primarily used for rhythm control, with reported success rates varying from 30% up to 95%. It may be especially effective as a second-line therapy after magnesium, beta-blockers or calcium channel blockers. Amiodarone can cause hypotension and QT prolongation. Longer-term use can cause pneumonitis, peripheral neuropathy and photosensitivity.
- Beta-blockers: typically utilised as rate control drugs; however, one study found 85% of patients on a non-cardiac surgical ICU will achieve rhythm control with an esmolol infusion. This could be because control of rate allows for spontaneous cardioversion. Beta-blockers can cause hypotension, particularly in underfilled patients with vasopressor requirements, in whom the AF is not the primary cause of the haemodynamic instability. In these patients a short-acting beta-blocker is preferred.
- Calcium channel blockers (CCBs): non-dihydropyridine CCBs (verapamil and diltiazem) are used for rate control but they can result in rhythm control in up to 62% of patients. They can result in hypotension so are typically used for stable acute AF.
- Magnesium: there are limited studies looking at magnesium. One RCT reported better rhythm control than amiodarone with 78% of patients achieving sinus rhythm when treated with a magnesium infusion aiming for a serum concentration of 1.5–2mmol/L. Other trials have found good success rates with the use of magnesium, and it has minimal side effects (potential to cause transient hypotension with a rapid bolus).
- Electrical cardioversion: there are limited studies for direct current cardioversion (DCCV) in critically ill patients. Some studies have reported 35% of patients being in sinus rhythm at 1 hour, and a smaller percentage still in sinus at 24 hours (despite amiodarone given prior to DCCV in 70% of patients).
- Digoxin: success for rhythm control in one study was found to be around 55%. Digoxin can be used for both rate or rhythm control and as it is a positive inotrope, is often used in unstable patients and in those with an impaired LV.

SBA Paper 5: Answers

In the patient in this question, he is still underfilled and haemodynamically unstable, and hence first-line treatment would be with fluid resuscitation, with correction of electrolytes. Dependent on the response, second-line treatments may then be required.

References
1. O'Bryan LJ, Redfern OC, Bedford J, et al. Managing new-onset atrial fibrillation in critically ill patients: a systematic narrative review. *BMJ Open* 2020; 10(3): e034774.
2. Holt A. Cardiac arrhythmias (combine with drugs). In: Bersten AD, Handy JM, Eds. *Oh's intensive care manual*, 8th ed. London: Elsevier; 2018: chapter 22: pp. 213–77.
3. Smith S, Scarth E, Sasada M. *Drugs in anaesthesia and intensive care*, 4th ed. Oxford: Oxford University Press; 2011.

● Answer 8: c

Fat embolism is the presence of fat globules within the blood and is common after trauma, but in most patients their presence has no physiological effects. A small proportion of people develop fat embolus syndrome (FES), characterised by respiratory compromise (in 96%), neurological dysfunction (in 59%) and a petechial rash (in 33%). The exact pathogenesis is not known, but it is thought that it is due to a combination of fat globules causing mechanical obstruction (particularly in the lungs) and an inflammatory response to the presence of fat globules having the potential to cause multi-organ failure. Inflammation also causes a prothrombotic state which activates the clotting cascade and increases the size of the fat emboli, causing more obstruction. Thrombocytopaenia and DIC can also be seen in FES.

Risk factors for FES are major traumatic injury with long bone fractures (particularly femoral shaft fracture), but it can also occur with severe soft tissue trauma, or with non-traumatic causes such as pancreatitis, sickle cell and osteomyelitis.

Diagnosis can be made using the Gurd criteria, with the presence of one major and four minor being consistent with a diagnosis of FES:

- Major criteria: petechiae in axillae or conjunctiva, hypoxia with bilateral changes on radiological imaging, cerebral signs unrelated to head injury.

- Minor criteria: tachycardia, pyrexia, retinal emboli on fundoscopy, fat in the urine, sudden decrease in haematocrit or platelets, increased erythrocyte sedimentation rate (ESR) and fat globules in the sputum.

Clinical presentation: from around 24 hours after injury, respiratory symptoms start to develop as the fat globules initially reach the lungs. This causes a tachypnoea secondary to irritation of the lung tissue followed by hypoxaemia and the development of an ARDS-type picture, with 44% of patients requiring mechanical ventilation. CT of the chest will classically show patchy ground-glass opacification, with a crazy paving pattern of smooth interlobar septal thickening. The neurological symptoms develop after the onset of respiratory symptoms as the fat emboli migrate to the brain, either through a patent foramen ovale (PFO) or as micro-emboli which pass through the pulmonary circulation into the left side of the heart.

Neurological symptoms include acute confusion, altered GCS, seizures and focal deficits, and can progress to cerebral oedema. MRI of the brain is the preferred imaging modality. A starfield pattern of fat micro-emboli, with multiple lesions throughout the grey and white matter may be seen. More severe symptoms appear correlated to the number of lesions.

A third of patients develop a petechial rash typically in non-dependent areas (face, neck, axillae); this is thought to be due to the low density of fat causing it to accumulate in non-dependent areas.

Other presentations can include a fever, cardiovascular effects (tachycardia, hypotension, myocardial ischaemia, RV failure, arrhythmias, pulmonary hypertension), retinopathy, renal and liver injury and haematological effects (anaemia, low platelets, coagulopathy).

Management of established FES is mainly supportive. Aspirin may be helpful and is used in the treatment of cerebral emboli causing neurological deficits. Early fixation of long bone fractures may reduce the risk of developing FES, but there is a lack of definitive data to support this.

References
1. Luff D, Hewson DW. Fat embolism syndrome. *BJA Educ* 2021; 21(9): 322–8.

SBA Paper 5: Answers

● Answer 9: a

Thrombotic microangiopathy (TMA) describes several conditions that present with thrombocytopaenia, microangiopathic haemolytic anaemia (MAHA) and end-organ damage (typically renal). The pathophysiology is that small vessels are occluded by platelet-rich thrombi which leads to the thrombocytopaenia, and the narrowing in the vessels causes mechanical haemolysis or MAHA. This pathological process, in addition to low platelets and anaemia, leads to a raised LDH, low haptoglobin and schistocytes and fragments are seen on a peripheral blood film (from the haemolysis). A negative Coombs test and normal clotting screen are usual.

The three main thrombotic microangiopathies are thrombotic thrombocytopenic purpura (TTP), Shiga toxin-mediated haemolytic uraemic syndrome (HUS) (also known as typical HUS) and atypical HUS (all other causes but mainly complement-mediated).

TTP is covered on page 50, Paper 1, Q17.

Shiga toxin-producing *Escherichia coli* (STEC-HUS) is the most common form of TMA. It more commonly occurs in children under the age of 5 and follows a clinical infection with *E. coli* (typically *E. coli* 0157:H7), causing bloody diarrhoea, vomiting and abdominal pain. In most patients the infection is self-limiting, but a small percentage will go on to develop HUS after around 7–10 days. The Shiga toxin produced by the *E. coli* (and *Shigella*), causes increased release of the ultra-large multimer of von Willebrand factor (UL-vWF) which is normally cleaved into smaller units by ADAMTS13. The ADAMTS13 cannot keep up with the UL-vWF being produced (despite normal levels and function of ADAMTS13), and increased platelet activation occurs. Other infections such as *S. pneumoniae* and HIV can trigger HUS by slightly different mechanisms. Treatment is mainly supportive with renal support as needed.

Atypical HUS is a TMA that occurs as a result of excessive alternative complement pathway activation. It can be congenital or acquired, triggered by infections such as Covid-19 and pregnancy. As well as supportive therapy, treatment is with eculizumab which prevents the cleavage of C5 into C5a and C5b.

Other rare causes of TMA include: drug-induced TMA (e.g. quinine, various chemotherapy agents), TMA post-solid organ and bone marrow transplant, malignancy, hypertension, autoimmune diseases (systemic lupus erythematosus, catastrophic antiphospholipid syndrome), glomerular disease.

References

1. Thompson GL, Kavanagh DJ. Diagnosis and treatment of thrombotic microangiopathy. *Int J Lab Hematol* 2022; 44(S1): 101–13.
2. Sarig G. ADAMTS-13 in the diagnosis and management of thrombotic microangiopathies. *Rambam Maimonides Med J* 2014; 5(4): p.e0026.
3. bestpractice.bmj.com. Haemolytic uraemic syndrome — symptoms, diagnosis and treatment. BMJ Best Practice, 2022 Available at: https://bestpractice.bmj.com/topics/en-gb/470.

● Answer 10: e

Necrotising fasciitis (NF) is a life-threatening surgical emergency. It is infection of the deep soft tissues that results in destruction of the muscle fascia and underlying fat. It can be classified according to the causative organism (type I–IV), anatomical location (Fournier's, Meleney's, etc.) or clinical presentation (fulminant, acute or insidious):

- Type I NF: polymicrobial infection with aerobic and anaerobic bacteria. Common organisms include *Clostridium* or *Bacteroides* in combination with *Enterobacteriaceae*.
- Type II NF: monomicrobial Gram-positive infection, typically due to Group A *Streptococcus* but also can be other streptococci or *Staphylococcus aureus*.
- Type III NF: monomicrobial Gram-negative infection. Common organisms are *Vibrio* species from salt water which tend to have a fulminant course with multi-organ failure within 24 hours if not treated or *Clostridium* species which are associated with gas formation in the tissues.
- Type IV NF: fungal infection, mainly *Candida* species and zygomycetes, in immunocompromised patients particularly after trauma.

SBA Paper 5: Answers

The presentation of NF is with erythematous skin in the affected area, with swelling often extending beyond the erythema, and pain which may appear out of proportion to skin changes in both severity and distribution. Initially the skin may appear relatively normal but in the latter stages becomes discoloured, with haemorrhagic bullae and necrosis evident. Systemic features include tachycardia, fever, hypotension and tachypnoea.

Laboratory-based scoring systems may be used to confirm the diagnosis of NF but should not be used to exclude it (due to variable sensitivity of between 43% and 80%). The Laboratory Risk Index for NF (LRINEC) uses six variables — CRP, WCC, Hb, Na^+, creatinine and glucose — to create a score of 0–13, with a score of 8 or over having a 75% probability for the presence of NF (the patient in question had a score of 10). Another diagnostic test is the 'finger sweep test', where a 2cm incision is made down to deep fascia (under local anaesthetic as a minimum). If there is minimal resistance to finger dissection in addition to a lack of bleeding, presence of necrotic tissue and greyish, murky 'dishwater' fluid from the wound, then NF is highly likely (sensitivity of 86%).

Urgent surgical debridement is the cornerstone of management of NF. It should be performed as early as possible and repeated as needed until there is no remaining necrotic tissue. Antibiotics play a vital role in the management of NF, but only as an adjunct to surgical debridement. Broad-spectrum antibiotics should be given as soon as possible, although ischaemia and hypoxia compromise antibiotic delivery to the infected area, so debridement of affected tissue must be prioritised to prevent further spread. Broad-spectrum antibiotics should initially be used until the causative organism(s) and their sensitivities are known. Tazocin® (piperacillin/tazobactam to cover anaerobes/Gram-negative organisms) in combination with clindamycin (to reduce toxin production) and vancomycin (to cover methicillin-resistant *Staphylococcus aureus* [MRSA]) are often chosen as empirical therapy but may vary due to local antibiotic resistance patterns and policies.

IVIg is no longer recommended for use in NF (for more information about IVIg please see page 81, Paper 1, Q47). Hyperbaric oxygen therapy (HBOT) is used in some centres for the management of NF (following surgical debridement) with the theory that an oxygen-rich environment may be toxic to obligate anaerobes (type I and some type III NF) and thus aids tissue healing. There is limited evidence for the use of HBOT for this indication, but it may reduce mortality from the initial event and the risk of requiring a major amputation. For most patients it would require transfer to a specialist centre, so it is often not a realistic early management.

References

1. bestpractice.bmj.com. Necrotising fasciitis — symptoms, diagnosis and treatment. BMJ Best Practice, 2024. Available at: https://bestpractice.bmj.com/topics/en-gb/3000241.
2. Misiakos EP, Bagias G, Patapis P, et al. Current concepts in the management of necrotizing fasciitis. *Front Surg* 2014; 1: 36.
3. Hoesl V, Kempa S, Prantl L, et al. The LRINEC score — an indicator for the course and prognosis of necrotizing fasciitis? *J Clin Med* 2022; 11(13): 3583.
4. Kazi FN, Sharma JV, Ghosh S, et al. Comparison of LRINEC scoring system with finger test and hstopathological examination for necrotizing fasciitis. *Surg J (N Y)* 2022; 8(1): e1–7.
5. Hedetoft M, Bennett MH, Hyldegaard O. Adjunctive hyperbaric oxygen treatment for necrotising soft-tissue infections: a systematic review and meta-analysis. *Diving Hyperbc Med* 2021; 51(1): 34–43.

● Answer 11: b

Acute pancreatitis is a mild disease in the majority, but 20–30% of patients will develop severe disease which has an in-hospital mortality of 15%. The diagnosis of pancreatitis requires two out of the three following elements: abdominal pain typical of pancreatitis (epigastric pain with or without radiation to the back), biochemical evidence of pancreatitis (serum lipase or amylase >3x upper limit of the normal range) and characteristic findings for pancreatitis on imaging of the abdomen.

The revised Atlanta classification of pancreatitis has three grades of severity:

- Mild acute pancreatitis: no organ failure and no local or systemic complications.
- Moderately severe acute pancreatitis: organ failure which resolves within 48 hours and/or local or systemic complications (without persistent organ failure).

- Severe acute pancreatitis: either single- or multi-organ failure that persists beyond 48 hours.

As well as being classified by severity, acute pancreatitis may be subdivided into two types based on pathophysiology: interstitial oedematous pancreatitis (the majority of cases) and necrotising pancreatitis (5–10% of cases). Several scoring systems to assess severity and mortality outcomes from pancreatitis are in common use:

- The Glasgow-Imrie score uses eight criteria with a point given to each present to indicate the presence of severe acute pancreatitis. It is scored at 48 hours after admission and a score of ≥3 is high risk for severe pancreatitis. Criteria used are: PaO_2 <7.9kPa, age >55, WBC >15 x 10^9/L, calcium <2mmol/L, urea >16mmol/L, LDH >600 IU/L, albumin <32g/L and glucose >10mmol/L.
- The Ranson criteria has two components. The first is used on admission to predict the likelihood of severe pancreatitis, where a score ≥3 of the following factors make severe pancreatitis likely: WBC >16 x 10^9/L, age >55, glucose >11.1mmol/L, AST >250 U/L and LDH >350 IU/L. The second part is assessed at 48 hours into admission and in combination with the first part provides a predicted mortality rate. Factors scored at 48 hours are: haematocrit drop >10% from admission, blood urea nitrogen (BUN) >1.79mmol/L increase from admission, Ca^{2+} <2mmol/L, arterial PaO_2 <7.7kPa, base deficit >4, fluid balance >6L.
- The Bedside Index of Severity in Acute Pancreatitis (BISAP) can be used during the first 24 hours to identify patients at a higher mortality risk with a score ≤2 equating to a mortality of 1.9% and scores of 3 or above with increasing mortality with each point scored. The criteria used are: BUN >8.92mmol/L, impaired mental status, age >60, presence of pleural effusion and ≥2 systemic inflammatory response (SIRS) criteria (HR >90/min, RR >20/min, temperature <36°C or >38°C and WCC <4 or >12 x 10^9/L). This score has a greater sensitivity than the others and a similar AUROC to APACHE II.
- Generalised severity of illness scoring systems such as APACHE II may also be used, although despite having a good sensitivity it is complex to calculate so less commonly utilised.
- The Balthazar scoring system is part of the scoring index used for grading acute pancreatitis based on the CT appearances and degree of pancreatic necrosis.

The management of acute pancreatitis is predominantly supportive, with management of the underlying cause where appropriate. Focus on fluid balance (will likely need high volumes initially and then further fluid based on clinical state), analgesia (pancreatitis is painful and patients often need IV opiates), glycaemic control, early enteral nutritional support if not eating and drinking, and attempts at prevention of organ dysfunction. If patients develop pancreatic fluid collections at a later stage, they may require endoscopic, percutaneous or open surgical drainage.

References

1. Leppäniemi A, Tolonen M, Tarasconi A, *et al.* 2019 WSES guidelines for the management of severe acute pancreatitis. *World J Emerg Surg* 2019; 14(1): 27.
2. Banks PA, Bollen TL, Dervenis C, *et al.* Classification of acute pancreatitis — 2012: revision of the Atlanta classification and definitions by international consensus. *Gut* 2013; 62(1): 102–11.
3. Wu BU. Prognosis in acute pancreatitis. *CMAJ* 2011; 183(6): 673–7.
4. MacGoey P, Dickson EJ, Puxty K, *et al.* Management of the patient with acute pancreatitis *BJA Educ* 2019; 19(8): 240–5.

Answer 12: c

Disseminated intravascular coagulation (DIC) is a syndrome that occurs secondary to several underlying conditions. Systemic activation of the coagulation occurs, resulting in clot formation in small- and mid-sized vessels leading to reduced blood flow and organ dysfunction. The consumption of platelets and clotting factors by clot formation results in thrombocytopaenia and low concentrations of clotting factors with risk of severe haemorrhage.

Causes of DIC include: severe infection (up to 35% will develop DIC), trauma, obstetric conditions (pre-eclampsia, placental abruption and pre-eclampsia), malignancy, organ destruction (e.g. pancreatitis), toxins (recreational drugs, snake bites) and severe liver failure.

No single blood test can diagnose DIC and a scoring system using four different tests in combination with a high clinical suspicion of DIC can be used to help guide diagnosis. Clinical suspicion should be based on the presence of an underlying condition known to cause DIC, decreasing platelet count and prolonged clotting times. The International Society on Thrombosis and Haemostasis (ISTH) revised their criteria in 2025 for the identification of overt

DIC (Table 5.13), and have added criteria for the identification of early-phase DIC in sepsis — sepsis-induced coagulopathy (SIC), with the aim or preventing progression to overt DIC in these cases. The SIC criteria include two lab tests and calculation of the SOFA score.

Table 5.13. ISTH overt DIC and sepsis-induced coagulopathy scoring systems.

	Score	Overt DIC	Sepsis-induced coagulopathy (SIC)
Platelet count (x 10^9/L)	2	<50	<100
	1	50–100	100–150
D-dimer	3	>7x upper normal level	-
	2	>3x upper normal level	-
PT prolongation(s)/INR	2	≥6s PT prolongation	INR >1.4
	1	3–6s PT prolongation	INR 1.2–1.4
Fibrinogen (g/L)	1	<1	-
SOFA score	2	-	≥2
	1	-	1
Total score for DIC		≥5	≥4

A score of ≥5 is compatible with a diagnosis of DIC. If the patient scores less than 5 but there is an ongoing high clinical suspicion of DIC, the score can be repeated in 1 to 2 days.

The primary management of DIC is treatment of the underlying cause, as without removal of the trigger the abnormal clotting activation will continue. If the patient has no major bleeding or thrombotic issues, they can continue to receive prophylactic low-molecular-weight heparin (LMWH). If the patient is actively bleeding, or if they need to undergo an invasive procedure, then blood products are indicated to correct to the following parameters: platelets >30–50 x 10^9/L, PT prolongation <3 seconds and fibrinogen >1.5g/L. Vitamin K may also be administered if deficiency is suspected. If the patient has overt thromboembolism or organ failure related to clots, then an unfractionated heparin infusion would be indicated.

In the scenario in question the patient has results consistent with DIC (clinical suspicion, an underlying trigger and a score of 6) but no active bleeding and no immediate need for an invasive procedure. In addition, she has inadequate management of the underlying cause of the DIC; therefore, the best treatment of her coagulopathy would be a change of antibiotics.

References

1. Levi M, Scully M. How I treat disseminated intravascular coagulation. *Blood* 2018; 131(8): 845–54.
2. Levi M, Toh CH, Thachil J, Watson HG. Guidelines for the diagnosis and management of disseminated intravascular coagulation. British Committee for Standards in Haematology. *Br J Haematol* 2009; 145(1): 24–33.
3. Iba T, Maier CL, Scarlatescu E, Levy JH. Introducing the new definition and diagnostic criteria of disseminated intravascular coagulation released by the International Society on Thrombosis and Haemostasis in 2025. *Semin Thromb Hemost* 2025; Aug 19. doi: 10.1055/a-2675-6068. Online ahead of print.

● Answer 13: b

The basics of acid-base balance are covered on page 309, Paper 4, Q7. Acidosis is either respiratory (caused by an increase in the $PaCO_2$) or metabolic.

Metabolic acidosis is commonplace in critical care and the result of an increase in endogenous acids, a decrease in acid excretion, administration of exogenous acids or a reduction in the strong ion difference (SID). The outcome for patients with acidosis is dependent upon the underlying cause of the acidosis, with lactic acidosis linked to poor outcomes and diabetic ketoacidosis to relatively good outcomes.

There are numerous anions that are not routinely measured but contribute to acidosis. The presence and impact of these anions can be assessed using an anion gap calculation as follows:

Anion gap = $(Na^+ + K^+) - (Cl^- + HCO_3^-)$

A normal anion gap is around 4–12mmol/L and is predominantly due to the presence of albumin and phosphate. If the anion gap is above 30mmol/L it will almost certainly be accompanied by an acidosis. The anion gap can by underestimated in hypalbuminaemia and so a correction formula should be used which is:

SBA Paper 5: Answers

Corrected anion gap = anion gap + [0.25 x (40 − albumin in g/L)]

Causes of a high anion gap metabolic acidosis (HAGMA) include:

- Excess endogenous anions: renal failure (phosphate, sulphates and urates), DKA (keto-acids), lactic acidosis secondary to sepsis, tissue hypoperfusion, liver disease, propofol infusion syndrome.
- Excess exogenous anions: citrate toxicity (citrate), aspirin overdose (salicylic acid), paracetamol (5-oxoproline), methanol ingestion (formic acid), ethylene glycol ingestion (oxalic acid).

A normal anion gap metabolic acidosis (NAGMA) is the result of a decrease in the SID and primarily occurs due to an increase in chloride. Causes include:

- Iatrogenic (often 0.9% saline administration).
- GI loss of bicarbonate-rich fluid (and accompanied chloride retention) in diarrhoea, ileostomy and pancreatic fistula.
- Reabsorption of chloride-rich fluid (ileal conduit urinary diversion), renal tubular acidosis (chloride retention and bicarbonate loss).
- Acetazolamide use (resulting in renal sodium and bicarbonate loss and chloride retention).

Use of the urinary anion gap can help to differentiate between renal and GI causes of NAGMA, and is calculated as follows:

Urinary anion gap = $(Na^+ + K^+) - Cl^-$

Renal causes result in a positive urinary anion gap; GI causes result in a negative (less than 0) urinary anion gap.

Regarding the patient in the question, there is a degree of respiratory acidosis, a normal anion gap but a significantly low SID present — likely due to administration of 0.9% saline — and this is the primary cause of the acidosis.

References

1. Park MAJ, Cave G, Freebairn RC. Metabolic acidosis in anaesthesia and critical care. *BJA Educ* 2024; 24(3): 91–9.
2. Nickson DC. Anion gap. Life in the fast lane (LITFL); 2020. Available at: https://litfl.com/anion-gap/.

Answer 14: c

Rib fractures are common in blunt chest wall trauma and contribute to 25% of deaths after trauma. Up to 20% of all trauma patients will have at least one rib fracture, and the greater the number of rib fractures, the higher the mortality rate. They are associated with long-term morbidity with two thirds of patients having ongoing pain at 2 years and a third being unable to return to their usual employment due to long-term sequelae from their rib fractures.

The most commonly fractured ribs are 4–10, which are not protected by the clavicle and shoulder girdle (unlike 1–3) and also have an anterior connection to the sternum (unlike 11 and 12 which are more mobile and therefore less likely to fracture). A flail segment is defined radiologically as the presence of three contiguous rib fractures in two or more places per rib, and clinically when an area of the chest paradoxically moves inwards during inspiration. The presence of a flail segment is associated with an increased mortality of up to 35%.

Rib fractures are often associated with damage to the underlying structures and are commonly associated with pneumothorax, haemothorax and lung contusions. They are also associated with a risk of later complications such as pneumonia and prolonged weaning.

The management of patients with rib fractures is predominantly supportive, with the use of multimodal analgesia, and regional techniques for patients with more severe injury or a higher risk of complications. Positive pressure in the form of CPAP or invasive ventilation may be necessary in significant chest trauma. Surgical fixation is an option and is becoming more commonplace, but there is a lack of consensus regarding the exact indications for fixation and the decision to operate is often dependent upon local expertise. NICE recommends fixation in patients with a flail chest who are requiring mechanical ventilation; in general, more than rib fractures and a flail segment requiring mechanical ventilation, symptomatic non-unions and significantly reduced lung capacity despite adequate analgesia should all be considered for surgery. Relative contraindications to fixation are a high likelihood of mechanical ventilation regardless of fixation (such as those with severe underlying lung contusions or high spinal cord injuries). Not all ribs require fixation with ribs 4–9 usually targeted; however, the fixation plan will be individualised to the patient's need.

SBA Paper 5: Answers

There are a few scoring systems that are used to estimate the likelihood of complications and mortality after rib fractures such as the Rib Fracture Score, Chest Trauma Score, RibScore and the STUMBL chest scoring system. The most significant risk factors for increasing mortality are increasing patient age, high number of rib fractures, pre-existing chronic lung disease, oxygen saturations on arrival to hospital and anticoagulant use prior to injury.

In this patient scenario, the patient had good enough underlying lung function to consider initial extubation, and probably failed due to mechanical issues from the flail segments in addition to poor pain management. Failed extubation due to rib fractures alone would be a strong indication for discussion and consideration of rib fixation. Changing the analgesia regime alone is unlikely to result in a significantly improved outcome and his oxygenation with positive pressure is acceptable so the other options are unlikely to be beneficial.

References

1. Williams A, Bigham C, Marchbank A. Anaesthetic and surgical management of rib fractures. *BJA Educ* 2020; 20(10): 332–40.
2. de Moya M, Nirula R, Biffl W. Rib fixation: who, what, when? *Trauma Surg Acute Care Open* 2017; 2(1): p.e000059.
3. National Institute for Health and Care Excellence (NICE), guideline IPG361. Insertion of metal rib reinforcements to stabilise a flail chest wall, 2010. Available at: https://www.nice.org.uk/guidance/ipg361/chapter/1-Guidance.

● Answer 15: d

In the updated form for the diagnosis of death by neurological criteria, there are a number of preconditions that must be met prior to testing. These include (and replace) the 'red flag' features that were in the previous guidance which originated from previous cases of misdiagnosis of brainstem death. Precondition 2 is of relevance here: there must have been a long enough period to exclude the potential for recovery. Brainstem death testing should not be undertaken less than 6 hours after the loss of the last brainstem reflex, and in a patient who has a hypoxic brain injury or are post-cardiac arrest you should not test before 24 hours after the loss of the last reflex. If the patient has been hypothermic (including therapeutic) then there should be at least a 24-hour observation period following rewarming (core temperature should be greater than or equal to 36°C) prior to testing. If there is any uncertainty about the possibility for recovery, then the observation time should be extended.

For further information on the diagnosis of death by neurological criteria please see page 247, Paper 3, Q34.

References

1. The Academy of Medical Royal Colleges (AoMRC) and the Faculty of Intensive Care Medicine (FICM). Form for the diagnosis of death using neurological criteria, 2025. Available at: https://ficm.ac.uk/sites/ficm/files/documents/2024-12/Form%20for%20the%20Diagnosis%20of%20DNC%20-%20adults%20and%20children%20over%202%20years%20-%20January%202025.pdf.

Answer 16: a

Intracerebral haemorrhage (ICH) is the cause of acute stroke in around 10% of cases but is responsible for more deaths (early mortality up to 40%) and higher disability adjusted life-years lost compared to ischaemic strokes. The majority (75%) of haemorrhagic strokes are intracerebral with the remainder being subarachnoid.

There are many risk factors for intracranial haemorrhage with the most common being: hypertension, older age, male sex, heavy alcohol use, anticoagulant use and pregnancy. Early imaging is vital to determine the aetiology as the management of haemorrhagic stroke differs significantly from that of ischaemic stroke:

- Blood pressure control: systolic blood pressure (SBP) of over 150mmHg should be actively lowered by no more than 60mmHg in the first hour and 90mmHg in total, aiming for a range of 130–150mmHg for 7 days after the initial bleed. There is no consensus regarding the choice of antihypertensive agent, but IV labetalol or nicardipine are often preferred in the early stages due to their rapid titratability. The use of venodilators may be harmful and reducing SBP to <130mmHg may worsen outcomes so both should be avoided. If the patient requires urgent neurosurgical intervention, then the safety of BP lowering is not well established and should be guided by the neurosurgeons. SBP management is not required in patients with large bleeds who are not surgical candidates.

SBA Paper 5: Answers

- Anticoagulation reversal: 20% of ICHs occur in patients taking oral anticoagulants. This group have a high risk of early haematoma expansion; therefore rapid reversal of the anticoagulant is a priority. Patients on warfarin should receive prothrombin complex concentrate (PCC) followed by vitamin K to prevent a rebound increase in the INR. Dabigatran can be reversed with idarucizumab, or if this is unavailable, PCC. Factor Xa inhibitors (e.g. apixaban) should be reversed with PCC, or andexanet alfa if available.
- Location of care: patients should be managed on a specialist stroke unit and discussed with a neurosurgeon unless the nature of the patient's bleed and pre-existing comorbidities warrants a palliative approach. If a patient has a bleed that is amenable to surgical intervention or symptomatic hydrocephalus, urgent transfer to a neurosurgical centre for ongoing management is indicated.
- Surgery: options include a decompressive craniectomy with or without haematoma evacuation (depending on the location) and external ventricular drain (EVD) insertion. Patients with posterior fossa bleeds or blood within the ventricles are at high risk of developing hydrocephalus and warrant EVD insertion if symptomatic. There is no clear evidence on which bleeds benefit from surgical intervention and the decision to operate is guided by the neurosurgical team.
- Supportive care: regular neurological monitoring for early detection of deterioration is vital. In all patients there should be glycaemic control (4–11mmol/L), saturation target management (aim for SpO_2 93–96% and avoidance of hyperoxia), maintenance of normothermia and control of any seizures (Keppra® and sodium valproate are commonly used). Adequate nutrition (via a nasogastric tube and feeding if needed) and VTE prophylaxis (with intermittent pneumatic compression stockings) should be provided with the avoidance of LMWH in the early stages following a bleed. Starting statins is not indicated.

References

1. bestpractice.bmj.com. Stroke due to spontaneous intracerebral haemorrhage — symptoms, diagnosis and treatment. BMJ Best Practice, 2024. Available at: https://bestpractice.bmj.com/topics/en-gb/3000109.
2. Greenberg SM, Ziai WC, Cordonnier C, *et al.* 2022 guideline for the management of patients with spontaneous intracerebral hemorrhage: a guideline from the American Heart Association/American Stroke Association. *Stroke* 2022; 53(7): e282–361.

● Answer 17: c

Clostridioides difficile infection (CDI) is a common hospital-acquired infection. It can be classified as non-fulminant disease — which is divided into non-severe CDI (WCC <15 x 10^9/L and creatinine <130µmol/L) and severe CDI (WCC >15 x 10^9/L and creatinine >130µmol/L) — or fulminant colitis (with hypotension, shock, ileus and megacolon).

Diagnosis of CDI is a two-stage approach. Initially, testing for the presence of glutamate dehydrogenase (GDH) enzyme in the stool takes place. GDH is produced by all *C. difficile* isolates, so a positive result indicates the presence of *C. difficile* bacteria but does not determine if they are toxin-producing. If the GDH test is negative the likelihood of CDI is very small. If the patient is GDH-positive, stool is then tested for *C. difficile* toxins A and B. If these are present, then infection is likely, and the patient should be treated as such. If the patient is GDH-positive but toxin-negative, they are only treated if symptomatic but do need to be barrier nursed as a minimum to prevent *C. difficile* transmission.

Treatment varies according to disease severity, but in all cases the likely causative agent should be stopped:

- Non-fulminant, non-severe CDI: can be managed with enteral antibiotics if it is the first presentation (usually metronidazole, vancomycin or fidaxomicin dependent on local resistance patterns); in recurring infection a repeat course of enteral antibiotics and consideration of bezlotoxumab (a monoclonal antibody that binds to toxin B) are indicated. In cases of repeated infection, a faecal transplant may be considered.
- Non-fulminant, severe CDI: fidaxomicin is preferred, but oral vancomycin can be used, with a faecal transplant second-line therapy.
- Fulminant disease: oral vancomycin is given at a higher dose; vancomycin enemas in combination with IV metronidazole are used if ileus is present. If there is no response to first-line therapy, escalation of antimicrobials to tigecycline and the addition of IV immunoglobulin (IVIg) may be considered (limited data but recommended in fulminant disease where surgery is not an option).

- Surgery may be required if the patient has evidence of toxic megacolon and fulminant CDI. A surgical opinion and CT of the abdomen should be considered in patients with the following features: hypotension, temperature ≥38.5°C, ileus or significant abdominal distention, altered GCS, peritonitis, WBC ≥20 x 10^9/L, lactate >2.2mmol/L, end-organ failure and failure to improve after 3–4 days of maximal medical therapy. Surgery is indicated in the following situations: colonic perforation or full-thickness ischaemia on CT, abdominal compartment syndrome, escalating vasopressor requirements (although this is associated with worse outcomes than surgery performed in patients without significant haemodynamic instability), worsening end-organ failure, WBC >50 x 10^9/L and lactate >5mmol/L.

This patient has a fulminant CDI and has received first-line therapy but continued to deteriorate with signs of an acute abdomen. The antibiotic choice suggested is not correct, and although IVIg may be indicated, if there is deterioration on a new antibiotic regime, the patient urgently needs a surgical review and abdominal imaging.

References

1. bestpractice.bmj.com. *Clostridium difficile*-associated disease — symptoms, diagnosis and treatment. BMJ Best Practice, 2025. Available at: https://bestpractice.bmj.com/topics/ en-gb/230.
2. Updated guidance on the diagnosis and reporting of *Clostridium difficile*. Available at: https://assets.publishing.service.gov.uk/media/5a7cc0c1e5274a2f304efdb0/dh_133016.pdf.
3. www.uptodate.com. *Clostridioides difficile* infection in adults: treatment and prevention. UpToDate, 2025. Available at: https://www.uptodate.com/contents/clostridioides-difficile-infection-in-adults-treatment-and-prevention.
4. www.uptodate.com. Surgical management of *Clostridioides difficile* colitis in adults. UpToDate, 2025. Available at: https://www.uptodate.com/contents/surgical-management-of-clostridioides-difficile-colitis-in-adults.

● Answer 18: a

Right ventricular dysfunction can occur in a wide range of clinical situations. The pulmonary circulation is a low-pressure system, and the RV is thinner with fewer muscle fibres and greater compliance than the left ventricle (LV).

As such, the management of RV failure differs significantly from LV failure. The causes of RV failure are varied and can be due to isolated RV failure or in combined RV and LV failure. The causes of RV failure can be classified as follows:

- Increased afterload: pulmonary embolism (the most common cause of isolated acute RV dysfunction), COPD (the leading cause of cor pulmonale), all causes of pulmonary hypertension, acute respiratory distress syndrome, obstructive sleep apnoea and interstitial lung disease, mechanical ventilation, congenital heart disease with RV outflow obstruction.
- Reduced contractility: RV myocardial infarction, myocarditis, cardiomyopathies (dilated, hypertrophic or arrhythmogenic RV).
- Abnormal preload: hypovolaemia/hypervolaemia (often in combination with other pathology), LV failure (failure of forward flow), pericardial tamponade, mechanical ventilation, left-right shunt.
- Other: arrhythmias, post-cardiac surgery, post-left ventricular assist device insertion and cardiac transplant.

The management of RV failure is via treatment of the underlying cause, reducing afterload and optimising RV filling as the RV is sensitive to haemodynamic imbalance:

- Reducing afterload: this is a key management aim but can be difficult to achieve. Interventions include minimising PEEP and airway pressures in ventilated patients, prevention of hypoxic pulmonary vasoconstriction by optimising oxygenation, avoidance of hypercapnia and acidosis, and use of inhaled and IV pulmonary vasodilators (in specific conditions).
- Optimise preload: optimisation of RV filling is important as an underfilled RV will result in reduced cardiac output. Accurate assessment of filling status is very difficult in RV failure, so fluid challenges should be given in smaller boluses (100ml at a time) with the response noted. Conversely, overfilling will impair both RV function and LV diastolic filling (and so cardiac output). Therefore, in overfilled patients, diuresis and fluid removal via CRRT may be required.
- Improve contractility and perfusion: systemic hypotension may result in reduced coronary perfusion, impaired myocardial contractility and

worsening RV function so the use of vasopressors to maintain MAP in well-filled patients is indicated. Inotropes can also improve RV contractility, with milrinone and dobutamine commonly used for this reason. Intra-aortic balloon pumps (IABPs) may be considered to augment coronary and systemic perfusion. There are also RV assist devices available that can be surgically inserted to improve RV outflow.
- Maintain rate and rhythm: a higher heart rate is preferred in RV failure as a shorter diastole limits the risk of overdistention of the RV and improves CO when stroke volume is limited. This must be balanced against LV function but is a consideration if starting inotropic agents. Sinus rhythm is ideal but often can be difficult to achieve as many patients with RV failure have chronic AF.
- Ventilation: unlike the LV which likes PEEP as it reduces the work of the ventricle, the RV does not! The use of invasive ventilation and application of PEEP can have markedly detrimental effects on RV dynamics and must be used judiciously in patients with known and established RV failure. Minimally invasive respiratory support — such as high-flow nasal oxygen — is well tolerated. The risks of any interventions must be balanced against the detrimental effects of hypoxia and acidosis on pulmonary vascular resistance. In an intubated patient the lowest possible PEEP should be used with Vt limited to 6ml/kg to minimise the peak airway pressures generated by invasive ventilation.

In this case the patient has had a RV infarct and is receiving mechanical ventilation with a high PEEP which will increase afterload. Although fluid status can be difficult to assess, the patient does not seem grossly underfilled. They may require diuresis at some stage; however, the most impactful first management step would be to decrease the PEEP in an attempt to improve haemodynamic status.

References

1. Murphy E, Shelley B. Clinical presentation and management of right ventricular dysfunction. *BJA Educ* 2019; 19(6): 183–90.
2. Arrigo M, Huber LC, Winnik S, *et al*. Right ventricular failure: pathophysiology, diagnosis and treatment. *Card Fail Rev* 2019; 5(3): 140–6.
3. Disselkamp M, Adkins D, Pandey S, Coz Yataco AO. Physiologic approach to mechanical ventilation in right ventricular failure. *Ann Am Thorac Soc* 2018; 15(3): 383–9.

Answer 19: b

Patients with haematological malignancies represent a small proportion of patients in critical care; however, 7% of all haematological malignancy-related hospital admissions involve a period of time in critical care. The complication rates for treatment of haematological malignancy are highest in patients following stem cell transplantation, with an ICU admission rate in this cohort of up to 14%.

Commonly encountered complications in patients receiving treatment for haematological malignancy include:

- Neutropenia: defined as an absolute neutrophil count of <1.5 x 10^9/L, with severe neutropenia being a neutrophil count of <0.5 x 10^9/L. Neutropenic sepsis (presence of severe neutropenia and a temperature >38°C) is a medical emergency requiring broad-spectrum antibiotics within an hour of presentation. The antibiotics used typically include an antipseudomonal agent (e.g. Tazocin®) and an agent to cover Gram-positive cocci infection (e.g. vancomycin). The source of the infection may not be initially evident, and a full septic screen should be undertaken and repeated until a source is identified. Granulocyte colony-stimulating factor (GCSF) can be used to promote neutrophil recovery, but not in cases where the total white cell count is elevated.
- Typhlitis (aka neutropenic enterocolitis): this presents as abdominal pain, fever and diarrhoea following chemotherapy in patients with severe neutropenia. It is thought that the chemotherapy causes bowel wall mucosal damage which in addition to thrombocytopenic-related gastrointestinal bleeding and colonisation of the bowel with pathogenic bacteria results in a colitis. Typical CT findings include bowel wall thickening, mesenteric fat stranding, bowel dilatation, mucosal enhancement and pneumatosis. Treatment is supportive with nasogastric tube drainage, IV fluids, nutritional support and broad-spectrum antibiotics. Surgery may be considered in cases of failed medical management but is associated with a high risk of associated morbidity and mortality.
- Tumour lysis syndrome: discussed in greater detail on page 127, Paper 2, Q10 and page 352, Paper 4, Q39.

- Leukostasis: hyperleukocytosis is defined as a WCC >100 x 10^9/L; symptomatic hyperleukocytosis is a medical emergency and referred to as leukostasis. It is most commonly seen in acute myeloid leukaemia but can also occur in other leukaemias and is due to increased blood viscosity causing obstruction of small blood vessels. The most common organ system involved is the central nervous system with symptoms such as visual changes, dizziness, tinnitus, confusion and sometimes coma seen. The respiratory system is also commonly affected with dyspnoea, hypoxia and diffuse changes on imaging occurring. Fever occurs in most patients with leukostasis; less common features include myocardial ischaemia, bowel ischaemia, renal failure, acute limb ischaemia and bowel infarction.
- Acute respiratory failure: this is a common reason for admission to critical care and is often due to infection which may be caused by a wide range of potential — and often atypical — pathogens. Other causes of respiratory failure include drug-induced pneumonitis, pulmonary oedema, graft vs. host disease, malignant lung infiltration and pulmonary haemorrhage.
- Graft vs. host disease (GVHD): this occurs after stem cell transplant (including bone marrow transplant and can be acute or chronic. In GVHD, the donor stem cells mount an immune response to the host cells causing systemic illness. Acute GVHD occurs within 100 days of the stem cell transplant. It affects the skin, liver and gut resulting in a skin rash, elevation in bilirubin and diarrhoea, with disease graded according to the severity of these three symptoms. Treatment is with additional immunosuppression, typically steroids plus other immunosuppressants as indicated. Chronic GVHD occurs at least 3 months after transplantation but may present several years after transplantation. It can affect almost any organ, and treatment is again with immunosuppression.

References

1. Fizza Haider S, Sloss R, Jhanji S, et al. Management of adult patients with haematological malignancies in critical care. *Anaesthesia* 2023; 78(7): 874–83.
2. www.uptodate.com. Neutropenic enterocolitis (typhlitis). UpToDate, 2025. Available at: https://www.uptodate.com/contents/neutropenic-enterocolitis-typhlitis.
3. www.uptodate.com. Hyperleukocytosis and leukostasis in hematologic malignancies. UpToDate, 2024. Available at: https://www.uptodate.com/contents/hyperleukocytosis-and-leukostasis-in-hematologic-malignancies.

4. Beed M, Levitt M, Bokhari SW. Intensive care management of patients with haematological malignancy. *Contin Educ Anaesth Crit Care Pain* 2010: 10(6): 167–71.

● Answer 20: b

Aspergillus is a genus of moulds that typically grows in decaying leaves but can also colonise buildings where it favours warm, damp or humid areas such as bathrooms or around windows. Testing for *Aspergillus* is via PCR of body fluid (typically bronchoalveolar lavage [BAL]), a beta-D-glucan performed on BAL or serum (although this is not specific to *Aspergillus* and will be positive in other fungal infections such as *Candida*) and a galactomannan test of any bodily fluid (which is more specific for *Aspergillus*).

Aspergillus infection in humans presents in one of several ways:

- Invasive aspergillosis: a progressive multisite pulmonary disease with cavitating lung lesions prominent. Disease may spread from the lungs to the brain and solid organs. Patients who are immunosuppressed, including patients receiving frequent treatment with steroids for chronic lung disease are at greatest risk of infection. It can also occur in patients with an intercurrent illness, as well as immunocompetent patients with a high spore load. Symptoms include shortness of breath, cough, haemoptysis, pleuritic chest pain, fever, malaise and resting hypoxia. Imaging demonstrates nodules (single or multiple) which may or may not have cavitation, patchy consolidation and ground-glass changes. The halo sign on CT is relatively specific for aspergillosis and is ground-glass opacity due to haemorrhage surrounding a pulmonary nodule or mass. Treatment is with voriconazole (or any azole) and organ-supportive measures as required.
- Allergic bronchopulmonary aspergillosis: a hypersensitivity reaction of *Aspergillus* colonisation of the airways in patients with asthma and cystic fibrosis. It presents as asthma exacerbations, and causes mucoid impaction in the bronchi, eosinophilic pneumonia and granulomatosis around the bronchi. Investigations reveal a raised serum eosinophil count and a raised total IgE. Imaging shows bronchiectasis most commonly affecting the upper and middle lobes in the central bronchi. Treatment is initially with steroids and antifungal agents.

- Aspergilloma: the development of a fungal ball of *Aspergillus* that collects in a pre-existing cavity such as an old TB cavity.

Tuberculosis (TB) is the main differential for aspergillosis and presents with cough, shortness of breath and haemoptysis. In patients with reactivated TB, the changes seen on imaging are typically in the apical and posterior segments of the upper lobes.

References

1. Carr C. Fungal infection. In: Bersten AD, Handy JM, Eds. *Oh's intensive care manual*, 8th ed. London: Elsevier; 2018: chapter 73: pp. 866–75.
2. bestpractice.bmj.com. Aspergillosis — symptoms, diagnosis and treatment. BMJ Best Practice, 2024. Available at: https://bestpractice.bmj.com/topics/en-gb/425.
3. www.uptodate.com. Epidemiology and clinical manifestations of invasive aspergillosis. UpToDate, 2025. Available at: https://www.uptodate.com/contents/epidemiology-and-clinical-manifestations-of-invasive-aspergillosis.
4. www.uptodate.com. Clinical manifestations and diagnosis of allergic bronchopulmonary aspergillosis. UpToDate, 2024. Available at: https://www.uptodate.com/contents/clinical-manifestations-and-diagnosis-of-allergic-bronchopulmonary-aspergillosis.

● Answer 21: c

A spontaneous breathing trial (SBT) can be performed using several different methods, but the underlying intention is to evaluate the patient for a period of time with limited or no respiratory support via their endotracheal tube (ETT) or tracheostomy tube to assess if they will manage once extubated or decannulated. There is no universal agreement on if, and when, a SBT should be used in weaning patients.

A SBT can be conducted by leaving the patient on a ventilator but reducing PEEP to a minimum (typically 5cmH$_2$O) and pressure support to zero (aside from tube compensation) or attaching external CPAP or a T piece with supplemental oxygen to the patient's ETT or tracheostomy. The patient should then be observed for a minimum of 30 minutes.

Patients undergoing a SBT should be ready to wean based on the following criteria: resolution of the underlying cause for respiratory failure, cooperative, comfortable, P/F ratio >26.6kPa or sats ≥90% on an FiO_2 of ≤0.4, PEEP ≤8cmH_2O, haemodynamically stable (HR ≤140/min, no or low-dose vasopressors, optimised fluid balance, SBP 90–160mmHg), adequate cough, minimal secretion load, able to initiate inspiration, afebrile.

If enough of these criteria are met that the clinician feels the patient is ready to wean, then a SBT can be commenced. It is important to observe the patient closely during the first few minutes in case of rapid failure and then continue for 30 minutes to assess tolerance of unsupported breathing. Criteria that suggest a successful breathing trial are as follows, but should be used in combination with clinical signs and symptoms:

- Respiratory rate <35/min.
- SBT well tolerated by the patient and they look comfortable at the end without any signs of increased work of breathing or distress.
- HR <140/min or less than a 20% increase in HR from the start of the SBT.
- O_2 sats >90% or PaO_2 >8kPa with an FiO_2 of <0.4.
- SBP between 80mmHg and 160mmHg or less than 20% increase in SBP from the start of the SBT.
- Rapid Shallow Breathing Index of <105 (see page 52, Paper 1, Q18).

A successful SBT does not guarantee extubation success as approximately 10% of patients passing a SBT will ultimately fail their extubation (often due to a failure to clear secretions). However, it is a valuable tool in the assessment of a patient's readiness for extubation but should always be used alongside clinical judgement.

References

1. Zein H, Baratloo A, Negida A, Safari S. Ventilator weaning and spontaneous breathing trials; an educational review. *Emerg Tehran* 2016; 4(2): pp. 65–71.
2. MacIntyre NR. The ventilator discontinuation process: an expanding evidence base. *Respir Care* 2013; 58(6): 1074–86.
3. Leaver S. Respiratory therapy techniques: IPPV-weaning techniques. In: Waldmann C, Rhodes A, Soni N, Handy J, Eds. *Oxford desk reference: critical care*, 2nd ed. Oxford: Oxford University Press; 2019: chapter 1: pp. 17–9.

SBA Paper 5: Answers

 Answer 22: a

Pulse oximeters use spectrophotometric techniques to measure the oxygen saturation of blood. This means that radiation (in the form of red and infrared light) is passed through a sample (typically the finger) and the amount of radiation absorbed indicates the composition of the sample. Two laws of physics describe how radiation is absorbed by a sample/solution:

- Beer's law: the absorption of radiation by a given thickness of a solution of a given concentration is the same as that of twice the thickness of a solution of half the concentration.
- Lambert's or Bouguer's law: each layer of equal thickness absorbs an equal fraction of radiation which passes through it.

In an oximeter, light of the wavelengths 660nm and 940nm is emitted; these wavelengths are absorbed to a different degree by oxyhaemoglobin and deoxyhaemoglobin. The amount of each wavelength emitted reaching the sensor on the opposite side of the probe (having travelled through body tissue) can then be used to determine the proportion of oxyhaemoglobin and deoxyhaemoglobin and thus oxygen saturation of the sample. A two-measurement oximeter will not be able to differentiate between oxyhaemoglobin and carboxyhaemoglobin (which is why standard pulse oximeters have limited use in carbon monoxide poisoning); however, specialist oximeters which measure multiple wavelengths of light are able to differentiate in this setting.

Several factors can affect the accuracy of pulse oximeter readings, the most notable of which is the effect of skin pigmentation, with darker skin tones having a higher risk of occult hypoxia (the SaO_2 will be lower than the SpO_2, so whilst the probe may read 92%, the SaO_2 may be <88%). The lower the SaO_2 and the darker the skin tone, the greater the disparity leading to a risk of missing significant hypoxia. Other factors that can also lead to inaccurate readings include: use of nail polish, henna tattoos, methylene blue or indocyanine green administration, and poor peripheral perfusion.

With reference to the other physical laws cited in the question:

- Henry's law states that the amount of a given gas dissolved in a given liquid at a given temperature is directly proportional to the partial pressure of the gas in equilibrium with the liquid.

- Charles' law is one of the three perfect gas laws and states that at a constant pressure the volume of a given mass of gas varies directly with the absolute temperature.
- Dalton's law states that in a mixture of gases the pressure exerted by each gas is the same as that which it would exert if it alone occupied the container.
- Fick's law states that the rate of diffusion of a substance across a unit area (such as a membrane) is proportional to the concentration gradient.

References
1. David PD, Kenny GNC. *Basic physics and measurement in anaesthesia*, 5th ed. Oxford: Butterworth-Heinemann/Elsevier; 2003.
2. Cabanas AM, Fuentes-Guajardo M, Latorre K, *et al.* Skin pigmentation influence on pulse oximetry accuracy: a systematic review and bibliometric analysis. *Sensors (Basel)* 2022; 22(9): 3402.

Answer 23: b

There is British Thoracic Society (BTS) guidance available on the management of pleural disease.

In the management of pneumothorax, the decision to insert a chest drain primarily depends on patient symptoms, specifically pain, breathlessness or physiological compromise. If they are asymptomatic then conservative management may be followed regardless of the size of the pneumothorax. If the patient has a secondary spontaneous pneumothorax (e.g. in the presence of lung disease such as COPD) it can be managed conservatively if the patient is asymptomatic, but the patient should remain in hospital for observation.

If the patient is symptomatic then assessment should occur for high-risk symptoms supporting chest drain insertion (assuming the anatomy and size of the pneumothorax means it is safe to insert one). These high-risk characteristics include: haemodynamic compromise (tension pneumothorax), significant hypoxia, bilateral pneumothorax, underlying lung disease, age ≥50 years with significant smoking history and haemopneumothorax. The management of patients who are symptomatic but without high-risk characteristics is via clinical judgement and includes conservative management, insertion of an ambulatory device, needle aspiration and traditional chest drain insertion.

SBA Paper 5: Answers

If pleural infection is suspected and the effusion is large enough that it may be safely aspirated, then a sample should be taken and analysed to guide management. A collection with a pH of ≤7.2 should be managed via chest drain insertion. If the pH is 7.21–7.39 and the LDH is ≥900 IU/L, then insertion of a chest drain should be considered especially if the effusion is a large volume, septated or has a low glucose.

These guidelines do not advise on traumatic pneumothorax management which should be guided by the patient's clinical state; for example, a small (<3cm depth at the hilum) traumatic pneumothorax without symptoms and other significant chest pathology may be managed conservatively. Management also considers other patient factors such as the requirement for positive pressure ventilation.

References
1. Roberts ME, Rahman NM, Maskell NA, *et al.* British Thoracic Society guideline for pleural disease. *Thorax* 2023; 78(Suppl 3): s1–42.
2. Tran J, Haussner W, Shah K. Traumatic pneumothorax: a review of current diagnostic practices and evolving management. *J Emerg Med* 2021; 61(5): 517–28.

Answer 24: c

Malnutrition in ICU patients is common with up to 56% of patients having evidence of malnutrition on admission to the ICU, and critical illness being a risk factor for the development of malnutrition. Assessment of patients for signs of malnutrition and guidance of ongoing nutritional support is a vital part of intensive care management. Generic scoring systems such as the Malnutrition Universal Screening Tool (MUST) score and the Nutritional Risk Screening (NRS) score highlight patients at risk of malnutrition but are not validated for use in critical care populations. The Nutrition Risk in the Critically Ill (NUTRIC) score was designed specifically for use in critical care patients, with a score of >5 indicating a high risk for malnutrition but has no nutritional parameters and displays large variability when compared to more traditional screening tools. Body Mass Index (BMI) is a commonly used assessment tool, with mid-upper arm circumference (MUAC) often used to estimate BMI and may be useful in patients with peripheral oedema where the BMI may not be accurate. All of the above are used to assess a patient's current nutritional state or risk of malnutrition.

Energy expenditure is the amount of energy that the patient is currently using and may guide how much energy (in kcal) the patient requires. The gold standard is indirect calorimetry which is based on the premise that all inhaled oxygen delivered to the tissues is utilised to oxidise fuels and all the CO_2 produced is recovered. The measured oxygen delivered and CO_2 expired within the ventilator circuit are then used to calculate the resting energy expenditure (REE). The ratio between the total delivered oxygen and the total CO_2 produced is called the respiratory quotient (RQ), a figure that varies based on the primary substrate being used for energy — 0.7 for fat, 0.8 for protein (or a mixed diet) and 1 for carbohydrates. The RQ can also be used to help guide feed composition for a given patient. Indirect calorimetry, although recommended by the European Society for Clinical Nutrition and Metabolism (ESPEN), is not currently widely available so in most cases feed is started at a standard rate of 20–25kcal/kg/day unless there is a risk of refeeding syndrome, when it will be started at a lower rate.

References

1. Singer P, Blaser AR, Berger MM, et al. ESPEN guideline on clinical nutrition in the intensive care unit. *Clin Nutr* 2019; 38(1): 48–79.
2. Mtaweh H, Tuira L, Floh AA, Parshuram CS. Indirect calorimetry: history, technology, and application. *Front Pediatr* 2018; 6: 257.
3. British Association for Parenteral and Enteral Nutrition (BAPEN) Malnutrition Universal Screening Tool, 2003. BAPEN. Available at: https://www.bapen.org.uk/pdfs/must/must_full.pdf.

Answer 25: e

Data can be broadly classified as being qualitative or quantitative.

Qualitative data can be nominal (divided into categories with no numerical order such as blood group) or ordinal (data that have an implicit order, such as ASA grading, where the difference between groups is not the same).

Quantitative data can be discrete (finite values such as number of children, or the score in a scoring system) and continuous (data that can take any value including fractions such as height, weight and BMI). Quantitative data can also be classified as a ratio (data which has 0 as its baseline value such as blood pressure) and interval (data that includes 0 as a point on a larger scale such as centigrade temperature measurement).

There is a hierarchy of the usefulness of data based on how well it can be statistically manipulated, where continuous data > ordinal data > nominal data.

References
1. Spoors C, Kiff K. Statistics for the anaesthetist. In: Spoors C, Kiff K, Eds. *Training in anaesthesia: the essential curriculum*. Oxford: Oxford University Press; 2010: chapter 24: pp. 561–72.
2. Cross M, Plunkett E. Statistical principles. In: Cross M, Plunkett E, Eds. *Physics, pharmacology and physiology for anaesthetists*, 2nd ed. Cambridge: Cambridge University Press; 2014: section 12: pp. 347–76.

● Answer 26: d

Rhabdomyolysis is the constellation of clinical symptoms and complications that occur due to large-volume muscle cell death. There are three categories of causes of rhabdomyolysis:

- Traumatic or direct muscle injury — such as crush injury, burns, compartment syndrome and immobilisation.
- Non-traumatic exertional — which may occur in normal muscle due to extreme exercise, heat stroke, seizures and in abnormal muscle due to myopathies, malignant hyperpyrexia and neuroleptic malignant syndrome.
- Non-traumatic non-exertional — such as alcoholism, drugs (amphetamines, cocaine), toxins (carbon monoxide), infection, electrolyte abnormalities, endocrinopathies (hyperthyroidism).

The symptoms of rhabdomyolysis are often dependent upon the underlying cause, but generic symptoms include muscle pain, weakness and swelling along with dark-coloured urine due to the presence of myoglobin (seen in less than 10% of cases). Patients are often hypovolaemic from fluid loss into injured muscle with several blood test abnormalities due to release of intracellular contents. These include hyperkalaemia, hyperphosphataemia, hyperuricaemia, markedly elevated creatine kinase (typically >5000 U/L for non-exertional and >10,000 U/L for exertional) and raised myoglobin. Myoglobin is a monomer released from muscle cells that is not significantly protein bound so quickly appears in the urine and can be detected on urine dipstick even if urine is not the classical 'cola colour'. Urine dip is usually positive for blood as the dipstick tests for peroxidase which is present in RBCs and myoglobin. Hypocalcaemia due to increased binding of calcium to phosphate and also entry into the damaged myocytes is often seen. Acute kidney injury is a very common complication of rhabdomyolysis and is multifactorial with hypovolaemia, tubular obstruction and tubular injury all contributory.

The management of rhabdomyolysis is predominantly supportive with fluid resuscitation and renal support if renal injury occurs. The goal with fluid resuscitation is for a urine output of 200 to 300ml/hr until CK levels are ≤5000 U/L and continuing to fall. Historically, sodium bicarbonate has been used as a replacement fluid; however, there is no compelling evidence of benefit over isotonic fluid resuscitation, and it may compound hypocalcaemia and cause intracellular acidosis in patients with decompensated respiratory failure or circulatory failure.

References

1. www.uptodate.com. Rhabdomyolysis: epidemiology and etiology. UpToDate, 2024. Available at: https://www.uptodate.com/contents/rhabdomyolysis-epidemiology-and-etiology.
2. Somagutta MR, Pagad S, Sridharan S, *et al*. Role of bicarbonates and mannitol in rhabdomyolysis: a comprehensive review. *Cureus* 2020; 12(8): e9742.
3. www.uptodate.com. Rhabdomyolysis: clinical manifestations and diagnosis. UpToDate, 2024. Available at: https://www.uptodate.com/contents/rhabdomyolysis-clinical-manifestations-and-diagnosis.
4. Lines SW, Lewington AJP. Dipstick test for myoglobinuria. *BMJ* 2008; 337 (dec02 1): a2789.

● Answer 27: c

A simplified flow chart of the clotting cascade with the mode of action of commonly used anticoagulants is shown overleaf (Figure 5.1). Arrows indicate activation and crosses inhibition.

SBA Paper 5: Answers

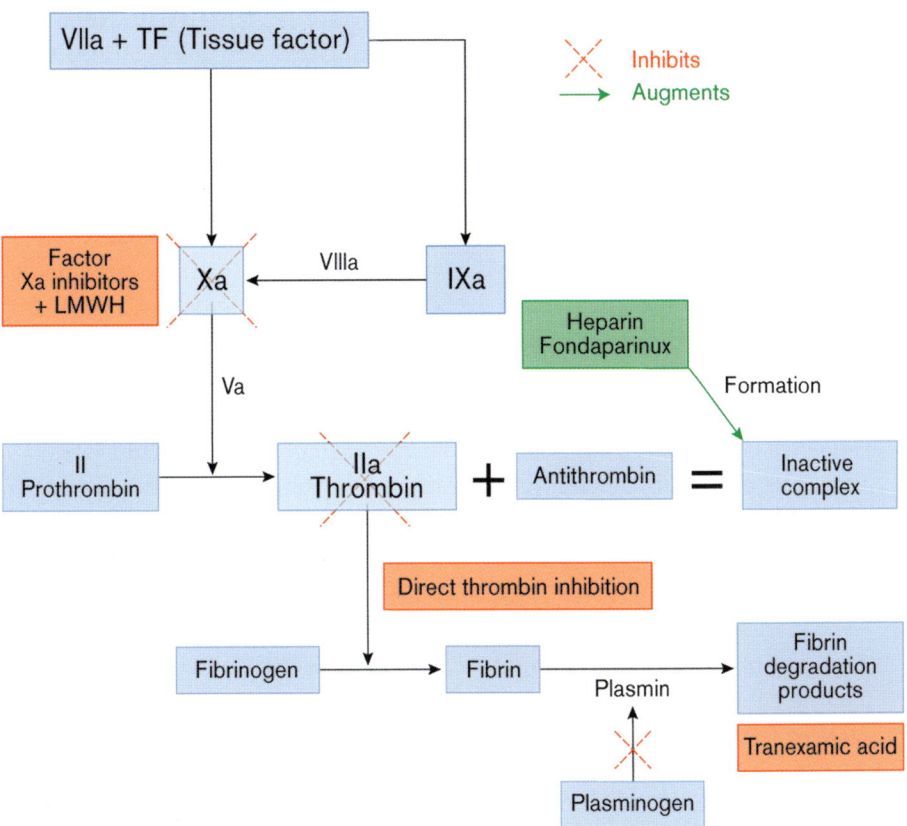

Figure 5.1. Simplified clotting cascade flowchart.

Direct oral anticoagulants (DOACs) — also known as non-vitamin K antagonist oral anticoagulants (NOACs) — work by two mechanisms:

- Direct thrombin inhibition: direct binding to thrombin which prevents the cleaving of fibrinogen to fibrin. They are available as intravenous preparations (bivalirudin and argatroban) and oral (dabigatran). Of note, dabigatran is 80–85% excreted renally so has a significantly increased half-life in renal failure.
- Direct factor Xa inhibition: direct binding to factor Xa which prevents the cleaving of prothrombin to thrombin. These agents are only available orally. Examples include rivaroxaban, apixaban and edoxaban.

Heparins: unfractionated heparin — a specific sequence of the heparin molecule binds to antithrombin, inducing a conformational change resulting in a ten-thousand-fold increase in activity. A smaller pentasaccharide sequence is responsible for antithrombin inhibition of factor Xa, and a longer sequence of 18 saccharides for antithrombin inhibition of thrombin. Low-molecular-weight heparin is smaller and so has a higher ratio of Xa inhibition: thrombin inhibition.

Fondaparinux is a synthetic version of the antithrombin-binding pentasaccharide sequence found in heparin and binds to antithrombin causing enhanced activity against factor Xa. It does not have any affinity for platelet factor 4 and is safe to use in heparin-induced thrombocytopaenia. For more information on HIT see page 210, Paper 3, Q2.

Warfarin acts on vitamin K-dependent compounds such as the coagulation factors II, VII, IX and X and the anticoagulant proteins C and S. The precursors of these factors are activated in the liver by a process linked to the oxidation of reduced vitamin K. Warfarin prevents vitamin K returning to its reduced form and thereby prevents these factors becoming activated.

References

1. Hunt BJ. Haematological drugs. In: Waldmann C, Rhodes A, Soni N, Handy J, Eds. *Oxford desk reference: critical care*, 2nd ed. Oxford: Oxford University Press; 2019: chapter 15: pp. 236–43.

2. www.uptodate.com. Direct oral anticoagulants (DOACs) and parenteral direct-acting anticoagulants: dosing and adverse effects. UpToDate, 2025. Available at: https://www.uptodate.com/contents/direct-oral-anticoagulants-doacs-and-parenteral-direct-acting-anticoagulants-dosing-and-adverse-effects.

● Answer 28: a

Constipation affects up to 70% of intensive care patients and is defined as the failure to open the bowels for 3 days. The causes of constipation in intensive care patients differs from the general patient population, with a combination of medication side effects and a reduction in normal physiological gut function due to a lack of a balanced diet, exercise and biofeedback frequently responsible.

Medications that cause constipation include opiates, anticholinergics, calcium channel blockers and neuromuscular blocking drugs (especially when given as infusions). Deep sedation is associated with constipation primarily from the high doses of opiates used. Although constipation is listed as a side effect of omeprazole, diarrhoea is a more commonly seen side effect in intensive care patients.

Non-pharmacological causes of constipation include delayed enteral nutrition, reduced mobility, electrolyte disturbances (hypercalcaemia, hypokalaemia), dehydration, abdominal surgery, spinal cord injury, nicotine withdrawal and severe illness.

Constipation commonly results in agitation and delirium and is associated with increased ICU length of stay, slower respiratory weaning and even increased mortality rates.

Management includes the prevention of modifiable risk factors where possible (e.g. use of sedation holds to minimise opiate sedation) and the use of laxatives. Local practice may vary but in general after 2–3 days of no bowel motion a laxative is added in. Laxative types include stimulant (senna), osmotic (lactulose), emollient (docusate) and bulk-forming (ispaghula husk). If there is rectal loading, an enema can be helpful and in certain conditions such as spinal cord injury regular manual dis-impaction or digital rectal stimulus is needed for a bowel motion to occur.

References

1. Kim MJ, Tatham KC. Gastrointenstinal drugs: constipation in critical care. In: Waldmann C, Rhodes A, Soni N, Handy J, Eds. *Oxford desk reference: critical care*, 2nd ed. Oxford: Oxford University Press; 2019: chapter 13: pp. 214–5.
2. Derangedphysiology.com. Constipation and ileus in the critically ill. Deranged physiology, 2025. Available at: https://derangedphysiology.com/main/required-reading/gastroenterology-and-hepatology/Chapter%20514/constipation-and-ileus-critically-ill.
3. Gacouin A, Camus C, Gros A, *et al*. Constipation in long-term ventilated patients: Associated factors and impact on intensive care unit outcomes. *Crit Care Med* 2010; 38(10): 1933–8.

Answer 29: d

Eye problems are common in patients in intensive care due to a number of factors. The normal protective mechanisms of the eye such as blinking, tear production and eye closure whilst sleeping can often be disrupted or absent. Direct trauma to the eyes may occur, as well as damage from exposure and drying of parts of the eye that are normally moist or covered by high flow of dry gases during facial oxygen and CPAP delivery. The eyes can also suffer from changes in fluid balance, with patients who have a very large positive balance developing conjunctival swelling (chemosis). This may be exacerbated by positioning, particularly during prone positioning. The eye can also develop infections either originating in the eye or disseminated to the eye from systemic infection, and as the patient is unable to report changes in visual acuity or pain in the eyes when they are sedated, this may result in a delay in diagnosis with the risk of sight loss.

One of the biggest risks to the eyes is with lagophthalmos or incomplete eyelid closure as this can lead to drying of the exposed eye, corneal erosion and ulceration. It is vital that eyelid closure is assessed regularly on the ICU and steps taken to protect the eyes.

SBA Paper 5: Answers

Lagophthalmos grading (and suggested protective measures) is as follows:

- Grade 0: lid completely closed (no intervention required).
- Grade 1: any conjunctival exposure but no corneal exposure (4-hourly lubrication of the eyes).
- Grade 2: any corneal exposure (4-hourly lubrication and taping of the lids with adhesive tape such as micropore) along the lash margin. Patients in the prone position should have this level of eye protection regardless of initial grading.

Along with regular review by nursing staff, eyes should be examined as part of a daily medical review and any concerning changes to the eye should prompt further investigation and discussion with an ophthalmologist. Bacterial colonisation of the eyes is common in patients who are ventilated for prolonged periods and may develop into a bacterial conjunctivitis. In the presence of corneal damage, potentially deeper infections with the potential for permanent eye damage including blindness can result. Invasive candidiasis can lead to eye involvement and an ophthalmology review is advised in cases of invasive candidiasis.

References

1. Hearne BJ, Hearne EG, Montgomery H, Lightman SL. Eye care in the intensive care unit. *J Intensive Care Soc* 2018; 19(4): 345–50.
2. Keighley C, Cooley L, Morris AJ, *et al*. Consensus guidelines for the diagnosis and management of invasive candidiasis in haematology, oncology and intensive care settings 2021. *Intern Med J* 2021; 51(Suppl 7): 89–117.

● Answer 30: b

The Vaughan-Williams classification is an established categorisation system for anti-arrhythmic medication based on mechanism of action. An expanded and updated version was proposed in 2018. The new classification is shown in Table 5.14.

Table 5.14. The Vaughan-Williams classification.

Class	Subclass	Mechanisms of action	Indications	Examples
0		*Hyperpolarisation-activated cyclic nucleotide-gated (HCN) channel pacemaker current blockade*	Angina and heart failure (HF), HR ≥70/min	Ivabradine
I		*Voltage-gated Na^+ channel blockers*		
	Ia	Prolongs refractory period and slows action potential (AP) conduction	SVT, AF, VT	Quinidine, disopyramide
	Ib	Slight reduction in refractory period, slows AP conduction	VT	Lidocaine, mexiletine
	Ic	Slows AP conduction but prolongs AP duration at high heart rates — wider QRS	SVT, AF, A flutter, VT	Propafenone, flecainide (also IVb)
	Id	Prolonged AP recovery	Angina and VT	Ranolazine
II		*Autonomic inhibitors and activators*		
	IIa	Non-selective β and selective β-1 adrenergic receptor inhibition	Atrial tachycardias, long QT syndrome	Non-selective β-blockers (propranolol, carvedilol), selective β-1 (atenolol, bisoprolol, etc.)
	IIb	Non-selective β-adrenergic receptor inhibition	CHB with fast ventricular escape rhythm	Isoproterenol
	IIc	Muscarinic M2 receptor inhibition	Bradycardia	Atropine, hyoscine
	IId	Muscarinic M2 receptor activators	Sinus tachycardia or SVT	Digoxin, pilocarpine
	IIe	Adenosine A1 receptor activators	SVT, AV nodal tachycardia	Adenosine, aminophylline
III		*K^+ channel-mediated*		
	IIIa	Voltage-dependent K^+ channel blockers	VT, tachycardia with WPW, AF	Amiodarone, dronedarone, sotalol, ibutilide
	IIIb	Metabolically dependent K^+ channel openers	Stable angina	Nicorandil
	IIIc	Transmitter-dependent K^+ channel blockers	Nil yet	In development
IV		*Ca^{2+} channel-mediated*		
	IVa	Surface membrane Ca^{2+} channel blockers	Angina, SVT, AF	Verapamil, diltiazem
	IVb	Intracellular Ca^{2+} channel blockers	Polymorphic VT	Flecainide, propafenone (also Ic)
	IVc–e	Drugs in development		
V		*Mechanosensitive channel blockers*		In development
VI		*Gap junction channel blockers*		In development
VII		*Upstream target modulators*		ACE inhibitors, ARBs, statins

References
1. Lei M, Wu L, Terrar DA, Huang CL-H. Modernized classification of cardiac antiarrhythmic drugs. *Circulation* 2018; 138(17): 1879–96.

● Answer 31: c

The European Society for Clinical Nutrition and Metabolism (ESPEN) issued updated guidance for nutrition in critical care patients in 2023. This recommended that medical nutrition therapy should be considered for all patients in the ICU (or likely to be in the ICU) for more than 48 hours due to the risk of malnutrition. If 70% or more of dietary needs can be met with oral nutrition then this can be the sole route of nutrition; if less, then nutrition will require supplementation. If oral intake is not possible, early enteral nutrition (EN) in the form of nasogastric (NG) feeding should be initiated within 48 hours of admission. Patients with the following conditions should receive early EN (assuming no contraindications — see below): receiving ECMO, traumatic brain injury, stroke, severe acute pancreatitis, post-GI surgery including abdominal aortic surgery, patients with an open abdomen, patients on neuromuscular blockade infusion, patients in the prone position and patients with diarrhoea.

EN should be delayed in the following patient groups: uncontrolled shock with poor tissue perfusion (can be started once shock is controlled), uncontrolled life-threatening hypoxia, hypercapnia or acidosis, patients with active upper GI bleeding, overt bowel ischaemia, high-output intestinal fistula (if feeding distal to the fistula cannot be delivered), abdominal compartment syndrome and gastric aspirate volumes over 500ml in 6 hours.

EN should be started at a lower dose in the following groups: therapeutic hypothermia (dose can be increased after rewarming), intra-abdominal hypertension but no compartment syndrome (unless EN is further increasing abdominal pressure) and acute liver failure.

Patients who cannot have EN should have parenteral nutrition (PN) implemented within 3 to 7 days of admission and PN should not be started until all reasonable efforts to establish EN have been undertaken. Early PN is indicated if a patient cannot have EN and is severely malnourished. EN should be delivered via a NG tube unless the patient is deemed to be at high risk of aspiration or if there is intolerance to gastric feeding (for example, in pancreatitis) when post-pylori feeding via a nasojejunal tube is indicated.

References

1. Singer P, Blaser AR, Berger MM, et al. ESPEN practical and partially revised guideline: Clinical nutrition in the intensive care unit. *Clin Nutr* 2023; 42(9): 1671—89.

Answer 32: e

Invasive candidiasis (IC) is the most common invasive fungal infection and accounts for over 60% of invasive fungal disease within the ICU. It is associated with a mortality of above 50%. Diagnosis is made via multiple positive cultures from normally sterile sites. Other diagnostic methods include *Candida* PCR testing of samples, mannan antigen and anti-mannan antibody testing, β-d-Glucan testing of bronchoalveolar lavage (BAL) or serum (not specific to *Candida*) and the use of scoring systems (typically more accurate for ruling out IC than confirming its presence).

Several factors are known to increase the risk of invasive candidiasis. The risk factors with the strongest association with the occurrence of candidaemia are prolonged antibiotic use of greater than 7 days (odds ratio OR of 47.5), prolonged ICU stay (OR 13.35), multifocal colonisation (OR 14.68), clinical sepsis (OR 8.11), recent abdominal surgery, especially if associated with an anastomotic leak (OR 7.37) and previous hospitalisation within 30 days (OR 4.11). Other risk factors include mechanical ventilation, urinary catheter insertion, use of TPN, central venous catheter placement (including PICC), steroid use, haemodialysis, pancreatitis, haematological malignancy, stem cell transplant and neutropenia.

Treatment is typically with an echinocandin such as anidulafungin, as fluconazole is ineffective in invasive candidal infection.

References

1. Gupta P, Gupta P, Chatterjee B, et al. Evaluation of *Candida* scoring systems to predict early candidemia: a prospective and observational study at a tertiary care hospital, Uttarakhand. *Indian J Crit Care Med* 2017; 21(12): 830–5.

2. Carr A. Fungal infections. In: Bersten AD, Handy JM, Eds. *Oh's intensive care manual*, 8th ed. London: Elsevier; 2018: chapter 73: pp. 866–75.
3. CDC Clinical overview of invasive candidiasis, 2024. Available at: https://www.cdc.gov/candidiasis/hcp/clinical-overview/index.html.

● Answer 33: b

Encephalitis is infection or inflammation of brain parenchyma which leads to focal neurological signs or an altered conscious level. It typically presents with fever, altered mental state, headache and seizures. An underlying cause is only identified in around 50% of cases, with viral infection the most common aetiology. Certain clinical patterns and imaging findings may be suggestive of different causative viruses in encephalitis. Examples of associated clinical findings include:

- Parotitis with mumps encephalitis.
- Flaccid paralysis evolving into encephalitis with West Nile virus.
- Hydrophobia and aerophobia with encephalitic rabies.
- Dermatomal pattern vesicles with varicella zoster.

Imaging findings (typically on MRI) that may suggest the underlying pathogen include:

- Temporal lobe involvement with the herpes simplex virus (can occur with other herpes viruses).
- Thalamus or basal ganglia involvement in Creutzfeldt-Jakob disease (CJD), tuberculosis and arboviruses (includes West Nile virus).
- Hydrocephalus suggests a non-viral aetiology.
- Multifocal supratentorial white matter lesions with post-infectious encephalitis.

Non-viral causes of encephalitis can be bacterial (*Neisseria meningitidis*, syphilis, *Listeria*, Leptospirosis, *Streptococcus pneumoniae*, typhoid), fungal (*Cryptococcus*, *Coccidioides*, *Histoplasma*, *Blastomycosis*, *Candida*), parasitic (*Toxoplasma gondii*, *Plasmodium falciparum* malaria, schistosomiasis), prion disease (CJD) or paraneoplastic and autoimmune (for more information see page 314, Paper 4, Q10).

Treatment is predominantly supportive but does also typically involve acyclovir initially due to the frequency of HSV infection as the cause of encephalitis. Once a causative agent is identified, other specific treatments (e.g. immune modulation for autoimmune encephalitis) may be indicated.

References

1. bestpractice.bmj.com. Encephalitis — symptoms, diagnosis and treatment. BMJ Best Practice, 2025. Available at: https://bestpractice.bmj.com/topics/en-gb/436.
2. www.uptodate.com. Viral encephalitis in adults. UpToDate, 2025. Available at: https://www.uptodate.com/contents/viral-encephalitis-in-adults.

Answer 34: a

Delirium is very common in ICU populations and is an independent predictor of morbidity (including long-term cognitive decline) and mortality. It is defined as an acute change in mental state with a fluctuating course, associated with inattention, reduced awareness and disorganised thinking. It is categorised as hypoactive (withdrawn with severe inattention), hyperactive (agitation, paranoid thinking, hallucinations) and mixed. The most common subtype is hypoactive delirium which is often unrecognised or misdiagnosed as depression. Hyperactive delirium is the least common subtype but most recognisable so is much more likely to be diagnosed and treated. Most intensive care units now include delirium screening as part of their daily patient reviews to improve recognition and treatment. A number of screening scores exist; a commonly used one is the CAM-ICU (Confusion Assessment Method for the Intensive Care Unit) which uses a four-stage approach looking at mental status, inattention, level of consciousness and disordered thinking to screen for delirium.

Risk factors for delirium can be divided into predisposing pre-existing patient factors (such as age >65, cognitive impairment, dementia, depression, liver impairment, long-term institutionalisation) and precipitating or casual factors (infection, anticholinergics, opiates, pain, polypharmacy, sleep disturbance, use of physical restraints, increased severity of illness).

The prevention and management of delirium should primarily focus on non-pharmacological interventions such as modification of possible precipitants (treatment of underlying disease, minimising polypharmacy, multimodal analgesia, etc.) and reorientation and protection of the patient's sleep-wake cycle. If this management approach is unsuccessful and the patient is a risk to themselves (typically with hyperactive or mixed delirium), pharmacological management options should be considered and include:

- Typical antipsychotics: haloperidol is a mainstay of delirium management in the ICU. It may result in QTc prolongation, autonomic effects and extrapyramidal effects and should be avoided in Parkinson's disease or patients with a traumatic brain injury (can result in worse cognitive outcomes).
- Atypical antipsychotics: olanzapine, quetiapine, risperidone may all be considered and have a lower incidence of extrapyramidal side effects. Olanzapine is the agent of choice for patients with traumatic brain injury. Quetiapine and risperidone are preferred in patients with dementia.
- α-2 agonists: clonidine and dexmedetomidine may spare the use of other sedative agents and are often used to help reduce other sedative infusions and substance withdrawal management (e.g. nicotine, recreational drugs).
- Benzodiazepines: may precipitate or worsen agitation with delirium so are reserved for use in patients with dangerous agitation where rapid tranquilisation is required to maintain the safety of the patient or staff. The exception to this is alcohol withdrawal where longer-acting oral benzodiazepines (e.g. chlordiazepoxide) are indicated in alcohol withdrawal without significant liver impairment, delirium or dementia. If patients cannot tolerate oral medication, or have significant liver impairment, delirium or dementia, then a shorter-acting agent such as lorazepam is preferred.

Encouraging sleeping at night is an important part of delirium management, and sedating antidepressants such as trazodone and mirtazapine may be used in this setting. Low-dose haloperidol may be helpful but benzodiazepines and other GABAnergic agents are not recommended.

Non-pharmacological measures are key in the management of hypoactive delirium, particularly the minimisation of polypharmacy and agents that suppress the central nervous system. Haloperidol can be used in patients with very distressing hallucinations but should be avoided otherwise.

References

1. Bourne R, Borthwick M. Neurological disorders: delirium. In: Waldmann C, Rhodes A, Soni N, Handy J, Eds. *Oxford desk reference: critical care*, 2nd ed. Oxford: Oxford University Press; 2019: chapter 23: pp. 394–6.
2. Vizcaychipi MP, Farag M, Watson E. Delirium. In: Bersten AD, Handy JM, Eds. *Oh's intensive care manual*, 8th ed. London: Elsevier; 2018: chapter 56: pp. 697–703.
3. Roberson SW, Patel MB, Dabrowski W, *et al*. Challenges of delirium management in patients with traumatic brain injury: from pathophysiology to clinical practice. *Curr Neuropharmacol* 2021; 19(9): 1519–44.
4. bestpractice.bmj.com. Alcohol withdrawal — symptoms, diagnosis and treatment. BMJ Best Practice, 2023. Available at: https://bestpractice.bmj.com/topics/en-gb/3000096.

Answer 35: c

Magnesium is a chemical element that has a very broad range of therapeutic indications and is available in a variety of formulations (as different magnesium salts) for different functions. When given orally it is useful for both acid reflux and for the management of constipation and can also be used for the correction of magnesium deficiency.

The most widely used formulation for intravenous administration is magnesium sulphate, with 1g equating to 4mmol of magnesium. It can be used for the following indications:

- Acute severe asthma (and life-threatening asthma): 1.2–2g given over 20 minutes in adults, and 40mg/kg up to 2g in children over 20 minutes.
- Prevention or management of eclamptic seizures: 4g loading dose over 5–15 minutes, followed by an infusion of 1g/hr for 24 hours; in the context of additional seizures occurring give a further 2–4g over 5–15 minutes.
- Treatment of torsade de pointes: 2g given over 10–15 minutes repeated once if needed.

- Neuroprotection of neonate in preterm labour: 4g given over 15 minutes then 1g/hr until birth or 24 hours whichever is sooner.
- Atrial fibrillation: magnesium is commonly given for atrial fibrillation in critically ill patients, often as an adjunct to other strategies and has been shown to be effective. See page 415, Paper 5, Q7 for more information.
- Correction of hypomagnesaemia: the dose varies based on the severity of the hypomagnesaemia, typically given 10–20mmols at a time.
- Postoperative pain: there is evidence that suggests it may be helpful for the reduction in postoperative pain as part of a multimodal approach.

In patients receiving therapeutic magnesium infusions (not for replacement), for example, in pre-eclampsia, levels should be measured every 6–8 hours. A magnesium level up to 4mmol/L is unlikely to cause significant toxicity. At a level of 4–5mmol/L, loss of patellar reflexes may be seen, 5–7.5mmol/L can be associated with respiratory depression and respiratory paralysis and at a level above 12.5mmol/L, cardiac arrest may occur.

References

1. National Institute for Health and Care Excellence (NICE); British National Formulary (BNF). Magnesium sulfate, 2022. Available at: https://bnf.nice.org.uk/drugs/magnesium-sulfate/.
2. Choi GJ, Kim YI, Koo YH, et al. Perioperative magnesium for postoperative analgesia: an umbrella review of systematic reviews and updated meta-analysis of randomized controlled trials. *J Pers Med* 2021; 11(12): 1273.
3. Hicks MA, Tyagi A. Magnesium sulfate. StatPearls [Internet]; 2023. Available at: https://www.ncbi.nlm.nih.gov/books/NBK554553/.

Answer 36: b

Human immunodeficiency virus (HIV) is a retrovirus that is transmitted through sexual intercourse, exposure to infected blood or vertical transmission from mother to baby. It carries a reverse transcriptase enzyme that allows it to be incorporated into the host's DNA. There are two variants,

HIV1 and 2, with HIV1 having a faster progression to AIDS and causing the most infections worldwide. HIV2 leads to lower levels of viraemia, a slower decline in CD4 count, a higher incidence in West Africa and areas with historic ties to West Africa.

The stages of infection (without treatment) are as follows:

- Primary infection, where up to 60% of people will be asymptomatic; those who are symptomatic may have fever, myalgia, lymphadenopathy, rash, meningoencephalitis. This stage encompasses from exposure to around 10–12 weeks post-exposure and includes seroconversion which is the development of detectable antibodies against the HIV antigens. The patient's viral load will peak during this stage typically at around 3–6 weeks, and at this stage positive patients are highly infectious but likely asymptomatic.
- Early HIV infection, where the CD4 count is typically over 500 cells/µL. This is often asymptomatic and can be defined as the latent period. This period can last anywhere up to 10 years (and occasionally longer).
- Intermediate infection is a CD4 count of between 200–500 cells/µL. If patients develop an acquired immunodeficiency syndrome (AIDS)-defining illness during this stage, they will be considered to have AIDS. If they do not develop an AIDS-defining illness they would be considered to have chronic HIV infection.
- Advanced HIV disease is defined in persons living with HIV with a CD4 cell count of <200 cells/mm^3 or presenting with a WHO stage 3/4* AIDS-defining illness. If a patient achieves immune reconstitution with treatment (CD4 >200 cells/µL) and they have no AIDS-defining illnesses, then they no longer are defined as having AIDS.
- AIDS-defining illnesses are opportunistic illnesses (infections and malignancies) that occur more frequently or severely due to immunosuppression. Examples include *Pneumocystis jirovecii* pneumonia (PJP), oesophageal candidiasis, recurrent bacterial infections, extrapulmonary tuberculosis, Kaposi's sarcoma, cerebral toxoplasmosis, invasive cervical carcinoma, disseminated non-tuberculous mycobacterial infection amongst others.

SBA Paper 5: Answers

Admission to critical care is most commonly due to respiratory failure, either from HIV-related causes such as PJP, or other non-HIV-related illness such as COPD and asthma in HIV-positive patients. Patients can be admitted for problems directly caused by immunodeficiency, from indirect complications of HIV such as complications from treatment, or for problems unrelated to HIV such as trauma, poisoning or post-surgery.

* WHO clinical staging of HIV/AIDS is for patients with confirmed HIV infection. It consists of grades 1–4, and each clinical stage contains certain conditions, for example, herpes zoster would be within clinical stage 2, oral hairy leukoplakia in stage 3 and PJP in stage 4.

References

1. Padiglione A, McGloughlin S. Human immunodeficiency virus/acquired immunodeficiency syndrome and the intensive care unit. In: Bersten AD, Handy JM, Eds. *Oh's intensive care manual*, 8th ed. London: Elsevier; 2018: chapter 69: pp. 830–5.
2. Burtle D, Marsh S, Matin N. Update on the management of patients with HIV infection in anaesthesia and critical care. *BJA Educ* 2023; 23(7): 264–72.
3. www.uptodate.com. The natural history and clinical features of HIV infection in adults and adolescents. UpToDate, 2023. Available at: https://www.uptodate.com/contents/the-natural-history-and-clinical-features-of-hiv-infection-in-adults-and-adolescents.
4. World Health Organization. Guidelines for managing advanced HIV disease and rapid initiation of antiretroviral therapy, 2017. Available at: https://iris.who.int/bitstream/handle/10665/255884/9789241550062-eng.pdf?sequence=1.

● Answer 37: e

The Resuscitation Council of the United Kingdom has an algorithm for the management of patients with bradycardia (Figure 5.2). The definition of shock is a BP <90mmHg, pallor, cold extremities, confusion or impaired consciousness. Myocardial ischaemia can be identified by the presence of typical ischaemic chest pain or evidence of ischaemia on a 12-lead ECG.

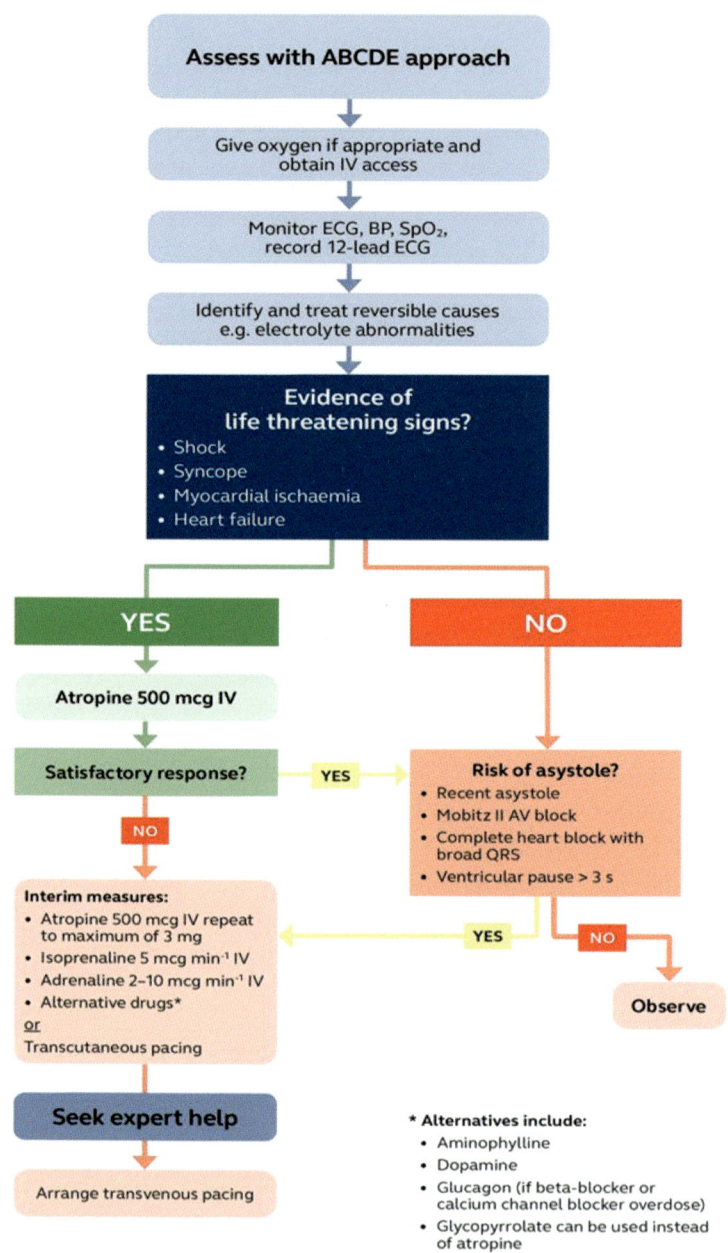

Figure 5.2. ALS bradycardia algorithm (with pulse). *Reproduced with permission from the Resuscitation Council UK.*

SBA Paper 5: Answers

● Answer 38: c

Cardiomyopathies are a heterogenous group of diseases characterised by structurally and functionally abnormal heart muscle in the absence of coronary artery disease, hypertension, valve disease and congenital heart disease which causes reduced cardiac function. Aetiology may be genetic or acquired and may be primary or secondary to a systemic disorder (such as sarcoid).

Cardiomyopathy is typically categorised based on phenotype, and whilst this presents the causes as separate entities, a patient may have a cardiomyopathy of mixed phenotype:

- Hypertrophic cardiomyopathy: increased left ventricle (LV) wall thickness (with or without increase in right ventricle [RV] wall thickness) that is not caused by abnormal loading of the heart. It is the most common inherited cardiomyopathy and has autosomal dominant inheritance. Hypertrophic obstructive cardiomyopathy occurs in 70% of patients. It predominantly causes diastolic dysfunction of the LV. Management focuses on maintaining sinus rhythm, keeping the heart rate slow to maximise diastolic filling time and in certain patients insertion of an implantable cardioverter defibrillator (ICD).
- Dilated cardiomyopathy (DCM): LV dilatation associated with a reduction in systolic function in the absence of abnormal loading of the heart (hypertension, valve disease, etc.). It is a common cause of arrhythmias and heart failure in young patients. Around two thirds of cases are idiopathic; other causes include post-viral, alcohol excess, neuromuscular disease, inborn errors of metabolism and genetic causes. Management is as for heart failure with the use of ACE inhibitors, diuretics, beta-blockers, pacing and ICD insertion. Heart transplantation may be considered in patients who can't be stabilised by medical therapy alone.
- Restrictive cardiomyopathy: restriction in LV and or RV function associated with normal or reduced diastolic volumes, normal or reduced systolic volumes and normal wall thickness. It is typically caused by infiltration or fibrosis of the myocardium, which can either be idiopathic or secondary to conditions such as sarcoidosis, haemochromatosis and amyloidosis. Systolic function is normal in early

stages of the disease, but diastole is impaired. Management focuses on maintenance of sinus rhythm, keeping the heart rate slow to optimise diastolic filling and patients may need an ICD.
- Arrhythmogenic right ventricle cardiomyopathy (ARVC): structural abnormalities (fibro-fatty replacement of cardiac myocytes) of the right ventricle associated with impaired function and arrhythmias originating in the RV. The LV can sometimes be involved. It is a genetic condition and is the cause of around 20% of sudden cardiac deaths in young people. Management is by pharmacological and electrical prevention of arrhythmias.
- Non-dilated left ventricular cardiomyopathy: patients have isolated LV dysfunction, and/or non-ischaemic scarring or fatty infiltration.
- Peripartum cardiomyopathy: patients present with severe heart failure during the third trimester or up to 6 months postpartum. It is usually a diagnosis of exclusion. Risk factors include pre-eclampsia, advanced age, multiple pregnancies, Afro-Caribbean ethnicity.
- Takotsubo syndrome: this is not a cardiomyopathy due to its transient nature, although sometimes it is referred to as stress cardiomyopathy. Classically there is transient apical LV ballooning with regional systolic dysfunction typically after a period of intense emotional stress.

References
1. Arbelo E, Protonotarios A, Gimeno JR, et al. 2023 ESC guidelines for the management of cardiomyopathies. *Eur Heart J* 2023; 44(37): 3503–626.
2. Ibrahim R, Sharkma V. Cardiomyopathy and anaesthesia. *BJA Educ* 2017; 17(11): 363–9.

Answer 39: b
When transferring a patient, part of the preparation includes checking all the equipment and ensuring you have a reliable power supply and an adequate amount of oxygen. Most transport ventilators display the amount of oxygen they are using per minute, but if not calculate the patient's oxygen usage, which then needs multiplying by double the time expected for transfer (to allow for increases in oxygen requirement during the journey or delays in the transfer).

Oxygen required for transfer = [(FiO$_2$ x minute ventilation L/min) + driving flow L/min] x [duration of transfer in minutes x 2].

In this patient, volume of oxygen required = [(0.5 x 10) + 2] x [30 x 2] = 7 x 60 = 420L.

A size D cylinder contains 340L of oxygen and an ambulance normally contains a large-capacity cylinder, but it is always wise to take as much oxygen as needed in cylinders in case the ambulance cylinder is running low.

References
1. Batchelor A. Intensive care unit organization and management: transfer of the critically ill patient. In: Waldmann C, Rhodes A, Soni N, Handy J, Eds. *Oxford desk reference: critical care*, 2nd ed. Oxford: Oxford University Press; 2019: chapter 34: pp. 622–4.

Answer 40: d

Local anaesthetics (LAs) work by passing through the phospholipid membrane of a nerve cell in its unionised lipophilic form. Inside the cell it is ionised and binds to the Na$^+$ channel preventing Na$^+$ influx into the cell and thus depolarisation. The potency of a local anaesthetic is related to its lipid solubility, the duration of action associated with the degree of protein binding and the onset of action related to the pKa (local anaesthetics are weak bases and so are mainly ionised at physiological pH — the higher the pKa the higher the proportion of ionised LA and the slower the onset).

Local anaesthetics can be esters (cocaine, procaine) or amides (lidocaine, bupivacaine, ropivacaine). Typically, amide LAs are used for regional anaesthesia such as epidurals, nerve blocks and wound catheters.

Lidocaine is a fast-onset LA with a moderate length of action. Within critical care it is used for anaesthetising the skin for procedures such as central lines and tracheostomies, and it is also used as an antiarrhythmic. It is rapidly metabolised by the liver, and the toxic dose depends on the route, but is typically 3mg/kg plain, and 7mg/kg when mixed with adrenaline.

Bupivacaine is a moderate-onset long-acting LA. It is available in 0.25% and 0.5% concentrations; these contain 2.5mg/ml and 5mg/ml, respectively. Within critical care it is commonly used for regional anaesthesia. The toxic dose is 2mg/kg, which when given as an infusion should not be given in less than 4 hours, so a maximum of 2mg/kg every 4 hours (to allow for metabolism). The S-enantiomer of bupivacaine is called levobupivacaine which is commonly used as it is less cardiotoxic. The maximum dose of levobupivacaine is 150mg as a single dose and 400mg over 24 hours (but often the dose of 2mg/kg is also used).

This patient is 50kg and hence the maximum safe dose is 100mg of bupivacaine, which would be 20ml of 0.5% or 40ml of 0.25%. You would not typically use lidocaine in this situation, but the maximum dose would be 150mg, which would be 15ml of 1% (as this is 10mg/ml).

References
1. Peck T, Hill A, Willliam M. *Pharmacology for anaesthesia and intensive care*, 3rd ed. Cambridge: Cambridge University Press; 2010.

● Answer 41: a

Acute coronary syndromes include ST-elevation myocardial infarction (STEMI), non-ST-elevation myocardial infarction (NSTEMI) (associated with a troponin rise) and unstable angina (no troponin rise).

The Universal Definition of Myocardial Infarction is:

- Type 1: acute atherothrombotic coronary artery disease precipitated by plaque disruption.
- Type 2: due to mismatch between oxygen supply and demand, e.g. vasospasm, sepsis, dissection, shock.
- Type 3: typical MI but patient dies prior to troponin being measured.
- Type 4a: due to PCI (troponin needs to be 5x normal to diagnose).
- Type 4b: stent thrombosis (standard troponin levels for diagnosis).
- Type 5: due to coronary artery bypass grafting — troponin 10x normal for diagnosis.

STEMI*: ST elevation of more than 1mm in two contiguous leads, except V2 V3 where — >2mm in men over 40 or >2.5mm under 40 and >1.5mm in women any age.

Management (based on NICE guidance): if presentation to the hospital is within 12 hours of symptom onset, then percutaneous coronary intervention

(PCI) should be undertaken within 90 minutes at an appropriate centre, or within 120 minutes of when thrombolysis could have been given at a non-PCI capable hospital. PCI should be considered if presenting after 12 hours of symptom onset but with evidence of ongoing chest pain. If a patient has had fibrinolysis but less than 50% resolution of ST elevation 60–90 minutes later, then rescue PCI should be considered.

NSTEMI and unstable angina management: PCI as soon as possible, within 24 hours if unstable (having had an out-of-hospital cardiac arrest, or in cardiogenic shock). Undertake the GRACE (Global Registry of Acute Coronary Events) calculator to assess the risk of further cardiovascular events, which guides onward management.

If there is an intermediate or a high risk on the GRACE calculator (mortality 3–9%) then PCI should be undertaken within 72 hours.

If there is a very high risk on the GRACE calculator (mortality >9%) then PCI should be undertaken within 2 hours.

All ACS patients should be loaded with aspirin and a P2Y12 receptor inhibitor such as ticagrelor or prasugrel; clopidogrel is less effective and should only be used if the others are not available or contraindicated. The need for an additional anticoagulant should be reviewed — typically bivalirudin for PCI or fondaparinux if PCI is not planned in the next 24 hours.

* It is likely that over the next few years we will be shifting to a different way of classifying MI as occlusive MI (OMI) and non-occlusive MI (NOMI). This is due to the limitations in the current classification which uses 'STEMI' as a marker for requiring revascularisation; however 25% of NSTEMI patients have acute coronary occlusion and delayed reperfusion in the group leads to higher mortality.

References
1. Byrne RA, Rossello X, Coughlan JJ, et al. 2023 ESC guidelines for the management of acute coronary syndromes. *Eur Heart J* 2023; 44(38): 3720–826.
2. National Institute for Health and Care Excellence (NICE), guideline NG185. Acute coronary syndromes, 2020. Available at: https://www.nice.org.uk/guidance/ng185/resources/acute-coronary-syndromes-pdf-66142023361477.

3. McLaren J, de Alencar JN, Aslanger EK, et al. From ST-segment elevation MI to occlusion MI: the new paradigm shift in acute myocardial infarction. *JACC Adv* 2024; 3(11): 101314.
4. Thygesen K, Alpert JS, Jaffe AS, et al. Executive Group on behalf of the Joint European Society of Cardiology (ESC)/American College of Cardiology (ACC)/American Heart Association (AHA)/World Heart Federation (WHF) Task Force for the Universal Definition of Myocardial Infarction. Fourth Universal Definition of Myocardial Infarction. *Circulation* 2018; 138(20): e618–51.

Answer 42: e

Shock is a pathological state in which there is insufficient delivery of oxygen and nutrients to the tissues, resulting in tissue hypoxia and potentially multi-organ failure and death. It is identified using findings from clinical examination and bloods tests, with the presence of hypotension (typically <90mmHg systolic), alteration in mental status due to brain hypoperfusion, oliguria and hyperlactataemia.

Shock is classified based on the pathophysiological mechanism:

- Hypovolaemic: depletion of the vascular reservoir, due to a sudden and profound reduction in blood volume due to major bleeding or over a longer period, for example, in the case of severe dehydration often secondary to diarrhoea and vomiting. In addition to the signs from the underlying cause, patients will have a prolonged capillary refill time (CRT), vasoconstriction with a high systemic vascular resistance (SVR) and low filling pressures. Management is with refilling of the intravascular volume, with blood products if the cause is bleeding and with balanced crystalloids if the cause is dehydration.
- Cardiogenic: due to failure of the heart to provide adequate cardiac output, either from pump failure or significant valve dysfunction. Causes for pump failure include cardiomyopathy, myocardial infarction, cardiac stunning (after MI or trauma), and sepsis (typically in combination with distributive shock). Patients will typically be very cool peripherally, with a raised JVP and a very low cardiac output on cardiac output monitoring. Management is with treatment of the underlying cause (for example, PCI in the case of MI) and then with pharmacological (inotropes) or mechanical (intra-aortic balloon pump, ECMO) cardiac support.
- Distributive: a combination of vasodilation causing reduction of blood flow to the organs and capillary leak, meaning fluid redistributes into the extravascular space giving intravascular hypovolaemia. This is the

type of shock seen in anaphylaxis and in sepsis and capillary leak syndrome. Patients will present with warm vasodilated peripheries, a normal or high cardiac output and evidence of reduced preload but failure or incomplete response to fluid boluses. Management is by treatment of the underlying cause and the use of fluid plus vasopressors to reverse the vasodilation.
- Obstructive shock: caused by obstruction of blood outflow from either the right or the left side of the heart (or both). The common causes include massive pulmonary embolus (PE) and cardiac tamponade. The patient presents with cool vasoconstricted peripheries, a dilated JVP and may have pulsus paradoxus. ECHO imaging is very useful in diagnosing obstructive shock and the likely cause. Management is with treatment of the underlying cause: thrombolysis or thrombectomy for PE and pericardiocentesis or surgery for cardiac tamponade.
- Neurogenic shock: injury to the cervical spinal cord can result in disruption of sympathetic outflow (sympathetic chain is T1–L2/3). Subsequent unopposed parasympathetic action leads to a picture of bradycardia and hypotension, due to vasodilation. Although this is predominantly seen in C-spine injuries, any injury above T6 can result in neurogenic shock. Causes other than injury include spinal anaesthesia ('high spinal' block), Guillain-Barré syndrome and neuropathies of the cervical and upper thoracic spinal cord. Management includes fluid resuscitation followed by vasopressors (ideally ones with a degree of β activity such as noradrenaline to avoid worsening bradycardia) along with management of the underlying injury/illness.

References

1. Day J, Voga G, Webster NR, *et al.* Shock. In: Waldmann C, Rhodes A, Soni N, Handy J, Eds. *Oxford desk reference: critical care*, 2nd ed. Oxford: Oxford University Press; 2019: chapter 27: pp. 490–501.
2. Dave S, Dahlstrom JJ, Weisbrod LJ. Neurogenic shock. StatPearls [Internet]; 2023. Available at: https://www.ncbi.nlm.nih.gov/books/NBK459361/.

● Answer 43: b

Cardiopulmonary exercise testing (CPET) is a reliable and objective way of testing patients' functional capacity, to help assess the likelihood of perioperative complications.

The patient has continuous 12-lead ECG monitoring (with ST segment analysis), oxygen saturation monitoring, non-invasive blood pressure and a closed breathing system allowing analysis of gas flows and volumes breath by breath. An exercise programme is then undertaken which consists of either cycling on a bike or using an arm bike, the work of which is then calculated based on the patient's height, weight, age and sex. This data is displayed in a nine-panel plot from which a variety of variables are calculated.

Not all patients are safe to undertake a CPET. Some absolute contraindications include patients with recent or active myocardial ischaemia, severe symptomatic valve disease, uncontrolled asthma, saturations on air of <85%, acute pulmonary embolus and uncontrolled heart failure.

The test begins with 3 minutes of baseline recording followed by unloaded pedalling for 3 minutes, and then a gradual increase in load at a predetermined rate until either the patient has to stop due to symptoms or fatigue or 100% of the work requirement is reached.

Ideally the patient would achieve maximal effort which will give accurate derived values of the anaerobic threshold (AT) and VO_{2peak} (VO_2 being oxygen consumption). Maximal effort is defined as: achieving >80% of predicted work in watts, achieving a HR of >80% predicted maximum (220 − age), achieving a respiratory exchange ratio (RER = VCO_2/VO_2) of >1.15. Patients may not reach maximal effort due to hypotension, arrhythmias, leg claudication, ST-segment depression, cardiac chest pain or fatigue.

There are many values and assessments that can be made from the nine-panel plot; however, for non-experts the two that are most useful are the AT and the VO_{2peak}:

- AT: this assesses the combined efficiency of the lungs, heart and circulation. As you exercise there is a point at which oxygen demand will exceed supply; at this point the muscle cells will start to produce ATP anaerobically, the anaerobic threshold. This produces lactate which is then buffered by bicarbonate resulting in increased CO_2 production, so the AT is the VO_2 at the point where the VCO_2 curve exceeds the VO_2 curve. The anaerobic threshold is usually reached around halfway through the test and will not vary with patient effort so is a reliable measure of a patient's functional capacity. An AT of under 11ml/kg/min is typically used as a trigger to consider postoperative critical care.

- VO_{2peak}: The VO_2 is equal to the cardiac output multiplied by the arterial-mixed venous oxygen difference and the maximum value achieved is the peak; this is effort-dependent so can vary depending on how hard the patient is pushing themselves during the test. This figure can also be improved by exercise, and there is growing interest in 'prehabilitation' or exercise training prior to surgery. There is not a fixed value for VO_{2peak} that is used as a cut-off for surgery or critical care admission and different hospitals will have specific protocols, for example, a VO_{2peak} of <20ml/kg/min in a patient undergoing elective abdominal aortic aneurysm surgery is associated with a higher mortality and postoperative complication rate.

References
1. Chambers DJ, Wisely NA. Cardiopulmonary exercise testing — a beginner's guide to the nine-panel plot. *BJA Educ* 2019; 19(5): 158–64.
2. Agnew N. Preoperative cardiopulmonary exercise testing. *Contin Educ Anaesth Crit Care Pain* 2010; 10(2): 33–7.

● Answer 44: b

Hepatorenal syndrome (HRS) is a complication of cirrhosis leading to functional circulatory changes in the kidney that reduce compensatory mechanisms and lead to a reduction in glomerular filtration rate. It is associated with a high morbidity and mortality.

HRS was historically defined as type 1 (rapid onset) and type 2 (refractory ascites); these terms have now been updated.

HRS-AKI (hepatorenal syndrome — acute kidney injury) has replaced type 1. It is diagnosed when there is an increase in creatinine (see stages below) in a patient with cirrhosis with ascites; there is no response to stopping diuretics and 2 days albumin therapy (1g/kg/day). There is absence of shock, no recent nephrotoxins and no signs of structural kidney injury. It is unusual for HRS-AKI to occur unprecipitated; common triggers include spontaneous bacterial peritonitis (SBP) and other infections and large-volume paracentesis (without albumin administration).

The staging of AKI within HRS-AKI is as follows:

- Stage 1: increase in creatinine by 26.5μmol/L or doubling from baseline, 1a creatinine <132μmol/L, 1b ≥132μmol/L.
- Stage 2: increase in serum creatinine 2–3 times baseline.
- Stage 3: increase in serum creatinine at least 3 times baseline or creatinine ≥353μmol/L with an acute increase of ≥26.5μmol/L or initiation of RRT.

HRS-NAKI (hepatorenal syndrome — no acute kidney injury), previously HRS type 2. There are two subcategories of HRS-NAKI:

- HRS-AKD (acute kidney disease) defined as an eGFR <60ml/min/1.73m^2 for <3 months without any other cause of kidney disease or a percentage increase in serum creatinine of <50% in the last 3 months.
- HRS-CKD (chronic kidney disease) defined as an eGFR <60ml/min/1.73m^2 for ≥3 months without any other cause of kidney disease.

In HRS-AKI, albumin is used for both prevention of AKI and first-line management (in addition to treating precipitants and managing risk factors — stopping nephrotoxic drugs, beta-blockers, diuretics). Albumin at a dose of 1g/kg/day for 2 days is used for all stage 1b and above AKI and for stage 1a if treatment of the precipitant and stopping risk factor medications alone does not resolve the AKI. Albumin has a variety of therapeutic mechanisms: volume expansion, positive cardiac inotropy, antioxidant and immunomodulatory properties. If there is no improvement with 2 days of albumin, then the next step is vasoconstrictor therapy. Terlipressin is first line, but noradrenaline can be used if terlipressin is contraindicated. Third-line treatment would be octreotide with midodrine (typically used where terlipressin is not available). Transjugular intrahepatic portosystemic shunt (TIPS) is typically a treatment for refractory ascites or uncontrolled variceal bleeding; however, it is being investigated as a possible treatment for HRS-

AKI. Liver transplantation is a treatment option for HRS-AKI and may reverse the renal injury or it may be decided to consider liver and kidney transplantation. Renal replacement therapy may be indicated for the management of fluid balance, uraemia or electrolyte derangements, but it does not improve survival and should ideally only be used as a bridge to transplantation (if this is an option). Extracorporeal liver assist devices have not yet been shown to improve survival.

References

1. Simonetto DA, Gines P, Kamath PS. Hepatorenal syndrome: pathophysiology, diagnosis, and management. *BMJ* 2020; 370: m2687.
2. bestpractice.bmj.com. Hepatorenal syndrome — symptoms, diagnosis and treatment. BMJ Best Practice, 2024. Available at: https://bestpractice.bmj.com/topics/en-gb/402.

Answer 45: c

Intermittent haemodialysis (IHD) works on the principle of diffusion. Blood flows in one direction along a semi-permeable membrane and dialysate fluid flows the opposite side of the membrane in the opposite direction and solutes move down the concentration gradient from blood into the dialysate fluid, and due to them flowing in the opposite direction the concentration gradient is maintained along the length of the membrane. The blood flow rates are much higher in haemodialysis (up to 400ml/min) resulting in rapid solute (and solvent-free fluid) clearance. When the patient has very high urea or severe metabolic disturbance, a rapid speed of solute removal can cause a disequilibrium syndrome which is due to sudden shifts in intracellular water content, including in the brain. Symptoms include nausea, vomiting, headache, seizures and coma. In unstable patients (like some patients in critical care), the rapid removal of fluid can result in severe hypotension and so IHD is not typically used for patients in critical care unless they are haemodynamically stable and have a positive fluid balance.

Indications for renal replacement therapy include hyperkalaemia, metabolic acidosis, volume overload, symptomatic uraemia and toxins. Hyperkalaemia will be corrected more rapidly with IHD as supposed to continuous renal replacement therapy (CRRT), but it is an indication for both. Toxicity from toxins that are water-soluble, with low protein binding and a low molecular weight and have a small volume of distribution, can be treated with IHD or

CRRT, but IHD will be more effective and rapid at clearance. Examples include methanol (and metabolites), ethylene glycol, salicylate, theophylline and lithium. Toxbase advises IHD followed by haemodiafiltration.

References

1. Forni LG, Ronco C. Renal therapy techniques. In: Waldmann C, Rhodes A, Soni N, Handy J, Eds. *Oxford desk reference: critical care*, 2nd ed. Oxford: Oxford University Press; 2019: chapter 3: pp. 69–79.
2. www.toxbase.org. TOXBASE — the primary clinical toxicology database of the National Poisons Information Service. Poisons-index-A-Z/l-products/lithium/. Available at: https://www.toxbase.org.

● Answer 46: d

There are several mechanisms of antibiotic resistance, some which are intrinsic to the bacteria type and some which are acquired:

- Outer cell membrane: Gram-negative bacilli have three layers to their cell wall and this outer membrane is relatively efficient at preventing beta-lactam antibiotics from penetrating through to reach the penicillin-binding protein on the innermost membrane. For beta-lactams to be effective they must pass through porin protein channels, and mutations that cause a reduction in these channels can cause acquired beta-lactam resistance. The impermeable outer member explains why *Pseudomonas spp.* is resistant to many beta-lactams.
- Alteration of target site: beta-lactam antibiotics bind to penicillin-binding proteins (PDPs) on the cell surface. Bacteria can develop an alternative pathway that means the cells can continue to multiply. In the case of MRSA, the PDP has been altered to PDP2 which is not inhibited by methicillin. This is also a mechanism of resistance for *Streptococcus pneumoniae*.
- Enzyme production: bacteria can start to produce enzymes which break down the antibiotics, for example, *Staphylococcus aureus* can produce β-lactamase which breaks open the β-lactam ring in the antibiotic inactivating it. Bacteria may also express enzymes which add a chemical group to an antibiotic, which inhibits its activity, for

example, *S. aureus* and *Pseudomonas spp.* can produce an enzyme which inactivates aminoglycoside antibiotics.
- Efflux mechanisms: bacteria can acquire a protein on their cell membrane which pumps the antibiotic back out of the cell. *Escherichia coli* can become resistant to tetracyclines via this mechanism and streptococci resistant to macrolides.

Resistance mechanisms can then be transmitted between bacteria by a number of different mechanisms:

- Transformation: bacteria take up 'naked' DNA (for example, from another lysed bacteria) and incorporate it into their genes. Often the whole gene for resistance is not taken up so it may result in an antibiotic having less effect on the bacteria.
- Conjugation: this is the transfer of plasmids between different bacteria by direct contact between the bacteria. Plasmids are circular portions of DNA which carry genes and can therefore carry a gene for a resistance mechanism and transfer this between bacteria.
- Transposons: these are DNA sequences that can move position within a genome or to and from plasmids and between bacteria. They can contain the DNA for a resistance gene and transfer this to a broad range of bacteria. This is likely how resistance to methicillin is transferred between *S. aureus* bacteria.
- Bacteriophages: these are viruses that only infect bacteria, but their DNA can be incorporated and therefore they can act as a method of resistance transfer between bacteria.

References

1. Munita JM, Arias CA. Mechanisms of antibiotic resistance. *Microbiol Spectr* 2016; 4(2): 10.1128.
2. Gillespie S, Bamford K. Resistance to antibacterial agents. In: Gillespie S, Bamford K, Eds. *Medical microbiology and infection at a glance*. Oxford: Blackwell; 2004: chapter 7: pp. 20–1.
3. www.uptodate.com. Beta-lactam antibiotics: mechanisms of action and resistance and adverse effects. UpToDate, 2023. Available at: https://www.uptodate.com/contents/beta-lactam-antibiotics-mechanisms-of-action-and-resistance-and-adverse-effects.

● Answer 47: c

Anaphylaxis is a medical emergency, and early recognition and administration of adrenaline is key. Signs of anaphylaxis include unexplained hypotension, bronchospasm, tachycardia or bradycardia, angioedema, cardiac arrest without an alternative cause and urticarial rash.

Management includes stopping or removing any possible triggers; chlorhexidine is an increasing cause of anaphylaxis and so should be washed off if anaphylaxis occurs. The dose for IM adrenaline is 500μg and is the route of choice for most practitioners; for those familiar with using IV adrenaline an initial dose of 50μg IV is recommended. Steroids and antihistamines have now been taken out of the guidelines by the Resuscitation Council UK as it is felt their inclusion was delaying administration of adrenaline; however, these can be given but only after adrenaline has been administered. A fluid bolus can be given for hypotension. Adrenaline boluses can be repeated every 5 minutes; after 3 boluses an adrenaline infusion should be considered.

Causes include foodstuffs, especially in young people, such as peanuts which account for 50% of fatal anaphylaxis episodes related to food. Medications are the cause of most anaphylaxis-related deaths. The commonest medication triggers are neuromuscular blocking agents (rocuronium predominantly), antibiotics (penicillin, teicoplanin), contrast media, chemotherapy agents and chlorhexidine.

References

1. Working Group of Resuscitation Council UK. Emergency treatment of anaphylaxis — guidelines for healthcare providers, 2021. Available at: https://www.resus.org.uk/sites/default/files/2021-05/Emergency%20Treatment%20of%20Anaphylaxis%20May%202021_0.pdf.
2. anaesthetists.org. QRH_3-1_Anaphylaxis_v.5. Available at: https://anaesthetists.org/Portals/0/PDFs/QRH/QRH_3-1_Anaphylaxis_v5.pdf?ver=2022-04-12-124225-493.

● Answer 48: c

In the UK, donation of organs after circulatory death represents an ever-increasing proportion of total donors. The use of donation after circulatory death (DCD) varies around the world, but there are established programmes across Europe and in Australia and the USA. DCD donors in the UK provide an average of 2.9 transplantable organs per DCD donor, compared to 3.5 from patients who donate after brainstem death (DBD). DCD donors can donate heart, lung, kidneys, pancreas and liver.

DCD can be categorised based on the Maastricht classification:

1. Uncontrolled, dead on arrival — typically in the emergency department.
2. Uncontrolled, unsuccessful resuscitation — typically in the emergency department.
3. Controlled, cardiac arrest follows planned withdrawal of life-sustaining treatments on the ICU.
4. Either controlled or uncontrolled, cardiac arrest in a patient who has been diagnosed dead by neurological criteria on the ICU.

In the UK, donations are only from category 3; other countries such as Spain also focus on category 1 and 2 patients.

References
1. ODT Clinical — NHS Blood and Transplant. Donation after circulatory death. Available at: https://www.odt.nhs.uk/deceased-donation/best-practice-guidance/donation-after-circulatory-death/.

● Answer 49: e

Organophosphorus insecticides can be highly toxic and are easily absorbed through the skin. The organophosphates used in chemical warfare are selected out to produce the most profound toxic effects. All organophosphates act by inhibition of neuronal acetylcholinesterase (AchE), which leads to excessive acetylcholine (Ach) at autonomic, central nervous system and neuromuscular junction sites.

The effect on parasympathetic receptors (cholinergic effects) are dominant early on in poisoning and can be remembered with the acronym DUMBBELS: **D**iarrhoea, **U**rination, **M**iosis, **B**ronchorrhea/bronchospasm, **B**radycardia, **E**mesis, **L**acrimation and **S**alivation.

Central nervous system effects occur in severe poisonings and include seizures, coma and respiratory failure. Toxicity at the neuromuscular junction results in fasciculations early on, followed by weakness. Delayed-onset neuropathy can occur 1–3 weeks after ingestion resulting in a painful peripheral paraesthesia and symmetrical motor polyneuropathy causing flaccid weakness affecting distal muscles.

Due to most of these agents being highly absorbable through the skin, it is important that staff caring for these patients prior to decontamination protect themselves with appropriate PPE (full-arm water-repellent gown and gloves). Once the patient has been decontaminated then standard PPE should be used. Management focuses on A–E assessment and management, early use of 100% oxygen and intubation if indicated, in addition to specific treatments.

Patients with cholinergic signs should have atropine immediately; 600μg boluses are sufficient in mild poisoning but patients are likely to need large doses. In severe poisoning, patients should receive 3mg straight away, and the dose doubled every 5 minutes until the lungs are clear, and the heart rate is above 80/min (the patient is then 'atropinised'). The patient may need an infusion of atropine at 20% of the initial dose required, per hour.

In addition to atropine, symptomatic patients should receive pralidoxime which reactivates the acetylcholinesterase enzyme and so works on treating both nicotinic and muscarinic symptoms. Pralidoxime therefore treats neuromuscular weakness, which atropine does not. This is given as an IV loading dose followed by an infusion for several days.

Agitation should be managed with benzodiazepines, as should frequent or prolonged seizures. Patients with severe poisoning should be managed in a critical care environment.

Fomepizole is used in methanol and ethylene glycol poisoning. It is a competitive inhibitor of alcohol dehydrogenase and so prevents toxic metabolite production.

Hydroxocobalamin is a form of vitamin B12 that is used to treat cyanide poisoning.

SBA Paper 5: Answers

Naloxone is a competitive antagonist at opiate receptors and is used in opiate/opioid overdose.

References

1. Toxbase.org. TOXBASE — the primary clinical toxicology database of the National Poisons Information Service. Poisons-index-A-Z/o-products/organophosphates. Available at: https://www.toxbase.org.
2. bestpractice.bmj.com. Organophosphate poisoning — symptoms, diagnosis and treatment. BMJ Best Practice, 2024. Available at: https://bestpractice.bmj.com/topics/en-gb/852.
3. www.uptodate.com. Organophosphate and carbamate poisoning. UpToDate, 2025. Available at: https://www.uptodate.com/contents/organophosphate-and-carbamate-poisoning.

Answer 50: d

Calcium has several functions within the body including membrane excitation, clotting factor activation, muscle contraction, endocrine and exocrine organ function and structural support in both cell membranes and bone. Calcium and phosphate homeostasis is via the action of three hormones, parathyroid hormone, vitamin D and calcitonin:

- Parathyroid hormone (PTH): this is produced by the parathyroid glands (four small glands in the thyroid) in response to decreased extracellular ionised calcium and by β-adrenergic stimulation. The chief cells in the parathyroid gland release the hormone and have Ca^{2+} receptors on their cell membrane which reduce PTH production when calcium levels are increased. Parathyroid hormone acts to increase ionised plasma calcium levels and decrease plasma phosphate levels. It does this via several mechanisms: increase the rate of bone resorption (via actions on osteocytes and osteoclasts), action on the renal proximal tubule to increase calcium reabsorption and decrease phosphate reabsorption and by increased formation of 1,25-dihydroxycholecalciferol (vitamin D).
- Vitamin D: cholecalciferol (vitamin D3) is produced in the skin by exposure to UV light; this is then hydroxylated in the liver to form 25-hydroxycholecalciferol and then in the proximal nephrons of the kidney, renal 1-α-hydroxylase (stimulated by PTH) converts it to

1,25-dihydroxycholecalciferol, otherwise known as vitamin D. Vitamin D raises plasma calcium and phosphate levels by promoting absorption from the small intestine. It also acts on the bone in combination with PTH to mobilise calcium and phosphate from the bone into the blood.
- Calcitonin: this is secreted by the parafollicular or C cells in the thyroid gland, in response to an extracellular calcium level of ≥2.4mmol/L. Calcitonin reduces plasma calcium and phosphate levels by inhibition of osteoclasts and by increasing renal excretion of calcium and phosphate and inhibition of 1-α-hydroxylase, hence reducing the synthesis of vitamin D.

References

1. Power I, Kam P. *Principles of physiology for the anaesthetist*, 2nd ed. London: Hodder Arnold; 2008.
2. Yu E, Sharma S. Physiology, calcium. StatPearls [Internet]; 2023. Available at: https://www.ncbi.nlm.nih.gov/books/NBK482128/.

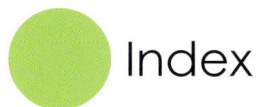 Index

A

Abdominal aortic aneurysm:
  - postoperative complications: p328, paper 4, Q20
Above cuff vocalisation: p37, paper 1, Q6
Acidosis: p426, paper 5, Q13
Action potential: p177, paper 2, Q48
Acute interstitial nephritis: p58, paper 1, Q24
Acute kidney injury:
  - classification: p218, paper 3, Q8
  - contrast-induced: p357, paper 4, Q44
  - drug alteration in AKI: p125, paper 2, Q8
Acute tubular necrosis: p34, paper 1, Q4
Adult life support:
  - after cardiac surgery: p73, paper 1, Q39
  - bradycardia: p461, paper 5, Q37
  - tachycardia: p245, paper 3, Q33
  - traumatic cardiac arrest: p226, paper 3, Q14
Alcoholic hepatitis: p337, paper 4, Q28
Alkalosis: p309, paper 4, Q7
Amniotic fluid embolism: p230, paper 3, Q18
Anaphylaxis: p476, paper 5, Q47
Antiarrhythmics: p451, paper 5, Q30
Antibiotics mechanism of action: p255, paper 3, Q42
Anticoagulants and neuraxial catheters: p258, paper 3, Q45
Antifungals: p357, paper 4, Q43
Antiplatelets: p172, paper 2, Q43
Antivirals: p156, paper 2, Q31

Aortic dissection:
- type A: p209, paper 3, Q1
- type B: p44, paper 1, Q12

ARDS:
- classification: p55, paper 1, Q21
- management: p31, paper 1, Q2

Ascites: p366, paper 4, Q50
Aspergillosis: p438, paper 5, Q20
Asthma:
- classification: p335, paper 4, Q26
- management adults: p48, paper 1, Q15
- management in paediatrics: p318, paper 4, Q13
- ventilation of: p124, paper 2, Q7

Atrial fibrillation:
- anticoagulation in: p241, paper 3, Q29
- management: p415, paper 5, Q7

B

Bacteria:
- Gram stain classification: p338, paper 4, Q29
- mechanisms of resistance: p474, paper 5, Q46
- MRSA: p266, paper 3, Q50
- PVL *Staph*: p47, paper 1, Q14

Blast injury: p77, paper 1, Q43
Blood transfusion:
- how each unit is made/stored: p343, paper 4, Q32
- special requirements (when irradiated, etc.): p162, paper 2, Q35

Botulism: p131, paper 2, Q11
Bronchopleural fistulas: p224, paper 3, Q12
Burns:
- airway burns: p304, paper 4, Q2
- assessment: p348, paper 4, Q36
- fluid management: p149, paper 2, Q26
- management: p54, paper 1, Q20 and p229, paper 3, Q17

C

Calcium: p64, paper 1, Q29 and p479, paper 5, Q50
Candida auris: p355, paper 4, Q42

Index

Capacity: p249, paper 3, Q35
Carbon monoxide: p163, paper 2, Q36
Cardiac output monitoring: p261, paper 3, Q47, p360, paper 4, Q46 and p364, paper 4, Q49
Cardiac tamponade: p413, paper 5, Q6
Cardiomyopathy: p463, paper 5, Q38
CAR T CRS: p41, paper 1, Q10
Caustic ingestion (acid/akali): p223, paper 3, Q11
Cerebral spinal fluid: p139, paper 2, Q18
Chemotherapy agents: p68, paper 1, Q34
Citrate overload: p42, paper 1, Q11
Citrate toxicity: p321, paper 4, Q15
Clostridioides difficile:
- management: p432, paper 5, Q17
- risk factors: p174, paper 2, Q45

Community-acquired pneumonia: p142, paper 2, Q21
Compartment syndrome: p63, paper 1, Q28
Constipation: p449, paper 5, Q28
CPET (cardiopulmonary exercise testing): p469, paper 5, Q43
Critical illness weakness:
- diagnosis: p323, paper 4, Q17
- risk factors: p237, paper 3, Q25

CRRT (continuous renal replacement therapy):
- access sites: p256, paper 3, Q43
- anticoagulation: p136, paper 2, Q16
- drug alteration in CRRT: p125, paper 2, Q8
- indications: p473, paper 5, Q45
- prescription: p252, paper 3, Q39

D

DAS guidelines — CICO: p168, paper 2, Q40
Data:
- distributions: p66, paper 1, Q32
- interpretation: p250, paper 3, Q36 and p444, paper 5, Q25
- outcome predictions (sensitivity and specificity): p147, paper 2, Q25

Delirium: p456, paper 5, Q34
Deprivation of Liberty Safeguards (DOLS): p234, paper 3, Q21

Diabetic ketoacidosis (DKA):
    - classification: p65, paper 1, Q30
    - management: p325, paper 4, Q18
Diarrhoea in the ICU: p254, paper 3, Q40
Direct oral anticoagulant (DOAC):
    - GI bleed management: p121, paper 2, Q4
    - mechanisms of action: p446, paper 5, Q27
Disorders of consciousness: p349, paper 4, Q37
Disseminated intravascular coagulopathy (DIC): p424, paper 5, Q12
Donation Action Framework: p171, paper 2, Q42
Drowning: p80, paper 1, Q46

E
ECG:
    - electrolyte derangement: p157, paper 2, Q32
    - long QT: p175, paper 2, Q46
Empyema management: p306, paper 4, Q4
Encephalitis:
    - autoimmune: p314, paper 4, Q10
    - infective: p455, paper 5, Q33
Encephalopathy grading: p240, paper 3, Q28
Endotoxins vs. exotoxins: p178, paper 2, Q49
Enteral nutrition: p453, paper 5, Q31
Extracorporeal membrane oxygenation (ECMO): p363, paper 4, Q48
Extubation: p52, paper 1, Q18
Eye care in the ICU: p450, paper 5, Q29

F
Fat embolism syndrome: p417, paper 5, Q8
Fire in the ICU: p167, paper 2, Q39

G
GI bleed in ICU risk factors: p315, paper 4, Q11
GPICS: p66, paper 1, Q31
Guillain-Barré syndrome:
    - aetiology: p340, paper 4, Q30
    - diagnosis: p137, paper 2, Q17

Index

H
Haemoglobinopathies: p235, paper 3, Q23
Hepatorenal syndrome: p471, paper 5, Q44
HHS (hyperglycaemic hyperosmolar state): p407, paper 5, Q3
HIT (heparin-induced thrombocytopaenia): p210, paper 3, Q2
HIV (human immunodeficiency virus):
    - diagnosis: p459, paper 5, Q36
    - treatment: p82, paper 1, Q48
HLH (haemophagocytic lymphohistiocytosis): p119, paper 2, Q3
Human herpes viruses: p332, paper 4, Q23
HUS (haemolytic uraemic syndrome): p419, paper 5, Q9
Hyperinsulinaemic euglycaemic therapy (HIET): p84, paper 1, Q50
Hypernatraemia: p329, paper 4, Q21
Hypersensitivity/allergic reactions: p72, paper 1, Q38
Hyponatraemia: p132, paper 2, Q12

I
Immune systems/immunoglobulins: p341, paper 4, Q31
Indirect calorimetry: p443, paper 5, Q24
Infective endocarditis: p238, paper 3, Q26
Intra-abdominal compartment syndrome:
    - classification: p165, paper 2, Q38
    - management: p231, paper 3, Q19
Intra-aortic balloon pump:
    - indications: p252, paper 3, Q38
    - trouble shooting: p70, paper 1, Q36
Intra-cerebral haemorrhage: p430, paper 5, Q16
Intra-cerebral pressure (ICP):
    - management of raised ICP: p46, paper 1, Q13 and p135, paper 2, Q14
Invasive candidiasis: p454, paper 5, Q32
IV immunoglobulin therapy: p81, paper 1, Q47

L
Lactate:
    - metformin-associated: p232, paper 3, Q20
    - type B2 acidosis: p336, paper 4, Q27
Legionella: p322, paper 4, Q16
Lemierre's syndrome: p225, paper 3, Q13

Leptospirosis: p126, paper 2, Q9
Liver disease:
    - acute liver failure:
- classification: p263, paper 3, Q48
- in pregnancy: p35, paper 1, Q5
- management: p319, paper 4, Q14
- transplant criteria paracetomol/non-paracetomol: p57, paper 1, Q23
    - chronic liver disease: p146, paper 2, Q24

Local anaesthetic toxicity: p465, paper 5, Q40
LVAD (left ventricular assist device): p143, paper 2, Q22

M

Maastricht classification: p476, paper 5, Q48
Magnesium: p458, paper 5, Q35
Major incident management: p122, paper 2, Q5
Major obstetric haemorrhage: p345, paper 4, Q33
Malignant hyperthermia: p311, paper 4, Q8
Mechanical assist devices: p143, paper 2, Q22
Mental capacity assessment: p249, paper 3, Q35
Motor neurone disease: p141, paper 2, Q19
Multiple sclerosis: p75, paper 1, Q41
Myasthenia gravis:
    - acute myasthenic crisis: p308, paper 4, Q6
    - considerations in the ICU: p155, paper 2, Q30
Myocardial infarction:
    - NSTEMI: p466, paper 5, Q41
    - STEMI: p218, paper 3, Q7
Myotonic dystrophy: p330, paper 4, Q22
Myxoedematous crisis: p313, paper 4, Q9

N

Necrotising fasciitis: p420, paper 5, Q10
Nephrotic syndrome: p71, paper 1, Q37
Neurological death testing: p305, paper 4, Q3 and p247, paper 3, Q34
Neuroprognostication: p161, paper 2, Q34
Never events: p179, paper 2, Q50
Notifiable diseases: p254, paper 3, Q41

Index

Nutritional requirements and assessment: p67, paper 1, Q33 and p443, paper 5, Q24

O
Organ donation (DCD): p136, paper 2, Q15
Organophosphate poisoning: p477, paper 5, Q49
Out-of-hospital cardiac arrest management: p228, paper 3, Q16

P
Pacemakers:
- permanent: p56, paper 1, Q22
- temporary: p404, paper 5, Q2

Paediatrics:
- acutely unwell infant: p117, paper 2, Q1
- cardiac arrest management: p234, paper 3, Q22
- consent: p60, paper 1, Q26
- neonatal collapse: p347, paper 4, Q35

Pancreatitis:
- aetiology: p245, paper 3, Q32
- management: p422, paper 5, Q11
- pancreatic fluid collections: p39, paper 1, Q8

Paracetamol:
- acute toxicity: p31, paper 1, Q1
- transplant criteria: p57, paper 1, Q23

Parenteral nutrition (or total parenteral nutrition [TPN]): p212, paper 3, Q3
Phaeochromocytoma: p141, paper 2, Q20
Phosphate: p236, paper 3, Q24
PJP (*Pneumocystis jirovecii* pneumonia): p306, paper 4, Q5
Pleural effusion: p251, paper 3, Q37
Pneumonectomy: p316, paper 4, Q12
Pneumothorax: p442, paper 5, Q23
PPE (personal protective equipment): p240, paper 3, Q27

Pre-eclampsia:
- classification: p59, paper 1, Q25
- management: p327, paper 4, Q19

PRIS (propofol-related infusion syndrome): p303, paper 4, Q1
Propanolol toxicity: p49, paper 1, Q16

Pulmonary embolus:
- management: p411, paper 5, Q5
- scoring systems: p362, paper 4, Q47

Pulmonary hypertension:
- definition: p175, paper 2, Q47
- management in the ICU: p227, paper 3, Q15

Pulse oximeter: p441, paper 5, Q22

R

Rapid sequence induction: p333, paper 4, Q25
Refeeding syndrome: p145, paper 2, Q23 and p222, paper 3, Q10
Renal transplant management: p117, paper 2, Q2
Renal tubular acidosis: p79, paper 1, Q45 and p134, paper 2, Q13
Rhabdomyolysis: p445, paper 5, Q26
Rib fractures: p428, paper 5, Q14
Right ventricular failure: p433, paper 5, Q18

S

SBT (spontaneous breathing trial): p439, paper 5, Q21
Scoring systems: p170, paper 2, Q41
Serious Hazards of Transfusion (SHOT): p351, paper 4, Q38

Shock:
- cardiogenic: p32, paper 1, Q3
- classification of: p468, paper 5, Q42

Spinal cord injury: p38, paper 1, Q7 and p61, paper 1, Q27
Spontaneous bacterial peritonitis: p83, paper 1, Q49
SSSS (staphylococcal scalded skin syndrome): p213, paper 3, Q4

Statistics:
- sensitivity and specificity: p147, paper 2, Q25
- type 1 and 2 errors: p346, paper 4, Q34

Status epilepticus: p353, paper 4, Q40

Stroke:
- ischaemic syndromes: p216, paper 3, Q6
- management: p216, paper 3, Q6

Subarachnoid haemorrhage:
- aetiology and management: p409, paper 5, Q4
- complications of: p173, paper 2, Q44
- grading systems: p74, paper 1, Q40

Index

Sustainability: p152, paper 2, Q28

T
Takotsubo cardiomyopathy: p463, paper 5, Q38
TEG/ROTEM: p149, paper 2, Q27
Tetanus: p76, paper 1, Q42
Thrombophilia: p257, paper 3, Q44
Thrombotic thrombocytopaenic purpura: p50, paper 1, Q17
Thyroid storm: p214, paper 3, Q5
TLS (tumour lysis syndrome):
- management: p352, paper 4, Q39
- recognition: p127, paper 2, Q10
Tracheostomy:
- emergency management: p152, paper 2, Q29
- insertion: p260, paper 3, Q46
Transfer: p464, paper 5, Q39
Transfusion triggers: p243, paper 3, Q31
Traumatic brain injury:
- management: p46, paper 1, Q13 and p135, paper 2, Q14
- monitoring of ICP: p220, paper 3, Q9
Tricyclic poisoning: p403, paper 5, Q1
Typhlitis: p436, paper 5, Q19

U
US physics:
- probes: p332, paper 4, Q24

V
Variceal bleed:
- management: p40, paper 1, Q9
- rescue therapies: p78, paper 1, Q44
Vasculitis: p53, paper 1, Q19
Ventricular tachycardia: p242, paper 3, Q30
Viral haemorrhagic fevers: p354, paper 4, Q41
Vitamins: p359, paper 4, Q45

W
Wernicke's encephalopathy: p160, paper 2, Q33
West zones: p264, paper 3, Q49